Comment on *Dump Your Toxic Waist!* from a reader

'What a fantastic book. *Dump Your Toxic Waist!* offers an invaluable insight into the causes of heart disease and how to prevent it. It's a witty and interesting read and keeps the reader engaged throughout. Even the 'non-reader' will find it hard to put this one down. If you have heart disease or want to make sure it doesn't affect you, read on and be entertained, educated and enthused to make lifestyle changes that may well be life saving for you.'

Denise Armstrong, Lifestyle Manager, Heart Research UK

Comments on *Stop that heart attack!* from readers

'An excellent read. This book is a must for absolutely anyone interested in heart health – as a reference, an inspiration, a good laugh and a new old friend!'

The Family Heart Digest

'The style is easy to read and there are plenty of humorous and personal anecdotes and some wonderful cartoons to make a serious issue an enjoyable read.'

Sara Stanner, British Nutrition Foundation

'Clear and readable, this book would be most suited to the well-motivated individual who is ready to make lifestyle changes.'

Sister Caroline Brennan, Cardiology News

'Dr Cutting writes well and the text is interesting.'

Dr Ric 70

Department of Cardiology, Conc

'It was a pleasure to read! I'm now going
information to the test . . . I'll be keeping it with

Suzanna Stuart

'The doctor offers hope for many healthy years to come if we use his knowledge and common sense and set ourselves attainable goals in exercise and adjusted diet. Thank you Dr Cutting for helping me to *Stop that heart attack!*'

Reviewed by Julia Westall, BCPA Journal

'I think that this book is really well set out and easy to read and has a mine of useful information.'

Prof Philip James, Rowett Research Institute, Aberdeen

'Concepts are well explained for the layman without being patronising and unusually for this type of book it is medically sound and gets the balance right.'

Professor Paul Durrington, Professor of Medicine, Manchester Royal Infirmary

'This is one of those books that once you start reading you really cannot put down. It ought to be on the reading list for every secondary school student . . .'

British Cardiac Patients' Association

I'm sure the general public will find it enlightening, humorous and educational. I am impressed with his nutritional knowledge.'

Azmina Govindji BSc, SRD, Consultant Nutritionist and Dietitian

'It is the best written book I have ever read . . . It is magnificent in every way.'

Dr Thomas White MD, retired General Practitioner

'Thank you for asking me to read this excellent book, I really enjoyed it! I too share the author's enthusiasm for healthy eating to stop heart disease. The book is easy to read for the motivated member of the public but also scientifically sound for the interested health professional . . . It is well written and is a pleasure to read with plenty of humour, common sense and personal anecdotes. I would highly recommend this book.'

Jacqui Lynas BSc, SRD, Specialist Lipid Dietitian

'This is an excellent book for those who are interested in unclogging their arteries, or getting down to their ideal weight for good, or controlling their blood pressure, or discovering a new vitality.'

The Family Heart Digest

'. . . an excellent, comprehensive book . . .'

Dr Chris Steele, TV Quick

'This is a brilliant book! I've found it invaluable. The clear explanations and humour make it such light reading, and so interesting. I can't speak too highly of this book.'

Rosemary A. May

'As a bus driver I have been trying for some time to get fit, unsuccessfully. I found this book both informative and easy to read. As a person who doesn't normally read, I found the humorous angle helped me to read on and finish the book.'

Stewart Holt

'I found myself wide awake at 3 am and unable to put the book down . . . This book should be compulsory reading at an early age.'

British Journal of Cardiology

'. . . thank heavens for Dr Derrick Cutting . . . recipes that won't take a week to prepare and are ideally suited to your average burger-loving Brit.'

Amanda Ursell, The Sunday Times

'This is an exceptional book . . . It does exactly what it says on the cover and provides successful and medically accurate strategies for a healthy and fulfilled life.'

Cardiology News

'. . . enjoyable, informative and can be highly recommended.'
Diabetes Research & Wellness Foundation

'. . . packed with information on how to live a longer, healthier life.'

Slimming Magazine

' . . . a comprehensive diet, fitness and lifestyle book . . . puts you in charge of your own health.'

My Weekly

'. . . highly recommended . . .'

Practice Nurse

'Congratulations! It is excellent, readable and even sometimes fun!'
Dr Rudolph Canepa-Anson, Consultant Cardiologist

Comments from people who have put Dr Cutting's plan to the test

'. . . this incredible and fascinating book . . . may well be the best investment I've ever made . . . I thought you might like to know how I fared with the new style of living and some recent tests . . . I am very pleased with the results of these tests, and believe it must be a great number of years since my blood fats and pressure were so good: and it is all mainly due to your brilliant book, thank you very much indeed.'

Patrick S.

'I was over 13 stone for many years. In fact I went up to 17 stone at one point. I was always dieting and losing a bit of weight, only to put it straight back on again. Since I went onto the diet Dr Cutting advises, I've stayed around my ideal weight of 9 st 2 lbs. It's over six years now. I'm delighted!'

Mary M.

'My cholesterol level was dangerously high at 7.6. Thanks to this easy-to-follow plan my average cholesterol is now 5.4 – and that's without drugs!'

Ali Osman S.

'It was three years ago that I gave up smoking and changed my diet with Dr Cutting's help. I recommend this plan to anyone who needs to do the same.'

Edward G.

'Having been to the doctor for a health MOT, I discovered that my cholesterol was over 8.0. Following the dietary principles in Dr Cutting's book (which I found easy to stick to) my cholesterol level reduced to 4.8 within 4 months. My GP was impressed by the improvement, and I was delighted that my diet had made such a difference.'

Dirk L.

Dump Your
TOXIC WAIST!

Lose inches, beat diabetes and stop that heart attack!

DR DERRICK CUTTING

CLASS PUBLISHING

Printing history
First published (as *Stop that Heart Attack!*) 1998
Reprinted with revisions 1999

WORCESTERSHIRE COUNTY COUNCIL	
451	
Bertrams	13.06.08
613.25	£14.99
WO	

Fourth edition (fully revised and expanded, as *Drop that Extra Waist!*) 2008

The information presented in this book is accurate and current to the best
of the author's knowledge. The author and publisher, however, make no
guarantee as to, and assume no responsibility for, the correctness or
sufficiency of such information or recommendation. The reader is advised
to consult a doctor regarding all aspects of individual health care.

The author and publisher welcome feedback from the users of this book.
Please contact the publishers.

Class Publishing, Barb House, Barb Mews, London W6 7PA, UK
Telephone: 020 7371 2119
Fax: 020 7371 2878 [International +4420]
email: post@class.co.uk
Website: www.class.co.uk

A CIP catalogue for this book is available from the British Library

ISBN Paperback 978 1 85959 191 8
Hardback 978 1 85959 201 4

10 9 8 7 6 5 4 3 2 1

Edited by Caroline Sheldrick

Cartoons by Peter Maddocks

Line illustrations and additional cartoons by David Woodroffe

Typeset by Martin Bristow

Printed and bound in Finland by WS Bookwell, Juva

Contents

Preface

This book began life as *Stop That Heart Attack!* which enjoyed three editions. From the outset, its popularity demonstrated the need for a medically accurate guide that's easy to read.

In the meantime, more and more research has highlighted the central role of abdominal fat in our Western plagues of diabetes and heart disease. Whether your primary aim is to have the profile of a beauty queen, or to lower your blood pressure, beat diabetes or avoid a heart attack, you cannot escape the crucial importance of ditching the abdominal fat that's undermining your metabolism.

Any book about losing fat must compete with 'The Seven-Day Miracle Beetroot Broth Diet That Will Change Your Life Forever'. The book you're looking at is for those who want the scientific evidence filtered and concentrated into an easy, practical plan that actually works.

No single 'superfood' holds the whole answer. For one food to impart health and weight loss when the rest of the diet is damaging and unbalanced would be a miracle indeed. How often I see a TV chef extol the health-giving virtues of an ingredient, only to follow it with a terrifying dose of salt or saturated fat.

It's hard to keep your eye on ten balls at once and in this book I was determined to do that so my reader doesn't have to. Here, then, is a scientifically sound but simple tool to lose inches from your waist and avoid the slippery slope to obesity, diabetes, high blood pressure and heart disease.

Acknowledgements

Readers of *Stop that heart attack!* have been a tremendous encouragement and if it weren't for their enthusiasm, this new book would never have been born. I am particularly indebted to Professor Paul Durrington, Azmina Govindji, Professor Philip James, Jacqui Lynas, Sue Phipps and Dr Richard Wray who read early manuscripts. Jacqui Morrel (formerly Lynas) made time in her busy schedule to read new material with her discerning dietetic eye.

Baldeesh Rai of H.E.A.R.T. UK kindly produced information on South Asian diets.

As ever, I am grateful to my wife, Heather, who faithfully converts my manuscripts into electronic data. Our teenage daughters, Serena and Christabel, have patiently tested a wide range of recipes and can always be relied upon for an honest opinion.

Derrick Cutting

Copyright

Notes

Calories

Reference to the number of 'calories' in food always means kilocalories (kcal). Strictly speaking, this should be written as 'Calories' with a capital C, but for easy reading we refer to kilocalories as 'calories'.

1 kcal = 1 Calorie = 1000 calories

1 megajoule (MJ) = 1000 kilojoules (kJ) = 239 kilocalories (kcal).

Abbreviations

g = grams; mmol/l = millimoles per litre;

oz = ounce; ml = millilitre; lb = pound weight.

Registered trademarks

Trade names are used in this book as examples only and do not imply any particular recommendation.

All-Bran, Corn Pops, Crunchy Nut Corn Flakes, Frosties, Rice Krispies and Special K are registered trademarks of The Kellogg Company

Acomplia is made by Sanofi-Aventis

Benecol is a registered trademark and produced for McNeil Consumer Nutritionals Ltd

Champix is made by Pfizer

Cheerios, Golden Grahams, Nesquik, Shredded Wheat and Shreddies are registered trademarks of Société des Produits Nestlé SA, Vevey, Switzerland

Columbus eggs are produced by Belovo

Flora pro.activ is a trademark of Van den Bergh Foods Ltd

Kwai is a registered trademark of Biocare

LoSalt is a trademark of Klinge Foods Ltd

miniCol is a registered trademark of the Emmi Group

Olean (olestra) is made by Procter and Gamble

Omacor is a registered trademark of Solvay Healthcare

Perfect Sweet (xylitol) is a Health by Nature Ltd product

Polydextrose is made by Pfizer

Quorn is a registered trademark of ICI Ltd

Reductil is made by Abbott

Ryvita is a registered trademark of Associated British Foods Ltd

Simplesse is made by Nutrasweet

Solo is a registered trademark of the Low Sodium Sea Salt Co.

Sugar Puffs is a registered trademark of Quaker Trading Ltd

Total is a registered trade mark of Fage Dairy Industry SA

Weetabix and Puffed Wheat are registered trademarks of Weetabix Ltd, Kettering, UK

Xenical (orlistat) is made by Roche

Zyban is made by Glaxo-Wellcome

Introduction

If you've been fighting a losing battle against flab and fatigue, you're certainly not alone.

Standard advice about diet has done nothing to avert the tidal wave of obesity that's now overwhelming the Western world. Indeed, the higher the volume has been turned up on dietary advice, the faster the fat has accumulated.

The chances are that you, like so many others, are locked into a metabolic vicious cycle. We now know that the fat behind an expanding waistline isn't just ugly and useless: it's metabolically toxic.

Yes, abdominal fat actively produces chemicals that upset your metabolism. These toxic messengers are known as adipokines, and their discovery provides the key to understanding – and escaping – the fat trap.

If your waist has gradually expanded (and you're not pregnant), adipokines will be at work. Their metabolic mischief leads to: unbalanced blood fats and cholesterol; formation of blood clots and fatty deposits in arteries; raised blood pressure; poor control of blood glucose and high insulin levels – resulting in the production of, yes, more abdominal fat! This is a truly vicious cycle.

No wonder you've struggled in vain to trim your tummy and recharge your battery!

This self-perpetuating metabolic malaise has come increasingly under the spotlight of research in recent years. The inescapable conclusion is that the build-up of toxic abdominal fat, which is central to the so-called 'metabolic syndrome', is the number one health issue for industrialised nations; this is what's fuelling our epidemics of uncontrolled weight gain, diabetes and heart disease; this is what underlies most sickness and premature death in the developed world.

And it's probably the answer to your own frustration with dieting, your struggle to find a lasting solution for sluggish mood and metabolism.

When you have metabolic syndrome, waist disposal is top priority. So how can you achieve that? Certainly, the conventional low-fat, high-carbohydrate diet has failed a lot of people – and we have good scientific evidence that it exacerbates some aspects of the metabolic syndrome.

Many sought an antidote to this in the Atkins Diet. But losing weight by avoiding helpful carbohydrates and eating more saturated fat is rather like curing work stress by staying at home and injecting heroin.

The answer lies in shifting the balance of nutrients. Some types of fat are very damaging while others are essential. When it comes to the helpful fats, the trick is to get the different fatty acids in the right proportions. Choosing the optimum quantity and quality of carbohydrate foods is crucial. Simultaneously adjusting the proportion of protein makes all the difference to appetite control – and hence to losing weight effectively without feeling hungry, tired or deprived.

This may sound complicated, but my 28-day plan will show you exactly how to do it until it becomes second nature. What's more, my revolutionary MUNCH method gives you a simple tool to get the balance just right – for good.

If you follow this plan to slim your waist and reverse the metabolic syndrome, not only will you look better and feel better, you will also be reducing your risk of diabetes, heart disease and cancer. That's not a bad start. But this book doesn't stop there. You'll find answers to questions you hadn't even thought of, especially about additional ways of reducing the risk of a stroke or heart attack – our biggest causes of death and disability.

Who wants to get old? In Western societies, arteries fur up and blood pressure rises as people get older. It doesn't have to be that way. We can learn from cultures in which people reach old age with unclogged arteries and lovely low blood pressures – completely free of heart disease. The lifestyle plan in this book can truly keep you young at heart.

Recent research has revolutionised our understanding of the way the body digests carbohydrate foods. Did you know that baked potatoes and wholemeal bread push up blood glucose faster than table sugar does? The glycaemic index of foods is interesting, but also extremely misleading. With this easy guide to glycaemic load, you can choose carbohydrate foods to help you lose weight, control diabetes and boost energy levels!

If you have diabetes, your risk of heart disease is hugely increased. Apart from controlling blood glucose, there are lots of vitally important ways to improve your health and protect your arteries. This book is full of them.

Of course, you may have heart disease already. Perhaps the first you knew about it was an unexpected heart attack or it may be that you suffer from angina. Either way, it's all the more important to slash your chances of having a heart attack in future. These pages tell you how to do just that.

It gets better. Doctors used to think that once arteries had been narrowed by a build-up of fatty deposits, there wasn't much you could do about it. Oh, you might slow down the artery-clogging process, but the idea of actually stopping it was wildly optimistic; to reverse the process would clearly be impossible. I bring good news! Several scientific studies have now shown that you can indeed start unblocking arteries again; when big enough changes are made, heart disease can be sent into reverse!

Research has also discovered more about free radicals – those unstable chemicals that go round damaging cells in your body. Over the years, free radicals on the rampage cause ageing, cancer and heart disease. But we have also learnt more about special substances in our diet – antioxidants – that can protect against free radical attack. You can't stop the clock, but you can slow it down – and keep your ticker happy.

Homocysteine is a substance linked with increased risk of strokes and heart attacks. Reducing your level with B vitamins sounds like a good idea, but wait till you read the shocking results of the latest research.

Do you have a hearty appetite for life? This isn't a book about giving up all the things you enjoy; it's about living life to the full. Too much of the advice about diet just tells you to cut down your favourite foods. But science has uncovered the fact that some foods are positively helpful when it comes to protecting your heart and circulation, and even avoiding cancer. You can discover here the secret of getting the right balance of helpful foods. Eating to your heart's content could give you a longer life, and more energy to enjoy it.

Do the new fat spreads really lower cholesterol or are they just gimmicks? What's the difference between soluble and insoluble fibre? Does fibre lower cholesterol? Is salt essential or dangerous? OK, so fish does you a power of good, but what if you hate fish? Is it true that garlic's good for you, or is that just an old wives' tale? Can alcohol protect your heart, and is red wine really better than other drinks? These are just a few of the basic questions about food that you will find answered here. This book is about scientific evidence, not unfounded theories.

No matter how compelling the evidence, it's of no use to you unless you can translate it into everyday eating and living. This is a practical book. You'll find tips on making a shopping list, understanding food labels, eating on a budget, and feeding children. You can find out how to eat out without doing yourself in. The recipes are simple and quick; good food must be convenient or most of us will never get round to eating it.

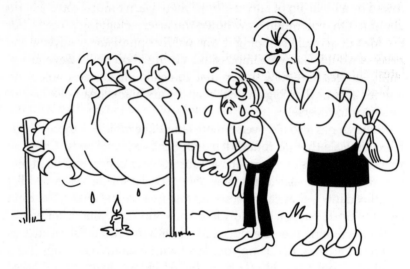

Good food must be convenient.

Have you been told you should reduce your cholesterol level? Perhaps you have tried to get your cholesterol down and been disappointed with the result. My book gives you a plan that will succeed where so many are failing – a plan to cut the 'bad' kind of cholesterol while looking after the 'good' sort.

Is there really any evidence that exercise prevents heart disease and, if so, what sort of exercise and how much of it is needed? Or could exercise bring on a heart attack? What's the best way to enjoy exercise if you're not a fitness fanatic? I'll sort out the facts from the fiction and show you how simply you can invigorate your life.

There is essential information for smokers here – and for non-smokers (who often find themselves smoking passively). If you're a smoker but would rather not be, why not make use of the plan in this book that's helped so many to become ex-smokers?

Like smoking, high blood pressure significantly raises your risk of stroke and heart disease. Some people need drugs to reduce blood pressure, but many could avoid the need for drugs if only they knew how. I explain a four-point plan to bring that pressure down.

Research shows a link between some forms of stress and increased rates of heart disease. Stress is a part of life, but it needn't be the death of you. You can put stress in its place with my simple stress-busting kit.

Weighing up risks can be tricky. You may have thought about taking hormone replacement therapy to cut your risk of heart disease and osteoporosis, but been worried and confused by reports about the dangers of HRT. This is an understandable dilemma – especially if you're a woman. Help is at hand with this straightforward guide to the latest findings of research.

Some risks are so big that urgent action is needed, while others are too small to bother about. You can get things in perspective with my ABC of assessing your risk. There's a ready reckoner of risk so you can check your chances of having a heart attack or stroke in the next ten years, and there's clear advice on how to get that risk right down!

If you already have heart disease, you urgently need this programme to cut the risk of a future heart attack. You may need drug treatment too. You'll find some essential information in Chapter 25, including the latest research findings on drugs used to lower cholesterol levels.

But if you simply want to lose inches from your waist and revitalise your metabolism, I firmly believe you are looking at the most accurate and effective guide available.

How to use this book

If you read this book from cover to cover, the picture will unfold in a logical sequence until it is complete. But I realise you may not want to read it like that. I won't be in the least offended if you focus on the parts you find most interesting. After getting your bearings in Chapter 1, you may want to go straight to Chapter 18 and on to the 28-day plan to start losing those inches. That's fine. You will certainly find things much easier, though, if you gain some understanding of glycaemic load from Chapter 6 on your way.

Key messages and action points are highlighted throughout the book. These will make it easier to skim sections without losing the thread. And, even if you do read every word, the boxes will help a great deal when you want to go back and revise.

The **Fat** chapter contains a lot of information. It's important information, but if it all seems a bit much at first, don't worry: let the key-message boxes help you through; you can always come back for more detail later. And, if you don't really like words at all, at least there are the cartoons to look at!

The **Action Plan** makes it easy to convert your new understanding into everyday living. The 28-day plan (Chapter 28) tells you exactly what to eat (because it can be really hard to convert general guides into effective action). If you think this is too rigid and you don't want to be told, you can still use the recipes and apply the unique MUNCH method to make up a balanced menu; you can adopt the plan in principle instead of following it to the letter. When you're presented with a loose guide, the converse isn't true: you can't use it prescriptively even if you want to. In other words, a prescriptive plan is more flexible than a general guide.

With the Action checklist you can see at a glance where action is needed – and reward yourself for the progress you've made. Useful addresses and books are listed in the appendices and the glossary provides a reminder of technical terms explained in the text.

I'd love to hear how successful you've been at changing your life and reducing your risk. Any suggestions for improving future editions would also be most welcome. You can write to me c/o Class Publishing, Barb House, Barb Mews, London, W6 7PA.

Do you want to break free from metabolic stagnation and lose deadly abdominal fat? Would you like to get down to your ideal weight for good? Are you interested in conquering diabetes, or unclogging your arteries, or controlling your blood pressure and cholesterol, or discovering a new vitality? If so, read on . . .

Chapter 1

The toxic bulge

LETHAL EPIDEMICS
SWEEP WESTERN WORLD

This sensational headline is no exaggeration. We are being engulfed by epidemics of obesity, diabetes and heart disease – all merciless killers.

Where does all this destruction come from? To track the origins of this metabolic plague, you may have to look no further than your waist. This is where it all begins for most of us. If your waist is even a little wider than it should be, forget 'love handles' and 'spare tyre': this is toxic tissue. It's not harmless flab, but a mass of metabolically malignant adipose tissue.

We now know that abdominal fat produces a range of noxious chemicals called adipokines that sabotage your metabolism. These chemical messengers act like spies carrying a false message. As a result, tissues become less sensitive to insulin – producing the condition known as 'insulin resistance' – and you lose control of your blood sugar; the pancreas has to pump out more insulin in order to get a response; insulin levels go up and a vicious cycle accelerates the accumulation of abdominal fat; blood pressure rises; the balance of blood fats and cholesterol is upset; blood clots form more easily and arteries clog up.

The metabolic syndrome (Chapter 18) used to be called 'Syndrome X', which makes it sound like a mysterious alien plot to wipe us out (and if it is, the aliens are enjoying a measure of success). If aliens had implanted a toxic mass in your belly, programmed to destroy you insidiously, wouldn't you be keen to get rid of it?

You may want to slim your waist so you can look good on the beach, or because you're fed up with buttons flying off your waistband. Quite understandable. Those are good enough reasons. But it's so much more important than that. Surely you want to do it in a way

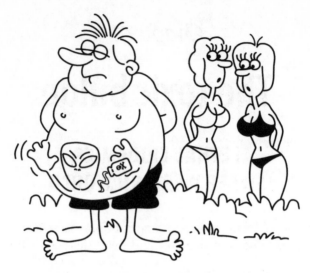

'Can you imagine getting a fat belly like his?'
'That would be like so totally alien to my nature.'

that keeps the weight off, blocking the vicious cycle and reversing the changes that lead to high blood pressure, diabetes, blood clots and heart disease.

That's what this book is all about.

◆ We have lethal epidemics of obesity, diabetes and heart disease in the Western world

◆ The metabolic syndrome is the association of an increased waist circumference with changes in body chemistry that can lead to diabetes and heart disease

◆ Excess abdominal fat is metabolically toxic, releasing chemical messengers called adipokines that are bad for arteries and set up a vicious cycle leading to more abdominal fat

◆ Reversing this vicious cycle is the key to correcting disordered metabolism, preventing diabetes and heart disease, and losing fat for good

Chapter 2

Fat, diabetes and heart disease

Can you really prevent diabetes?

Type 1 diabetes occurs in children and young people when the pancreas fails to produce enough insulin. The onset is usually dramatic and unexpected. We don't have a way of preventing this type of diabetes and it has to be treated with injections of insulin.

Type 2 diabetes is quite different. This is the kind that is afflicting the Western world on an epidemic scale and is linked to obesity – or, more particularly, fat around the tummy. It arises because tissues become less responsive to insulin, forcing the pancreas to work harder and push out more insulin to reduce blood glucose. It is sometimes called 'late-onset diabetes' to distinguish it from Type 1. But the shocking truth is that it often comes on much earlier now, and I have had to diagnose it in children in my own practice.

This type of diabetes does not have a dramatic onset. You may notice that you are getting more thirsty and passing more urine, but many adults have Type 2 diabetes without knowing it. And it's really bad for the arteries – especially if poorly controlled – and hurtles you towards diseases of the heart and circulation. This kind of diabetes is preventable.

A group of researchers put this to the test in a controlled trial published in the *New England Journal of Medicine*. The study involved 3234 people who were at increased risk of developing diabetes (because they had raised blood glucose levels) but who didn't have the condition at the start of the trial. Some of the people were given daily treatment with a drug called metformin which enhances the body's response to insulin and is used to *treat* diabetes. A second group were given a placebo (inactive) tablet. The third group improved their lifestyles – eating a better diet, losing weight, and undertaking moderate exercise for 150 minutes a week.

The metformin tablet did well, achieving a 31% reduction in new cases of diabetes compared with the dummy tablets. But the lifestyle change was far more effective, producing a 58% reduction.

What if you already have diabetes?

Another study, published in 2005, suggested that big enough changes in diet, combined with moderate exercise, can actually reverse Type 2 diabetes in people who already have it. This is far more controversial: the general view is that once you have diabetes, you can't get rid of it.

The fact is that after three weeks of this programme, half the people had normal blood tests. Had the doctor been assessing them for the first time at that point, they would not have been diagnosed with diabetes. Whether they had actually eradicated their diabetes or simply controlled it beyond detection, it was extremely worthwhile and would have achieved a massive reduction in the risk of eye complications, kidney problems and heart disease.

We're all heading that way

Over the years, the definition of diabetes has changed to include people with lower levels of blood sugar. That's because research has shown that the problem – the slippery slope to complications – begins at a lower threshold.

Even if you don't have diabetes, it is highly likely that you have features of the metabolic syndrome, or pre-diabetes as it is sometimes called. The term is used to describe the association of excess abdominal fat, raised blood pressure, reduced sensitivity to insulin and unbalanced blood fats (lipids). Recent research has increasingly identified this cluster of features as the root of our Western epidemics. It has become clear that even mild features operating together pave the way to future disaster, so current definitions of the metabolic syndrome embrace a very high proportion of the population (see page 313).

The diet and lifestyle fostered by our culture could be aptly described as *diabolic* – not only of the devil but also inducing diabetes through the metabolic syndrome.

Most of us are on a slide heading through the metabolic syndrome to diabetes or heart disease or both. The good news is, you can get off.

- ◆ Type 1 diabetes comes on suddenly in children and young people; it's treated with insulin injections

- ◆ Type 2 diabetes, which is epidemic, is very bad for the heart and arteries; it comes on gradually and many adults don't even realise they have it; it's preventable

- ◆ A key feature of Type 2 diabetes and the metabolic syndrome (or pre-diabetes) is 'insulin resistance', leading to poor control of blood glucose

- ◆ Most of us are on a slide heading towards diabetes and heart disease – but you can get off

What is heart disease?

Coronary heart disease is the single biggest killer in the UK. And it's not a male disease: it kills about one in six women and one in five men. OK, you have to die of something, but many are struck down in the prime of life. And statistics for deaths are only part of the story: many are living with heart disease.

'I feel as I always have, except for an occasional heart attack.'

ROBERT BENCHLEY (1889–1945)
Groucho Marx Grouchofile, **1976**

When it really happens, it's not funny, is it?

Don's story

It was 4 am. Don had been dreaming. It was a nightmare. He was trying to get up – trying to escape from a huge brute of a man who was sitting on his chest. He woke and realised it was just a dream. Or was it? It felt as though an elephant was on his chest. The pain got more intense as he came to. It was a crushing, endless pain; he could hardly breathe.

Don woke his wife, June. She could see at once that he was ill – very ill. He was pale, almost grey, and beads of sweat were running down his face. She called an ambulance. Don felt sick. He was afraid. He couldn't stand the pain a moment longer. The ambulance was there in minutes. The paramedics were very efficient; they set up a drip, put Don on a monitor, and knew exactly what to do. Soon, Don was being wheeled on a trolley into the hospital. June waited anxiously outside the treatment room. Everyone was very busy. A doctor confirmed it was a heart attack and that they were doing everything they could. Then, more doctors in white coats ran into the treatment room.

Forty minutes later, a doctor came out and June feared the worst. The doctor's strained face broke into a faint smile. It had been a close call, but Don must be a fighter, the doctor explained. The following hours would be critical. They were going to move Don to the coronary care unit where he would be in the best possible hands.

Don went on to make a full recovery from his heart attack, but it took Don and June a long time to come to terms with what had happened. Don had always been so well before this; there had never been any hint of heart disease. This had come totally out of the blue.

Gradually, Don came to understand what had happened to him. He realised that, unless he made some changes, it was all too likely to happen again – perhaps with a more tragic outcome. He had heart disease, but he didn't want another heart attack.

June was a great support. She didn't just help Don change his lifestyle: she changed hers as well. At first she did this to encourage Don, but then she learnt that it was vital for her too; she learnt that far more women were dying of heart disease than of breast cancer. Not only that, she discovered to her surprise that eating and living better gave her a new vitality and made life more enjoyable.

Don was heartened to find out that making the right changes could halt the progress of his heart disease and reduce his chances of another attack. He was delighted when he went on to discover a plan of action that could actually undo some damage – a plan to send heart disease into reverse!

What is a heart attack and why does it happen?

A sudden, unexpected heart attack is one of the commonest ways that heart disease shows up. But, although the attack is sudden, the run-up to it has taken years.

Figure 1 shows a human heart. The heart is made of a marvellous muscle that just keeps pumping blood round the body, day in, day out (and even while the rest of you is asleep, of course). To do this marathon task, it needs a constant supply of blood itself.

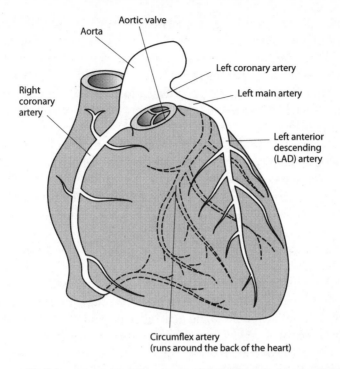

Figure 1 The human heart. The coronary arteries surround the heart muscle and send branches into the muscle, delivering blood containing oxygen. They start from the aorta, just above the aortic valve. Dotted lines indicate the arteries running around the back of the heart.

Blood is delivered to the heart muscle by the coronary arteries. In Western societies, because of our faulty diet and lifestyle, it is normal for arteries to become narrower as the years go by. The process starts in childhood.

This narrowing of arteries is the result of fatty, cholesterol-laden deposits (often called 'atheroma', which means 'porridge') forming on the smooth artery lining. The hardening ('sclerosis') of these fatty deposits of atheroma produces tough 'plaques' inside arteries. You can see why the gradual hardening and furring up of arteries is called 'atherosclerosis'.

Coronary atherosclerosis – the formation of fatty plaques in the heart's vital coronary arteries – builds up silently for years before it makes itself felt.

Figure 2 shows how atherosclerosis constricts the passage inside a coronary artery. Obviously, this reduces the rate at which blood can be delivered to the working heart muscle. Perhaps you remember Poiseuille's formula from your school physics, which indicated that the rate at which liquid flows in a tube depends on the fourth power of the radius – although it doesn't apply where there's turbulence. But if you neither remember nor care, suffice it to say that a little narrowing causes a huge increase in resistance to flow – a little constriction but a lot of friction.

That's not all. And don't worry, we don't need any physics for this next bit. The craggy surface of an atherosclerotic plaque is liable to become damaged; when this happens, the damaged area is plugged by the smallest blood cells (platelets), setting off a clot (or thrombus). A small clot could merely add to the size of the plaque – accelerating the process of atherosclerosis. But a bigger clot can completely block the artery and this is called coronary thrombosis – one of the names for a heart attack.

Sudden blockage of a coronary artery is the immediate cause of a heart attack. This is normally the result of coronary thrombosis; occasionally a lump of clot or plaque may break off and move downstream until it lodges at a narrow section, causing a total obstruction.

Of course, the sudden blockage of a coronary artery means that the part of the heart muscle that was supplied by that artery is at once deprived of blood and oxygen. That hurts! But, because the heart is an

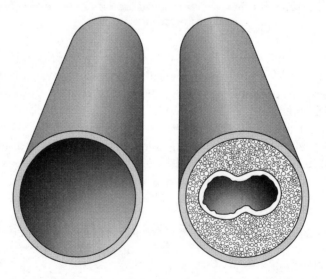

Figure 2 Build-up of atheroma deposits in the arteries gradually blocks the flow of blood.

internal organ, you don't feel the pain where the heart is; pain is referred, usually to the chest, but sometimes to the shoulder, arm, neck or jaw. Small heart attacks can be painless ('silent').

Muscle can't survive without blood and the affected area of heart muscle dies. If this is only a small area, the victim has a good chance of a full recovery; the damaged part heals with a small scar that doesn't interfere with the work of the heart. When more heart muscle is knocked off, it causes sudden death in some cases and, in others, an incomplete recovery because the heart has lost some pumping power.

So this is what a heart attack is: the death of a bit of heart muscle – big or small. As you know, we doctors don't like using simple words (in case our patients think we're simple too). Another name for heart muscle is 'myocardium' and another term for the death of a tissue deprived of blood is 'infarction'. So we prefer to call a heart attack a 'myocardial infarction' (MI).

Sometimes a heart attack is followed by an abnormal rhythm to the heartbeat (arrhythmia), or a cardiac arrest, in which the heart stops altogether.

What's angina?

You now understand how the narrowing of coronary arteries by atherosclerosis restricts the flow of oxygen-rich blood to the working heart muscle. If the heart muscle doesn't get enough oxygen to fuel the work it's doing, it hurts. This pain is called angina (sometimes 'angina pectoris', which means angina in the chest).

Angina, like the pain of a heart attack, is usually a heavy or tight pain but it's much less intense than most heart attacks. Mind you, the intensity of angina varies enormously from a dull ache to a severe pain 'like a vice round the chest' and some heart attacks are written off as 'indigestion'. Not surprisingly, because it's coming from the heart muscle, angina pain is felt in the same areas as the pain of a heart attack – typically across the front of the chest, but sometimes in the shoulder, arm or jaw. Of course, angina is the pain of unhappy heart muscle – not dying heart muscle.

When angina behaves in a predictable way – when you know, for example, that walking a little too fast up that slight slope to the newsagent will bring it on – it's called stable angina. Sometimes angina is unpredictable, perhaps striking unexpectedly while you're sitting in a chair or lying in bed; this is called unstable angina.

There is always the possibility that a period of unstable angina will be followed by a heart attack. So if your angina starts coming on more frequently or without provocation, speak to your doctor straight away: you may need a short spell in hospital to settle it down.

What is acute coronary syndrome?

A bout of persistent chest pain arising from the heart could turn out to be a heart attack or a bad episode of unstable angina. The doctor might say the patient has 'acute coronary syndrome'. (And the patient might say, 'What's cute about it?')

Having done an ECG, it may be some time before the doctor receives the results of blood tests showing whether the heart muscle has been damaged or not. Troponins are proteins in the cells of the heart muscle; levels in the blood are extremely low unless heart muscle has been damaged. Within 12 hours of a heart attack, raised troponin levels can be detected in the blood. Heart muscle is not damaged by unstable angina and a troponin blood test will be negative. In the same way, blood is sometimes tested for 'cardiac enzymes' to check for muscle damage, but troponin is more specific to the muscle cells in the heart.

'Acute coronary syndrome', then, is a term that covers both an attack of unstable angina (with no damage to the heart muscle) and a heart attack (in which heart muscle is injured).

Are there different kinds of heart disease?

Yes. There are various forms of heart disease – some very rare, others not so rare. You can be born with faulty heart valves. Some older folk have damaged heart valves because of rheumatic fever in childhood. Then there are several forms of cardiomyopathy, in which the heart muscle is abnormal.

But the only kind of heart disease most people need worry about is coronary heart disease, which causes heart attacks, sudden death, and angina. When people speak of 'heart disease', this is what they mean because everything else is uncommon by comparison. This is the epidemic that grips the Western world.

How can I escape the epidemic?

That's what this book is all about. Don's heart attack struck after years of silent atherosclerosis. You will learn how properly balanced nutrition, without deprivation, can put paid to that. But thrombosis is just as important; without that crucial clot, Don's heart attack would not have happened. It's not just a question of luck. You'll discover how the way you live and eat can stop those clots cropping up where they're not wanted. More remarkable still, you will find out how putting all parts of this plan into action can actually start unclogging arteries that have been clogging up for years – something doctors once took to be impossible.

And it goes well beyond your heart. When clogging and clots get to the arteries of the brain, rather than the coronary arteries, the result is a stroke. When the legs are affected, pain on walking (claudication), and even amputation, can follow. Narrowing of arteries to the penis causes erection problems. The plan in this book will look after all your arteries, but it goes much further than that.

A healthy circulation is the lifeblood of a vital body. Looking after your arteries could give you a new lease of life.

◆ Heart attacks strike unexpectedly

◆ Arteries have been clogging up for years before a heart attack

◆ The narrowing and hardening of arteries is called atherosclerosis

◆ Atherosclerosis in coronary arteries reduces blood flow to heart muscle

◆ When the heart muscle goes short of blood, angina results

◆ A heart attack occurs when a blood clot (thrombosis) blocks a coronary artery

◆ This book reveals how to stop atherosclerosis and thrombosis

Chapter 3

The diabolic slide

The epidemic

Almost a quarter of all deaths in the United Kingdom are caused by coronary heart disease. No other single disease claims so many of our lives.

And yet, in rural areas of developing countries you would be hard pressed to find a single case of coronary heart disease; it is virtually unknown. But when groups of people adopt westernised diets and lifestyles, heart disease appears.

You don't have to live the life of a rural African to escape heart disease; in some industrialised countries it is much less of a problem than in the UK.

Why are some groups of people plagued by an epidemic of heart disease and others not? Why does one person die from a heart attack at 40 and another live to 95? Scientists investigating these questions have identified certain characteristics that increase your chances of getting heart disease. These characteristics are called 'risk factors'. Here are some important risk factors:

- High blood cholesterol;
- High blood pressure;
- Smoking;
- Diabetes;
- Being overweight;
- Lack of exercise.

Every one of these risk factors can be reduced or, in some cases, completely overcome. Here are some more:

- Age – the older you are, the greater the risk;

- Male sex – women are at lower risk before the menopause;

- Family history – heart disease in a close relative under 60.

These are risk factors you cannot change. (There is no evidence that a sex change will reduce your risk.)

In the Seven Countries Study (1980), Professor Ancel Keys investigated the diets and cholesterol levels of men aged between 40 and 59 from Japan, Greece, Yugoslavia, Italy, The Netherlands, the United States and Finland. The 111579 men were studied for 15 years; during this time there had been 2288 deaths and there were big differences between the countries. Important findings were:

- Groups of people with low cholesterols had low rates of heart disease;

- High death rates were linked with high intakes of saturated fat;

- Low death rates were linked with consumption of olive oil.

How important are risk factors like raised cholesterol, high blood pressure, smoking and diabetes? When you hear about new risk factors coming to light, it makes you wonder whether we're concentrating on the wrong things. Perhaps the real answer has yet to be discovered.

A huge global study, led by Canadian researchers, found that most heart attacks can be predicted from a handful of risk factors that are easy to measure. The INTERHEART study, published in *The Lancet* in 2004, spanned 52 countries in Africa, Asia, Australia, Europe, the Middle East and North and South America. The investigation compared 15152 patients admitted to hospital suffering their first heart attack with matching controls – people without heart disease who were from the same town, and of the same age and sex, as the heart-attack victims.

Over 90% of heart attacks could be accounted for by nine risk factors. And the top five risk factors – abnormal blood lipids (i.e. cholesterol and related substances), smoking, diabetes, high blood pressure, and excess abdominal fat – were responsible for 80% of the risk.

This is a remarkable and very significant finding because it gives us the key to prevention of nearly all heart attacks – across the globe, in both sexes. It puts paid to the idea that many heart attacks arise mysteriously, unexplained by known risk factors.

The other factors were lack of exercise, not eating fruit and vegetables every day and stress; moderate alcohol consumption was mildly protective (see Chapter 11).

Clearly, risk factors are interrelated. For example, eating plenty of vegetables and exercising will help to tackle high blood pressure and excess abdominal fat. Shedding abdominal fat can improve the balance of blood lipids.

INTERHEART demonstrated that excess abdominal fat – the toxic bulge – indicates heart risk better than BMI (a measure of total weight in relation to height).

The crucial role of blood lipids is inescapable: many studies have found that groups of people with low cholesterol levels have low rates of heart disease. INTERHEART showed that, across the globe, people living in towns generally have a balance of blood fats that puts them at some risk of heart disease. As people change from their traditional rural culture to the urban lifestyle of the developed world, they get onto the diabolic slide: they accumulate abdominal fat; the metabolic syndrome appears; diabetes and diseases of the heart and circulation take off.

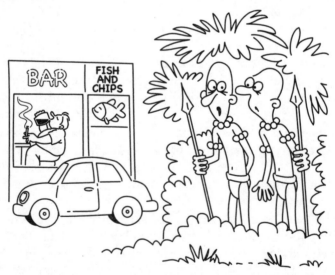

'I can't wait to move to town, get a job and become just like him.'

Alarmingly, INTERHEART found that the average age for that first heart attack was ten years younger in Africa, the Middle East and South Asia than other regions of the world. No doubt, this heralds epidemics of Western diseases among those abandoning their protective traditions in favour of self-destructive urban lifestyles.

In South Japan, largely because of their diet, the average cholesterol level is very low. As a result, heart disease is rare even though smoking and high blood pressure are common. (Of course, smoking is still very damaging to the health of the Japanese smoker.) In this sense, raised cholesterol is the 'essential' risk factor; without this, a population is not plagued by heart disease even if other risk factors are present.

When the Japanese migrate and eat Western diets, their cholesterols rise and they start getting heart disease. So bang goes the theory that it's all down to genetics.

◆ Heart disease kills more people in the UK than any other single disease

◆ 90% of heart attacks are accounted for by nine risk factors

◆ The top risk factors are: cholesterol, smoking, diabetes, blood pressure and abdominal fat

◆ When the Japanese migrate and eat Western diets, they get heart disease

◆ 'Normal' UK cholesterols would be high in Japan

Does that mean I needn't bother if my cholesterol's OK?

No. In a country with a very low average cholesterol level, heart disease is uncommon. Assessing the risk in an individual person is different – especially an individual from a country plagued by the metabolic syndrome, diabetes and heart disease. For a start, a 'normal' cholesterol level in the UK would be relatively high in, say, Japan. Also, as you read this book, you will learn about lots of ways that a good diet can protect you apart from bringing down your cholesterol level.

Your personal risk of heart disease is influenced enormously by other risk factors such as smoking and blood pressure. Your cholesterol level is of fundamental importance but you cannot judge your risk by looking at cholesterol on its own.

You cannot judge risk by cholesterol alone

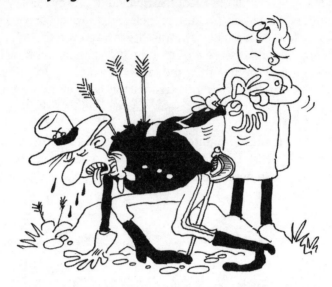

'That's odd . . . his cholesterol was fine.'

Chapter 4

Cholesterol and lipids explained

'. . . Explaining metaphysics to the nation – I wish he would explain his explanation.'

LORD BYRON (George Gordon, 6th Baron Byron), (1788–1824)
Don Juan, 1819–24 canto 1, dedication st. 2

What is cholesterol?

Cholesterol is a glistening white fatty or waxy substance. Chemically speaking, it is a sterol. It is found in people and animals but not in plants (so when the label on a vegetable margarine says 'Contains no cholesterol', this is a statement of the obvious and would be equally true of any purely vegetable product).

We could not survive without a certain amount of cholesterol because we need it to make cell membranes and various hormones, as well as bile salts and vitamin D. But we don't need any in our food – otherwise vegans would be in trouble – because the body makes its own cholesterol.

What do you mean by 'lipids'?

'Lipids' is really a posh word for fats – and fat-like substances such as waxes. The key thing about lipids is that they cannot be dissolved in water; it takes an organic solvent – like the dry-cleaning fluid needed to shift that duck fat from your dinner jacket.

When a doctor talks about your lipids, he is referring to the levels of cholesterol and triglycerides in your blood. A triglyceride is a naturally occurring fat (formed by the combination of one molecule of glycerol with three fatty acid molecules). Most of the fat we eat is in the form of triglycerides and this is also the form in which fat is stored in our bodies.

Cholesterol on the move

Of course, cholesterol has to be transported in the bloodstream from where it is made (the liver and small intestine) to the places where it is needed. This presents the body with a problem; big lumps of fatty cholesterol, which don't mix with water, would soon gum up the works and bring the circulation to a standstill.

To get round this, lipids are carried in tiny particles called lipoproteins. These lipoproteins act like a detergent, surrounding minute globules of cholesterol with a wetting agent and preventing them from clumping together.

The good, the bad and the ugly

Having a high blood cholesterol level increases your risk of getting heart disease. But some of the cholesterol in the blood is not harmful at all. Cholesterol carried in high-density lipoprotein (HDL) is being taken away from body tissues, including artery walls, and back to the liver. In fact the higher your level of this HDL-cholesterol, the lower your risk of heart disease. That's why HDL-cholesterol is sometimes called 'the good cholesterol'.

Most of the blood cholesterol is carried by low-density lipoprotein (LDL). This LDL-cholesterol is being transported the other way – from the liver to other parts of the body. Having a high level of LDL-cholesterol in your blood increases your risk of heart disease because it leads to the formation of fatty deposits in arteries. No surprise, then, that LDL-cholesterol is often called 'the bad cholesterol'.

And the ugly? Believe me, the fatty lumps of atheroma that block up arteries and lead to heart attacks and strokes are very ugly. So, remember:

LOW-density lipoprotein (LDL) cholesterol should be LOW;

HIGH-density lipoprotein (HDL) cholesterol should be HIGH.

What should the total cholesterol level be?

In 1986, the American Multiple Risk Factor Intervention Trial (MR FIT) studied over 361 000 men and showed that, throughout the range 3.9–7.8 mmol/l, the higher the cholesterol level, the higher the death rate from coronary heart disease.

Table 1 Serum cholesterol levels in England

Total cholesterol (mmol/l)	Men %	Women %
<5.2 (normal)	31	29
5.2–6.5	41	39
6.5–7.8	21	22
>7.8	7	10
mean	**5.8**	**6.0 mmol/l**

Data from *Health Survey for England*, 1994 © Crown copyright.

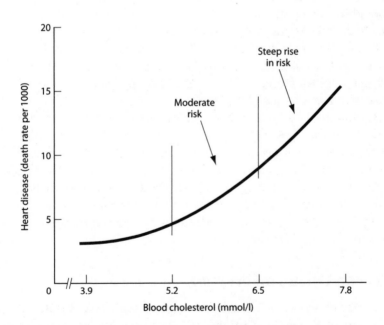

Figure 3 Cholesterol levels and death rates for coronary heart disease. The MR FIT study showed that, as cholesterol levels rose, so did the death rate.
©1996, The Lancet Ltd.

On this basis the lower your cholesterol, the better. The value of 5.2 mmol/l was chosen as the ideal maximum because above this level the rise in heart disease becomes noticeably steeper (see Figure 3).

Dangerously low?

It's worth mentioning that in the MR FIT study the total mortality – deaths from all causes – began to rise again as the cholesterol level dropped below 4.14 mmol/l, even though deaths from heart disease continued to fall. Some other studies have shown the same trend. In fact, there is an increased incidence of cancer among groups with very low cholesterols.

This alarming observation naturally led to the fear that very low cholesterol levels might be dangerous. Don't worry. We now know that cancers can cause the low cholesterol level – not vice versa. Rapidly growing cancers use up cholesterol. In any study of several thousand people with very low cholesterol levels, inevitably some will already have cancer; this will increase the total mortality of the group. But a low cholesterol level cannot cause cancer. And, if you are lucky enough to find your cholesterol is very low, it is most unlikely to be due to cancer! As you would expect, people (such as the Chinese and Japanese) who have average cholesterol levels around 4 mmol/l do not have higher overall cancer rates than groups of people with higher cholesterols (even though different groups of people have more of one type of cancer and less of another).

There have been many studies demonstrating that when cholesterol levels are lowered, either by diet or by drugs, the rates of coronary heart disease fall. Some of these appeared to show extra deaths from other causes, including violence, among those treated with drugs. This was a niggling concern until several major trials using the drugs simvastatin and pravastatin were carried out. In these, lowering cholesterol achieved big reductions both in coronary deaths and in deaths from all causes.

An important test of the drugs

The West of Scotland Coronary Prevention Study (WOSCOPS) published in 1995 included 6595 men aged 45–64 with raised cholesterol levels (average 7.0 mmol/l) but no past history of a heart attack. Each man was randomly allocated to one or the other of two groups (just as if a coin had been tossed). Half the men were given the cholesterol-lowering drug pravastatin and the other half were given placebo (dummy) tablets so that neither the men nor their doctors knew who was taking the active drug and who wasn't until the code was broken at the end of the five-year trial. (This 'randomised, placebo-controlled, double-blind' design is a standard way of eliminating bias in clinical trials.)

Giving pravastatin for five years had reduced the risk of:

- Heart attack by 31%;

- Death from any cause by 22%.

◆ A 'fasting lipid' test measures your cholesterol and triglycerides

◆ LDL-cholesterol can clog arteries; the level should be low

◆ HDL-cholesterol is moving away from artery walls; the level should be high

◆ As the total cholesterol level rises, so does the risk of heart disease

◆ Most people in the UK have a raised cholesterol; the average is 5.9 mmol/l

◆ A total cholesterol of 5.0 mmol/l or less is recommended

◆ A cholesterol level of 4 mmol/l would be better still

Should we all be taking a drug, then?

After all, the majority of people in the UK have blood cholesterols above the recommended level – and even further above the Japanese average. Wouldn't it make sense to put everyone on a drug like pravastatin if it could cut down heart attacks by one-third?

OK, it costs a few hundred pounds a year to keep one person on pravastatin 40 mg daily (the dose used in WOSCOPS). And you'd have to treat something like 110 people for five years before you saved one life. But how do you value a human life?

Convinced? Personally, I think there is something quite obscene about the idea of drugging the population *en masse* to try to prevent a disease that results from poor diet and lifestyle. (But if you already have heart disease, there is probably a strong case for taking a statin drug; this is discussed in Chapter 25.)

I would much rather reduce my risk of heart disease by enjoying the rich variety of a healthy diet than try to offset the damage of a poor, unbalanced diet with drugs. Wouldn't you? If so, read on.

FOOD

'Food is an important part of a balanced diet.'

FRAN LEBOWITZ,
Metropolitan Life, 1978

'I'd rather die young than live on a diet of lettuce and boiled fish,' you say. Who wouldn't? In any case, you would probably die prematurely from boredom and malnutrition on such a diet. We are designed to enjoy our food, so how can a boring diet be really healthy? And yet, so many health promotion messages are negative: 'Don't eat this'; 'You mustn't have that'. You could be forgiven for thinking that if you enjoy it, it must be bad for you. Not so!

There is a great abundance and variety of enjoyable foods, which will help you to ward off ageing processes and maintain a healthy heart and circulation, so why leave room for unhelpful foods?

It is confusing when experts disagree with each other about the healthy diet and keep changing their minds. Now we are told to eat less salt. Next week it may be pepper!

Well I quite understand how newspaper headlines can give this impression. I am looking at one which says 'Sunday Roast is Healthier than a Salad'. There is nothing in the article to justify this eye-catching headline even if a Greek salad and garlic bread may contain more fat than some English dishes. And here's a newspaper report that claims that 'there is as much protection against heart disease in a piece of milk chocolate as in a glass of red wine'. How many readers settled down to a winter of red wine and chocolate in a new health drive? The advice seems to change daily.

'Journalism largely consists in saying "Lord Jones Dead" to people who never knew Lord Jones was alive.'

G K CHESTERTON,
The Wisdom of Father Brown, 1914

Chlamydia: beastly bug or red herring?

You may have seen newspaper reports suggesting that, at last, the real cause of heart disease has been found – infection with Chlamydia. Chlamydia belong to a group of microscopic organisms that can't really decide whether to be viruses or bacteria. Strains of *Chlamydia trachomatis* have earned the group a bad name by causing sexually transmitted diseases and eye infections.

For some years medical scientists have been looking at a possible link between another member of the family (*Chlamydia pneumoniae*) and heart disease. Also, a bacterium known to cause duodenal ulcers (*Helicobacter pylori*) has attracted some scientific limelight after Mendall and colleagues reported a connection with coronary disease in 1994. Such theories are quite difficult to sort out as half the population have Helicobacter infection anyway – usually with no symptoms.

It could well be that the mild inflammation resulting from years of infection with these bugs triggers increased risk factors for coronary heart disease. On the other hand, it could be that social conditions (since childhood) increase the risk of infection *and* of heart disease. A study by Wald and colleagues, published in the *British Medical Journal* in 1997, was designed to minimise the effect that social differences might have on the result; no link was found between Helicobacter infection and death from coronary heart disease.

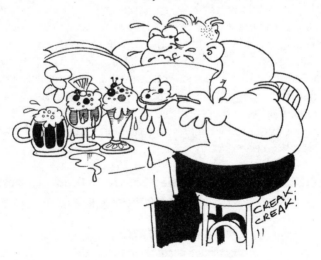

'I see they've found the bug that causes heart disease.'

Back to fact

In fact, there is an overwhelming consensus about healthy eating, which is founded on firm evidence. In this book, we will be dealing with scientific evidence – not dreary dogma and not gimmicks. You will discover how to apply the evidence – how to make changes that will enrich your life and protect your heart.

No doubt you have heard that we should eat less fat, sugar and salt but more fibre. Put like that it sounds rather negative: cut down three tasty things and increase one boring one. It doesn't help if your image of fibre is a bowl of bran.

The reality of healthy eating is quite different. We can translate nutritional wisdom into everyday eating that is far more enjoyable and satisfying than the average British diet. First, we need to know more about what our food is made of.

The nutrients in our food can be divided into these important categories:

1 protein;
2 fat;
3 carbohydrate;
4 vitamins and minerals.

Protein

Unlike fat and carbohydrate, protein doesn't have a whole chapter of its own in this book, but you will hear more about it later. Recent research has shown how protein can help you lose weight and slim your waist.

Much of our body is made of protein and we need a regular supply in our food for the growth and repair of body tissues.

Proteins are large molecules constructed from hundreds or thousands of small units called amino acids. Each amino acid consists of carbon, hydrogen, oxygen and nitrogen. When protein is digested in the intestine, it is broken down into amino acids again and these are absorbed into the bloodstream and used to make new proteins for the body's maintenance and construction programme.

Some of the amino acids are called 'essential' because the body is unable to make them; they must be supplied in the diet. Proteins that contain adequate quantities of all the essential amino acids are known as 'high biological value' (HBV) proteins. Those deficient in one or more essential amino acids are termed 'low biological value' (LBV) proteins.

Animal foods (meat, poultry, fish, dairy products, eggs) provide HBV protein while many plant foods contain LBV protein. Amino acids lacking in one plant will be present in another and, provided complementary foods are combined (such as pulses with grains), even a vegan need not go short of any amino acids.

◆ There is strong evidence for the importance of good food in preventing heart disease

◆ A good diet is not a boring diet

◆ The secret of success lies in the balance of nutrients

◆ To begin with, fat and carbohydrate must be balanced

Chapter 5

Fat

A fatuous phrase

If you need to lower your blood cholesterol level, the doctor advises a 'low-cholesterol diet', right? Wrong! Well, some doctors have been heard to use that fatuous phrase.

Many people imagine that the main change you should make if your cholesterol is too high is to eat less cholesterol. In fact, if it were possible merely to eat less cholesterol, it would achieve very little, but a 'cholesterol-lowering diet' is far more to the point. For a start, eating less saturated fat can make a big difference to the amount of cholesterol in your blood.

◆ Just eating less cholesterol makes little difference

◆ Eating less saturated fat lowers blood cholesterol

◆ The high fat content of UK diets increases heart disease and cancer

◆ Heart attacks are caused by atherosclerosis and thrombosis; saturated fats increase both

---

Get your fats straight

Fats in our food are made up of various 'fatty acids'. These fatty acids are divided into three main groups according to their chemical structure as shown in Table 2.

Now if all this detail about fat seems a bit heavy, don't worry. It's like that when you're dealing with fat; it does seem a bit heavy at first (but don't forget it actually floats on water). This is just necessary

Table 2 Types of fatty acids and their sources

Saturated fatty acids (SFA, saturates)	The molecule has no room for any more hydrogen atoms. It is SATURATED with hydrogen	Lauric	Coconut oil, palm kernel oil
		Myristic	Coconut oil, dairy products
		Palmitic	Palm oil, dairy products, meats
		Stearic	Cocoa butter, meats
Mono-unsaturated fatty acids (MUFA, mono-unsaturates)	There is only ONE area of the molecule that is not saturated with hydrogen atoms	Oleic	Olive oil, rapeseed oil, meat, fish
Polyunsaturated fatty acids (PUFA, polyunsaturates)	There is MORE THAN ONE area of the molecule with room for extra hydrogen	Linoleic	Corn oil, sunflower oil, soya bean oil
		Linolenic	Linseed oil
		Eicosapentaenoic	Fish
		Docosahexaenoic	Fish

preparation before we lift off. The book gets easier to read as we go along – honestly.

Table 2 shows some fatty acids that you gulp down every day, without even a thought for their names. As you see, some of the names give you a clue as to where you'd find the fatty acid.

The fatty acid content of oils depends on the variety and maturity of the seed or nut as well as growing conditions. Fatty acids do not account for 100% of the weight of a fat; the fat in foods also contains substances such as phospholipids and sterols.

Animal, vegetable or mineral?

You will often hear that saturated fat comes from animals while the polyunsaturated and mono-unsaturated fats come from vegetable sources. I don't want to make life complicated, but this really is too

Table 3 Fatty acid content of fats and oils

Oil/fat	Total fat (g/100 g)	Saturates g/100 g	Mono-unsaturates (g/100 g)	Polyunsaturates (g/100 g)	Trans fatty acids (g/100 g)
OILS					
Coconut oil	99.9	86.5	6.0	1.5	trace
Corn oil	99.9	14.4	29.9	51.3	trace
Olive oil	99.9	14.3	73.0	8.2	0
Palm oil	99.9	47.8	37.1	10.4	Trace
Peanut oil	99.9	20.08	44.4	31.0	Trace
Rapeseed oil	99.9	6.6	59.3	29.3	Trace
Safflower oil	99.9	9.7	12.0	74.0	Trace
Sesame oil	99.7	14.6	37.5	43.4	Trace
Soya oil	99.9	15.6	21.3	58.8	Trace
Sunflower oil	99.9	12.0	20.5	63.3	trace
Walnut oil	99.9	9.1	16.5	69.9	trace
SPREADING FATS					
Butter	82.0	52.1	20.9	2.8	2.9
	79.3	34.6	36.2	5.4	12.2
Margarine, soft, polyunsaturated	82.8	17.0	26.6	36.0	6.7
60% fat spread, polyunsaturated	60.8	11.3	18.1	28.6	3.3
60% fat spread with olive oil	62.7	11.3	36.4	12.5	6.0
Flora pro.activ low-fat spread	35.0	9.0	8.0	17.5	0.5
20–25% fat spread, not polyunsaturated	25.5	6.8	14.0	3.4	3.9
COOKING FATS					
Dripping, beef	99.0	50.6	38.0	2.5	4.4
Ghee, butter	99.8	66.0	24.1	3.4	Significant levels but no reliable data
Ghee, vegetable	99.4	48.4	37.0	9.7	1.1
Lard	99.0	40.3	43.4	10.0	Trace
Suet, shredded	86.7	49.9	30.4	2.2	4.0 (estimated)

Data from McCance and Widdowson's *The Composition of Foods*, 6th edition, 2002 (with additional manufacturer's data).

Fatty acids do not account for 100% of the weight of fat, which also contains substances such as phospholipids and sterols.

simple. There are some very important exceptions. Palm oil and coconut oil contain a lot of saturated fatty acids (see Table 3). So, when a food label lists 'vegetable oil' as an ingredient, beware! This could mean anything from highly desirable olive oil (70% mono-unsaturates) to unhelpful coconut oil (85% saturates). If it were olive oil, the label would probably say so. On the other hand, you may find that a bottle labelled 'vegetable oil' contains pure rapeseed oil – or a blend of soya, rapeseed and corn oils. You do need to know what you're getting.

However shaky your biology, you probably realise that fish are animals, not plants, but oily fish are a rich source of the special polyunsaturated fatty acids, eicosapentaenoic acid (EPA) and docosahexaenoic acid (DHA). They don't roll off the tongue but they can be a joy to eat and we'll learn more about them in Chapter 8.

More fat please. We're British

**'If you want to eat well in England,
eat three breakfasts.'**

—————

W SOMERSET MAUGHAM

Most people in the UK are eating far too much fat. If you don't want to be swallowed up in the epidemic of heart disease, your fat intake should be well below average.

In a typical UK diet, about 40% of the calories come from fat. The Department of Health's expert committee (COMA), reporting in 1994, recommended that this be reduced to 35%. The reduction was to be made by cutting down *saturated fat*. Reports by COMA in 1991 and 1994 set a target of 10% of calories for people's saturated fat intake (a significant reduction on the actual average of 16%).

Don't get confused here. You might be thinking, 'I don't eat anything like 40% fat!' Having 40% of your calories as fat does **not** mean that 40% of the weight of your food is fat. Fat is 'energy-dense': a little fat gives a lot of energy. Much of the fat we eat is hidden in processed foods. Meals with no visible fat can push you above the 35% mark in no time. Needless to say, when fat is obvious (as in greasy sausages and chips, pork crackling or cream cakes) your fat intake can shoot beyond the 40% level – and a lot of that will be saturated fat.

Slashing saturated fat is the cornerstone of the cholesterol-lowering diet because the body lowers blood levels of the harmful cholesterol (LDL-cholesterol) when it receives less saturated fat.

It has become clear that the different saturated fatty acids in our food don't all have an equal effect when it comes to raising cholesterol. In fact, stearic acid doesn't seem to raise it at all.

Most of the research highlighting the evils of saturated fatty acids has focused on their damaging tendency to raise LDL-cholesterol. But that's only part of the story. Fatty acids have a wide range of metabolic effects apart from altering LDL levels. Your chances of developing a thrombosis (blood clot in the circulation), suffering from an infection, or contracting cancer will all be influenced by different fatty acids. Individual saturated fatty acids may have a mixture of helpful and harmful effects; some raise the level of protective HDL-cholesterol at the same time as increasing dangerous LDL.

We put a man on the moon decades ago, but we still have a lot to learn about the different effects of fatty acids you eat every day.

Some saturated fatty acids may be more benign than others, but foods contain a mixture of fatty acids. So the only practical course is to cut down on all foods with a high content of saturates.

◆ A 'low-fat spread' containing 40% fat is still a very high-fat food

◆ A healthy diet does not mean lots of sunflower margarine or spread

◆ Too much polyunsaturated fat could be harmful; it may lead to damaging oxidation of LDL

A fat lot of good

To meet legal requirements, something labelled 'butter' or 'margarine' will contain a standard amount of fat (about 81 g/100 g) but there are important differences in the types of fat used. A 'low-fat spread' containing 40% fat (40 g/100 g) is still a very high-fat food.

Many people have got the message that a healthy diet means eating sunflower margarine – or reduced-fat spread. Certainly, changing from butter to a low-fat spread high in polyunsaturates is a good idea. Replacing saturated fat with polyunsaturates helps to lower blood cholesterol. This does not mean, as some people seem to think, that polyunsaturated fat is so good for you that you should have as much as possible!

Increasing your intake of linoleic acid (that's the polyunsaturated fatty acid in sunflower, safflower, soya bean and corn oils) can help to lower the blood cholesterol level. Unfortunately, large amounts of polyunsaturated fat may have some unwanted effects, such as increasing oxidation of LDL, which could put more fatty deposits in arteries. The real problem is that we do not know of any natural population that uses linoleic acid extensively, so we cannot be certain how safe it is to use it as a major source of energy. Government guidelines recommend that this type of fat should contribute no more than 6% of the total calorie intake. Sparing use of a low-fat sunflower spread is no problem at all.

A lot of good fat

'. . . and you can enjoy the fat of the land.'
_____

Genesis 45:18,
New International Version

Mono-unsaturated fat, on the other hand, features prominently in the olive oil-rich Mediterranean diet which is associated with low rates of heart disease.

If you eat less saturated fat and replace it with carbohydrate, the chances are your LDL-cholesterol level will fall. That's good. Sadly, your HDL-cholesterol level will probably come down too and that's bad. Replacing some of that carbohydrate with mono-unsaturated fat (from olive oil and almonds, for example) helps to preserve your HDL. Mono-unsaturates have the edge over polyunsaturates when it comes to maintaining HDL levels.

Studies also suggest that, unlike polyunsaturates, mono-unsaturates protect LDL against damaging oxidation.

The 1991 COMA report recommended that we obtain 12% of our energy from mono-unsaturated fatty acids, but the 1994 report did not give a figure; increasingly experts debated whether we should replace saturated fat with mono-unsaturated fat or carbohydrate.

> ### ACTION POINTS
>
> ◆ Beware 'vegetable oil'! It could contain lots of saturated fat
>
> ◆ Cut down on all foods with a high content of saturates
>
> ◆ Avoid hard margarines; they contain lots of trans fatty acids
>
> ◆ Avoid foods with 'hydrogenated vegetable oil' – especially when it's near the top of the ingredients list

What about 'trans fatty acids'?

I have already mentioned sunflower spread and there are also palatable spreads containing high levels of mono-unsaturates – no doubt excellent choices if you must spread fat on your food. In addition to the olive oil suggested by their name, these spreads are likely to be derived from rapeseed oil; in fact rapeseed oil is usually the main ingredient. But a word of caution: although lower in fat, in some ways a margarine (or reduced-fat spread) may not be as good for you as the oil from which it is made. Changing the oil from a liquid into a spread involves 'hydrogenation' – adding hydrogen atoms to some of those spare places on the fatty acid molecules. 'Hydrogenated vegetable oil' is a term you will often see on food labelling; you should regard it as similar to saturated fat and keep your intake to a minimum.

Another important point about this process of hydrogenation is that it results in some **trans fatty acids**. Now a trans fatty acid is a chemical variant of the more natural form of the fatty acid molecule. The natural form of the molecule is called cis, but the trans version has part of its structure twisted round to produce a different shape (see page 40). Think of a trans molecule as someone with the lower half of his body twisted round until his bottom faces forwards. Obviously, he'd have to put on his underpants and trousers back to front (not so much transvestite as TRANS-pants-SITE).

You can see the problems that this unnatural arrangement might cause in the everyday life of a fatty acid, and a little metabolic mayhem would not be surprising. He couldn't sit next to cis to watch TV and would probably end up standing; trans fatty acids are straight but the natural, cis molecule is bent at the double bond.

The percentage of saturated and trans fatty acids in a hard margarine is likely to be much higher than in a soft margarine or spread. A margarine made from hardened vegetable fats might contain 15% trans fatty acids compared with only 0.7% in a low-fat sunflower spread.

There is mounting evidence that high levels of artificially produced trans fatty acids in the diet are harmful. Several studies have shown that when people eat more trans fatty acids, LDL-cholesterol goes up and HDL-cholesterol goes down – a very undesirable combination. To make matters worse, trans fat increases the risk of thrombosis. In 1993, Willett and colleagues reported findings from the Nurses' Health Study, which involved 85 000 women. The women who ate more trans fatty acids were more likely to have heart disease. Less than 2% of your calories should come from this type of fat, so watch those processed cakes and biscuits as well as margarines (see Table 4).

What are 'essential fatty acids'?

Most people in the UK eat far too much fat but we all need some. A completely fat-free diet would be virtually impossible to achieve, but

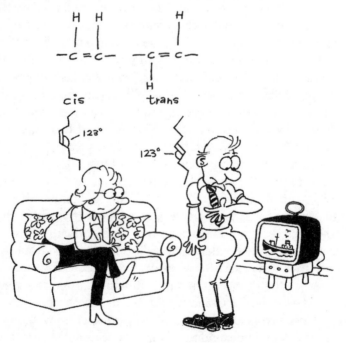

cis and trans isomers of an unsaturated fatty acid.

Table 4 Recommendations for population intakes of fat

TYPE OF FAT	CONTRIBUTION TO TOTAL ENERGY INTAKE	
	WHO Expert Consultation (2003)	UK recommendations (COMA 1991, 1994, 1998)
Total fat	15–30%	No more than 33%
Saturated	Less than 10%	No more than 10%
Omega-6 polyunsaturated	5–8%	No further increase from 6%
Omega-3 polyunsaturated	1-2%	0.2 g/day (1.5 g/week)
Trans	Less than 1%	No more than 2%

also very dangerous. Linoleic acid (from the omega-6 fat family) and alpha-linolenic acid (from the omega-3 family) are called 'essential' because the body cannot make them from other fatty acids. If you follow the guidelines in this book – and make sure your diet includes enough cereal grains (for omega-6 fats) and fish (for omega-3 fats) – you will have all the fatty acids you need.

If you are a vegan, seeds, nuts and cooking oils are important sources; it is helpful to use olive oil, or rapeseed oil (rather than sunflower, safflower or corn oil) to reduce the proportion of linoleic acid in your fat intake. (Vegans sometimes get as much as 60% of their fat in the form of linoleic acid and at this level it can interfere with the body's ability to make the 'fish oil' docosahexaenoic acid, which is not included in the vegan diet.)

If it's 'good fat', can I have as much as I want?

The 1994 COMA report specifically considered diet and cardiovascular disease (diseases of the heart and circulation). It recommended replacement of fats rich in saturates with those rich in mono-unsaturates, as long as the total fat intake does not provide more than 35% of calories. The committee recommended increased consumption of fish, vegetables, fruit, potatoes and bread.

The **total** amount of fat in your diet (saturates, polyunsaturates, and mono-unsaturates) – and not just the **type** – makes a difference to your risk of heart disease (not to mention your weight). Dr Miller and colleagues have found that higher-fat diets increase the risk of blood clots by affecting the activity of an important clotting factor (factor VII). Indeed, it seems that even one very high-fat meal increases the risk of thrombosis – so it's not just a question of your average intake over the week.

For convenience, we often talk of eating less 'saturated fat', but do remember that all fats in our diet are a mixture of different fatty acids (see Table 3). What we need to do is to select foods that have a very low content of saturated fatty acids.

◆ Trans fatty acids raise harmful cholesterol, lower helpful cholesterol and increase the risk of thrombosis

◆ A balanced diet, including cereal grains, seeds, nuts and fish, contains the fatty acids you need – even without adding cooking oils or fat spreads

◆ If you are a vegan, use olive oil or rapeseed oil

◆ 'Friendly fat' is found in olive oil, rapeseed oil, some nuts, avocados and fish

◆ Eating *too much* fat increases thrombosis risk

Fat chance of enjoying a healthy meal then?

How can I enjoy my food if I'm worrying about the percentage of saturated fat in it? Don't worry. Once you've learnt a few basic principles, you will find it easier and easier to select low-fat foods that provide the foundation of your low-fat diet. Be more relaxed about good sources of mono-unsaturated fatty acids (e.g. olive oil, rapeseed oil, hazelnuts, almonds, avocados) and include some oily fish (e.g. sardines, pilchards, mackerel, herring, salmon). This approach will provide the right balance of fats and soon becomes second nature.

To learn those principles, let's look at the major sources of fat in our food.

Dairy products

Milk

'Things are seldom what they seem,
Skim milk masquerades as cream.'

SIR W S GILBERT, *HMS Pinafore*, **1878**

Milk is an excellent source of important nutrients like protein, calcium and vitamins but it also makes a big contribution to the nation's saturated fat intake. Whole, fresh milk is about 4% fat, two-thirds of which is saturated. This may not sound very much but you must consider the quantity of a food you consume as well as the percentage of fat it contains. If you used milk like a condiment – just sprinkling a few drops on your dinner – the amount of fat would be insignificant, but a pint a day is a different matter.

The answer is to use skimmed or semi-skimmed milk. I thoroughly recommend skimmed milk (but not for children under five). This provides all the protein and calcium of whole milk but virtually no fat at all. Yes, it does taste different, but most people soon get used to this if they give themselves a chance. If you really feel you cannot adapt to skimmed milk, semi-skimmed will give you half the fat of whole milk. (Remember: too many compromises will undermine your efforts to make an impact on heart disease risk.) Even then, I recommend skimmed milk for cooking (including sauces and custard) because the chances are that you won't notice the difference in taste.

Another great advantage of fully skimmed milk is that you can buy it in powder form. Provided you reconstitute it in advance (by mixing with water in a pint jug and leaving it in the refrigerator until it is cold) you would never know it hadn't come from a bottle. I hate the thought of making the milkman redundant, but it is a great convenience to stockpile skimmed milk powder when it is on special offer in the supermarket; you need never run out of milk and you don't have to remember to cancel the milk when you go on holiday.

ACTION POINT

◆ Use skimmed milk. It contains all the goodness of whole milk – without the fat

Cream

Cream is no help to you at all when it comes to eating a low-saturated fat diet (see Table 5).

Table 5 Fat content of creams

Type of cream	Total fat content
Single	19%
Whipping	39%
Double	48%

Two-thirds of the fat in cream is saturated. It is best to exclude cream completely from your regular diet, then you can feel free to enjoy it on that special occasion. (Special occasions arise occasionally – not every weekend.)

Low-fat yoghurt (e.g. 1% fat) and very low-fat yoghurt (e.g. 0.1% fat) are good substitutes if you enjoy them, but they are not to everyone's taste. Greek yoghurt has a much creamier flavour but, being 7–9% fat, should be used sparingly. (Fat-free versions are now available but the creamy flavour is reduced accordingly.) Cows' 'strained' Greek yoghurt is about 9% fat, whereas the 'set' variety is only 4% fat. Typically, a 'set' sheeps' yoghurt would be 7.5% fat.

Fromage frais (8% fat) and virtually fat-free fromage frais (0.1% fat) are acceptable substitutes for cream. I particularly recommend vanilla-flavoured virtually fat-free fromage frais. (Try saying this five times quickly. Good: now you're ready to ask for some when it doesn't appear on the supermarket shelf.) If you have this instead of cream with strawberries on a summer's day, you won't feel deprived at all. If nothing but cream will do, at least dispensing it from a spray can bulks out the fat with a bit of air.

Be wary of cream substitutes based on vegetable oil, as they may still contain a lot of saturated fat.

◆ Virtually fat-free fromage frais is a useful alternative to cream; 'synthetic cream' is not

Cheese

**'Poets have been mysteriously silent
on the subject of cheese.'**

G K CHESTERTON

Like cream, most cheeses have a high fat content, two-thirds of which
is saturated (see Table 6).

Table 6 Fat content of cheeses

Variety of cheese	Typical fat content
Brie	27%
Camembert	23%
Cheddar	34%
Cheddar – reduced fat	15%
Cottage cheese	4%
Cottage cheese – reduced fat	1.5%
Parmesan	33%
Pecorino	33%

Clearly, cottage cheese is an exception to the general rule and is a
genuinely low-fat cheese (although two-thirds of the fat is still saturated). Be careful about 'lower fat' or 'reduced fat' cheeses because,
while they will contain less fat than the traditional version, they are
still likely to be high-fat foods. If you like Cheddar, miniCol is a great
alternative; the dairy fat has been replaced with wheatgerm oil, making it low in saturates but high in polyunsaturates and plant sterols.

◆ Cottage cheese is a low-fat food. Half-fat cheddar is still a fatty food

Quark (typically 0.2% fat) is a soft white cheese and you can use it freely. I wouldn't want to eat it by the lump as if it were delicious Boursin. You could spread it on bread instead of butter when making savoury sandwiches but it is especially useful when cooking a whole variety of recipes that call for cream cheese or even cream.

Parmesan and pecorino are useful cheeses because they have a high flavour-to-fat ratio. Small quantities grated into a dish will add a lot of flavour and not much fat.

So, don't stint on dairy products. Skimmed milk and a variety of products with a similar fat content (e.g. buttermilk, very low-fat yoghurt, virtually fat-free fromage frais, quark) are invaluable to the cook. They contain all the calcium and protein of full-fat products – without the fat. When you discard the fat, some fat-soluble vitamins go with it, but skimmed milk powder is fortified with vitamins A and D.

ACTION POINTS

◆ Save cream for really special occasions

◆ Use: virtually fat-free fromage frais, very low-fat yoghurts, quark and buttermilk

---

Meat and meat products

This group of foods is a rich source of protein but also of fat – much of it saturated. British cuisine places too much emphasis on meat. A mound of flesh dominates the plate while one or two demoralised vegetables pay homage at the margin. Six ounces of meat or poultry a day is a sensible limit and, of course, it is quite possible to be a healthy vegetarian.

Red meat
If you want to include red meat in your diet, buy lean cuts and trim off all visible fat. Typically, roast shoulder of lamb would be over 25% fat, while roast lean topside of beef would be less than 5% fat (see Table 7).

'The fat was so white, and the lean was so ruddy.'

OLIVER GOLDSMITH (1728–1774),
The Haunch of Venison, 4

As well as trimming fat before cooking, it is often worth draining or skimming off fat during or after cooking. Minced meat can conceal a lot of fat. Buy the leanest mince you can get or, better still, select lean meat and ask the butcher to mince it. Even then, browning the mince in a non-stick pan, transferring it to a sieve, and drying it with paper kitchen towelling before proceeding with the recipe will get rid of a lot of redundant fat. Another approach is to refrigerate a finished dish and carefully remove all the hardened fat from the surface before reheating.

So remember: SLIM, TRIM, and SKIM. Select SLIM meat; TRIM before cooking; SKIM after cooking.

Table 7 Fat content of meat and meat products

Meat/meat product	Total fat (g/100 g)	Saturates (g/100 g)	Mono-unsaturates (g/100 g)	Poly-unsaturates (g/100 g)
Beef				
Mince (microwaved)	17.5	7.6	7.7	0.7
Mince (stewed), extra lean	8.7	3.8	3.8	0.3
Topside (roast)	12.5	5.2	5.7	0.6
Topside (roast), lean	6.3	2.6	2.8	0.3
Lamb				
Breast (roast)	29.9	14.3	11.4	1.4
Breast (roast), lean	18.5	8.6	7.0	0.9
Loin chops (grilled)	22.1	10.5	8.4	1.3
Loin chops (grilled), lean	10.7	4.9	4.0	0.6

Table 7 Fat content of meat and meat products (*cont'd*)

Meat/meat product	Total fat (g/100 g)	Saturates (g/100 g)	Mono-unsaturates (g/100 g)	Poly-unsaturates (g/100 g)
Pork				
Loin chop (roast)	19.3	7.0	7.8	3.1
Loin chop (grilled), lean	6.4	2.2	2.6	1.0
Leg joint (roast)	10.2	3.6	4.4	1.4
Leg joint (roast), lean	5.5	1.9	2.3	0.7
Chicken				
Breast in crumbs (fried)	12.7	2.1	5.3	4.6
Breast, no skin (grilled)	2.2	0.6	1.0	0.4
Leg quarter, with skin (roast)	16.9	4.6	7.8	3.2
Light meat (roast)	3.6	2.1	3.4	1.5
Turkey				
Skin, dry (roast)	40.2	13.2	15.6	8.8
Breast, no skin (grilled)	1.7	0.67	1.0	0.3
Light meat (roast)	2.0	0.7	7.8	0.5
Dark meat	6.6	2.0	3.4	1.7
Duck				
Meat, fat and skin (roast)	38.1	11.4	19.3	5.3
Meat only (roast)	10.4	3.3	5.2	1.3
Meat products				
Beefburger (grilled)	24.4	10.7	11.4	0.5
Sausage, pork (fried)	23.9	8.5	10.3	3.5
Pork pie	25.7	9.7	11.0	3.2

Data from McCance and Widdowson's *The Composition of Foods*, 6th edition, 2002.

Fatty acids do not account for 100% of the weight of fat, which also contains substances such as phospholipids and sterols.

Game

Game (for example venison, rabbit and pheasant) is generally less fatty than farm animals – the four-legged ones, anyway.

Poultry

**'Long as there is chicken and gravy on your rice
Ev'rything is nice.'**

JOHNNY MERCER, 'Lazybones', 1932

Properly prepared, chicken and turkey can make a delicious contribution to a low-fat diet. Remove the skin and any visible fat (otherwise the fat content may be trebled). For many recipes, it is convenient to buy skinless chicken breasts (e.g. 2.2% fat) or skinless turkey breasts (e.g. 1.1% fat). Thigh meat has a higher fat content (typically 3.5% for turkey thigh). Extra lean turkey mince is an excellent, lower-fat alternative to minced beef in anything from burgers to bolognese.

You can even buy smoked turkey rashers which taste just like bacon but are only 1% fat. Do yourself some good with a cooked breakfast – turkey rashers, mushrooms and tomatoes cooked in a tiny amount of olive oil or rapeseed oil. But you do need to ration those rashers on account of their salt content.

Meat products

Beware unidentified frying objects. What's in a sausage? For a start, it's unlikely to be packed with lean meat when a bit of cheap fat makes the filling go so much further. In fact, sausages, salami and samosas, pies, pâtés and pasties are all disastrously loaded with fat. If you can't identify it, best not buy it.

Meat substitutes

Tofu, or soya bean curd, is widely used in Japanese cuisine. If you have never met it, you are probably rather wary but, once you have become acquainted, you will find it a very versatile alternative to meat or dairy products. Using soya protein in place of animal protein helps to lower the total blood cholesterol and LDL-cholesterol. Their large intake of soya, and various other vegetables and grains, may help to explain why oriental men have such low rates of prostate cancer (until they change to Western diets).

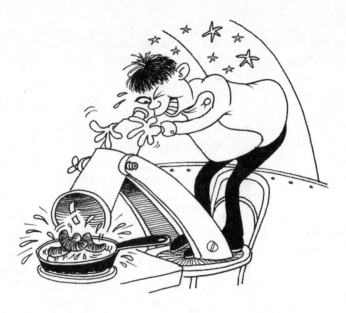

Beware unidentified frying objects.

Unlike most plant proteins, the protein from soya beans contains all the essential amino acids – making it a very good meat substitute from the nutritional point of view. Even if you dislike great lumps of soya masquerading as meat, you will probably find one or two packs of soya mince invaluable when you want to knock up a quick 'chilli con carne' – without the meat.

Quorn is a low-fat, high-protein meat substitute made from a fungus (like mushroom) and egg white. It has a chicken-like texture and will take on the flavour of any sauce in which it is cooked.

Of course, you can always compromise by using meat substitutes together with meat as a way of reducing the fat content of a dish.

ACTION POINTS

◆ Avoid processed meat products (such as sausages, salami, meat pies and pâté). They contain lots of saturated fat

◆ Quorn, tofu and soya mince can be used with meat to reduce the fat content of a dish

Fats and oils

Of all the fatty foods in our diet, this group is the fattiest. After all, any cooking oil will be 100% fat. The term 'oil' merely indicates that it is a liquid at room temperature. Adding large quantities of pure fat to your food will not help you to achieve a low-fat diet so these products should always be used as sparingly as possible.

Often, when a traditional recipe calls for added fat, you can leave the fat out altogether with very satisfactory results. On other occasions, a little fat makes all the difference – when roasting potatoes, for example. You could produce an ultra low-fat version by cooking in vegetable stock. I much prefer to toss the parboiled potatoes in a little preheated olive oil or rapeseed oil and roast them in a very hot oven until crisp and golden. The result is exquisite and will do you nothing but good.

You will note that I do not suggest using a little lard! Choose an oil with a high content of mono-unsaturated fatty acids and a low content of saturates. Olive oil meets the criteria, being about 70% mono-unsaturates and 14% saturates. It is a good first choice because of its track record: Mediterranean countries, with olive oil at the heart of their cuisine, have low rates of heart disease.

Rapeseed oil is an excellent choice too. In fact, it has a lower saturate content than olive oil and is about 60% mono-unsaturates but it cannot claim the track record of olive oil.

You see, the wild rapeseed plant contains a lot of erucic acid – a mono-unsaturated fatty acid, but one which we have no experience of eating in large quantities. It would be an unwise experiment to start eating large amounts of erucic acid; it might be good for us – but it might not.

Commercial production of rapeseed oil had to await the selection of a variety with very low levels of erucic acid. Don't worry. The rapeseed oil on your supermarket shelf will be a low-erucic acid variety; the high mono-unsaturate content is all down to oleic acid – exactly the same fatty acid as in olive oil. So I have every confidence in rapeseed oil (and it certainly stands beside the olive oil in my kitchen) even though it cannot yet claim to have been tried and tested through the centuries like olive oil. Mind you, as well as oleic acid, rapeseed oil is a good source of alpha-linolenic acid, which is in the same family as fish oils. The Japanese on Kohama Island and the people of Crete eat diets rich in alpha-linolenic acid and have remarkably low rates of heart disease.

Rapeseed oil has the advantage of being much cheaper than olive oil and it is also one of the main crops produced by British farmers.

It may be that the name puts people off rapeseed oil. It's very popular in the USA but they call it canola oil. After all, 'sunflower' conjures up positive images of a summer's day and 'olive' probably reminds you of a nice girl. A more cuddly name to replace 'rapeseed' might double its popularity overnight. Perhaps a manufacturer should run a competition to rename the oil: the promotion would be a heartening boost for British farming and for the beleaguered British heart.

Olive oil or rapeseed oil will meet most of your culinary requirements and it is not essential to buy any other oils or fats. If you want the flavour of olive oil (for example in salad dressing) extra virgin olive oil is useful. An oily salad dressing can give you an awful lot of fat, so, even if it is friendly fat, go easy. If you don't want an olive oil flavour (for example when making flapjack) select olive oil with a light flavour; the fatty acid content is similar but the taste is delicate. Of course, an alternative would be to use rapeseed oil. Other oils with a significant proportion of mono-unsaturated fatty acids are peanut oil (also called groundnut or arachis oil) and grapeseed oil.

Table 8 divides some common fats and oils into three groups. Those rich in mono-unsaturates are recommended and it is best to avoid completely those with a high saturated fatty acid content. Sparing use of fats and oils containing a high proportion of poly-unsaturates is acceptable. DO NOT re-use oils after cooking; reheating can oxidise polyunsaturated fats, making them more damaging to blood vessels.

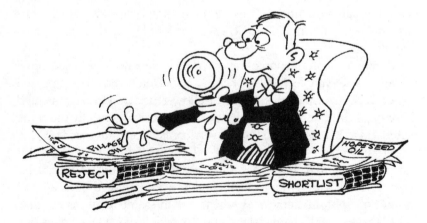

Perhaps we should have a competition to rename rapeseed oil.

ACTION POINTS

◆ When cooking oil is needed, use a little olive oil or rapeseed oil

◆ Don't re-use cooking oils

Table 8 Fats and oils

High in mono-unsaturates	High in polyunsaturates	High in saturates
Olive oil	Sunflower oil	Palm oil
Rapeseed oil	Corn oil	Coconut oil
Peanut oil	Safflower oil	Butter
'Olive oil' spread	Soya oil	Lard
	Walnut oil	Dripping
	Sesame seed oil*	Suet
	Sunflower spread	Margarines

*Sesame seed oil contains a reasonable helping of mono-unsaturates (37%)
as well as polyunsaturates (44%).

Hard margarines are particularly to be avoided. Not only do they contain high levels
of saturated fatty acids but also of trans fatty acids which may be even more damaging
(see page 39).

What about baking if olive oil and rapeseed oil are the only fats in your kitchen? Most recipes that call for a hard fat work perfectly well if you use oil instead. The general rule is to replace 4 oz (100 grams) of butter or margarine with 5 tablespoons (75 ml) of oil. Oil works extremely well in biscuits, cakes and bread. It is even possible to use oil in pastry and crumble but you may prefer a reduced-fat spread (high in mono-unsaturates) which is suitable for baking. You can mix oils; replacing some of the rapeseed oil in your flapjack with peanut oil will give it a more nutty flavour.

ACTION POINT

◆ Adapting recipes: for every 4 oz (100 g) of butter or margerine use
   5 tablespoons (75 ml) of rapeseed or olive oil

So remember:

● the traditional fat in a recipe often can be left out altogether;

● if you need to use fat:

   ▪ choose an oil rich in mono-unsaturates;

   ▪ use as little as possible.

What about my bread and butter, then? If you cannot contemplate life
without putting butter on your bread, you had better learn to spread
it thinly. A scraping of reduced-fat spread (high in mono- or polyunsaturates) would be preferable, but most people could surprise
themselves by discovering how happily they adapt to new habits. I
love toast and marmalade. An intervening layer of fat is entirely
superfluous. The French habit of eating unbuttered bread with a meal
is a healthy one.

The new fat spreads – a spreading revolution?

If you were on Mars or in a monastery at the time, you may have
missed the launch of the new fat spreads – Benecol and Flora pro.activ
– specially formulated to lower blood cholesterol levels.

These spreads belong to a new group of products known as 'functional foods' – foods that are claimed to do more for you than merely
supply tasty nourishment. We are likely to see many more functional
foods in the future. (What would you think of a contraceptive cheese,
or a sandwich spread that makes tax returns seem interesting?)

The new fat spreads have had prominent places in the media, but
what role, if any, do they have in our fight against heart disease?

Benecol products contain plant stanols while Flora pro.activ is fortified with plant sterols. Sterols occur naturally in the cell membranes
of plants and animals. (Cholesterol itself, which is found only in animals, is a sterol.) It has been known since the 1950s that plant sterols

can lower blood cholesterol levels. Stanols are produced by adding hydrogen to sterols and have a similar effect.

Sterols and stanols reduce the absorption of cholesterol from the intestine. (We normally absorb about half the cholesterol in the intestine; eating one of these products cuts that in half so we absorb about a quarter.) This raises an obvious question: do they still work if you are eating a low-cholesterol, low-fat diet?

A study by Denke was reported as showing that stanols weren't effective in men on a low-fat diet. But it probably wasn't the low-fat diet that reduced the effect of the stanols: it's much more likely that the stanols didn't work properly because they were given in gelatine capsules. Sterols and stanols work better when delivered with a fatty food so a spread is ideal. Indeed, two studies published in the *American Journal of Clinical Nutrition* in 1999 showed that stanols (dissolved in margarine) effectively lowered LDL-cholesterol in people eating low-fat, low-cholesterol diets.

You see, these products don't just reduce absorption of the cholesterol you eat. Some cholesterol that you make in your liver passes into the intestine before being absorbed into the bloodstream. Sterols and stanols reduce absorption of this cholesterol too, so it's not surprising that they lower blood cholesterol levels even when there's very little cholesterol in the diet. (Actually the body responds to this reduced absorption by making more cholesterol – but not enough to prevent a drop in blood cholesterol.)

To achieve a 10–15% reduction in LDL-cholesterol, you need to eat 2 g of plant sterol or stanol a day; this amount is added to the average daily portion of spread. Eating more than the recommended amount is unlikely to lower your cholesterol further.

Middle-age spread?

The average reduction in LDL-cholesterol produced by 2 g of sterol or stanol a day depends on the ages of the people studied. The average fall in LDL-cholesterol is 0.54 mmol/l in people aged 50–59, 0.43 mmol/l in those aged 40–49, and 0.33 mmol/l in those aged 30–39. So if you divide the average age by 100, it tells you the expected drop in LDL-cholesterol in mmol/l.

This is a very worthwhile reduction (especially when you consider how easily it's achieved) and amounts to a 25% cut in coronary risk. (Although the drop in cholesterol is smaller in a 35-year-old than in a 55-year-old, there is still a 25% risk reduction because raised cholesterol is a relatively more important risk factor in the younger person. The difference between relative risk and absolute risk is explained in Chapter 25.)

Are these spreads safe? They seem to be and Flora pro.activ has been approved under the EU Novel Foods regulations. One concern is that sterols and stanols reduce absorption of the antioxidants beta-carotene and vitamin E, but this isn't a problem if you eat enough fruit and vegetables. On current evidence, these products wouldn't normally be recommended for pregnant women or for children under five.

Of course, these spreads cost a lot more than standard fat spreads. That's because you need 2500 tons of vegetable oil to extract one ton of sterol. In middle age, you might be glad to spend about half the cost of a daily paper on staying alive, instead of saving up for a lavish funeral.

If you're in the habit of spreading fat on your bread, switching to Flora pro.activ or Benecol could be a wise move. But if, like me, you ditched that layer of fat long ago, what will you gain from adding 20 g of fat spread to your daily diet? Middle-age spread?

Nuts

**'I am Charley's Aunt from Brazil,
where the nuts come from.'**

BRANDON THOMAS (1857–1914),
Charley's Aunt

Nuts are nutritious. They are high-protein foods but they also have a very high fat content so this is a convenient place to deal with them. Nearly all the fat in coconut is saturated. You can see from Table 9 that, if you went nuts, a pile of brazils would give you a hefty dose of saturated fat as well.

Generally, though, nuts are quite helpful to your heart. Including some walnuts in a low-fat diet can lower blood cholesterol levels, according to a study published in the *New England Journal of Medicine* in 1993. Almonds too have been shown to have a cholesterol-lowering effect.

An investigation on over 30 000 Seventh-Day Adventists found that those who ate nuts frequently (more than four times a week) had about 50% fewer heart attacks than those who indulged infrequently (less than once a week).

You don't have to belong to a particular religious group to benefit from nuts. You could be a nurse. Findings of the Nurses' Health Study on over 86 000 women were published in the *British Medical Journal* in 1998. Women who ate nuts at least five times a week had a 35% lower risk of coronary heart disease than those who rarely ate nuts.

Mind you, sorting out the real cause of such observations is always a tough nut to crack. It could be that frequent nut eaters have generally healthier lifestyles; perhaps it's because they also eat more fruit and vegetables, smoke less, and take more exercise that they have less heart disease. Researchers have concluded that when all

Table 9 Fat content of common nuts

Type of nut	Total fat (g/100 g)	Saturates (g/100 g)	Mono-unsaturates (g/100 g)	Poly-unsaturates (g/100 g)	Trans fatty acids (g/100 g)
Almonds	55.8	4.4	38.2	10.5	0
Brazil nuts	68.2	16.4	25.8	23.0	0
Cashew nuts (roasted)	50.9	10.1	29.4	9.1	0
Chestnuts	2.7	0.5	1.0	1.1	0
Coconut (creamed block)	68.8	59.3	3.9	1.6	0
Hazelnuts	63.5	4.7	50.0	5.9	0
Macadamia nuts	77.6	11.2	60.8	1.6	0
Peanuts	46.0	8.7	22.0	13.1	0
Pecan nuts	70.1	5.7	42.5	18.7	0
Walnuts	68.5	5.6	12.4	47.5	0

Data from McCance and Widdowson's *The Composition of Foods*, 6th edition, 2002.

Fatty acids do not account for 100% of the weight of fat, which also contains substances such as phospholipids and sterols.

these 'confounding factors' are stripped away, the kernel of truth remains: nuts do offer some protection against heart disease. How?

In a nutshell, they contain more friendly fat than unfriendly – apart from coconut, that is. Walnuts are a good source of the essential polyunsaturated fatty acid alpha-linolenic acid (related to fish oil). Almonds and hazelnuts major on mono-unsaturates. Nuts also supply important antioxidants, including vitamin E. They are rich in L-arginine which boosts production of protective nitric oxide – vital to the normal function of the smooth lining of artery walls (endothelium).

Laboratory experiments have thrown some light on the effects of nut eating (apart from cholesterol reduction) that could be protecting Seventh-Day Adventists and nurses from heart disease. Eating a handful of walnuts can block some of the damaging effects of saturated fat, according to research published in the *Journal of the American College of Cardiology* in 2006.

After volunteers ate a meal high in saturated fat, the endothelium didn't function properly and there was an increased level of inflammatory molecules. These unwanted changes were prevented by eating 40 g of walnuts (about eight shelled nuts). When olive oil was used instead of walnuts, it also reduced inflammatory molecules, but it didn't boost endothelial function.

So, it's well worth shelling out on a few walnuts, almonds and hazelnuts. Eating them raw is particularly beneficial, whether in muesli or on salads, or on their own as a snack. Use them to replace other sources of protein and fat, and don't just add them to a bad diet! Remember that lots of calories come with the fat in nuts so, if keeping your weight down is a problem, nuts won't help you to crack it. Chestnuts are the exception that proves the rule: they contain very little fat. Enjoy roast chestnuts whenever you want but shy away from coconut.

◆ Apart from chestnuts, nuts are very high in fat

◆ Avoid coconut; it's loaded with saturated fat

◆ Other nuts give you more friendly (unsaturated) fats

◆ Eating a few walnuts, almonds or hazelnuts may help your heart

Snack foods

**'My wife's on a strict fast again.
She won't eat a thing – except fast food.'**

ANON.

We all have a little gap to fill between meals sometimes. That's where snack foods come in. If you choose the wrong ones, you'll overshoot your saturated fat allowance before you can say 'Jack Sprat'.

If you want lots of sugar with your fat, you'll get that in chocolate, pastries and commercial cakes and biscuits. Heavily salted fat is conveniently packaged as potato crisps, corn snacks etc.

Normal crisps are over 30% fat, while reduced fat versions may be about 25% fat – and, when one-quarter of the total weight is fat, you cannot pretend it's a low-fat snack. There are now some appealing lower fat options, but remember that most savoury snacks are still bristling with salt.

Unfortunately, factory-made cakes and biscuits frequently utilise hydrogenated vegetable oil and, as a result, contain significant quantities of trans fatty acids – which may be more damaging to your arteries than saturated fatty acids.

Fresh fruit is an ideal snack. Make sure it is either washed thoroughly or peeled. Many vegetables, like carrots, celery, mangetout peas or sugarsnap peas, make great gap-fillers too.

Dried fruits (such as apricots, pears, prunes, raisins, dates and figs) are available – ready to eat – in convenient, resealable packs. Next time you get that irresistible urge, try a handful of nuts and raisins instead of a chocolate bar – hardly a low-calorie snack, but most of the fat is friendly.

It's not the chocolate in most 'chocolate bars' that's the problem, but the lack of it. The cocoa bean is a rich source of minerals and flavonoid antioxidants (see page 108); the confectionery product you buy probably isn't. Processing usually strips away the good stuff and adds unhelpful sugar and fat.

A small piece of good quality dark chocolate, containing perhaps 85% cocoa solids, might actually do you some good. Try breaking one segment (usually 10 g) into four equal 'squares', and each of these into four; allow one little piece at a time to melt slowly in your mouth. Once you have acquired the taste, anything paler and sweeter just won't seem chocolatey enough. But beware: if you can't limit yourself to savouring a few small pieces, the excess fat and calories will do more harm than good.

Of course you like to have cakes and biscuits sometimes and, if you make them yourself, you can enjoy them without worrying about saturated and trans fatty acids. It may sound strange but, in many cakes, prune purée can be used instead of fat, and the results are excellent . When fat is required, select rapeseed oil or lightly-flavoured olive oil.

◆ Making your own cakes and biscuits can avoid saturated and trans fatty acids

◆ When baking, you can often replace fat with prune purée

◆ Reduced-fat crisps still contain lots of fat (and salt)

◆ Suitable snacks include: fruit, dried fruit, carrot sticks, sugarsnap peas; Japanese rice crackers, mackerel pâté on pitta bread, home-cooked poppadums and popcorn; home-made sandwiches, cakes and biscuits

---

When you have friends round for drinks, you will no doubt offer them crisps and other traditional, high-fat snacks. Why not include some healthier options as well? Japanese rice crackers have a relatively low fat content. Poppadums cooked by immersion in hot oil are obviously very fatty but they are surprisingly acceptable when cooked dry on a paper towel in the microwave (e.g. 40–60 seconds on high power). I still prefer the genuine, high-fat article but, if you cook them yourself in rapeseed oil, as a very occasional treat, at least you know what fat you're getting. Popcorn is a variety of maize, a good wholesome grain, which is usually coated in butter or hydrogenated vegetable oil. Try popping it yourself in a covered saucepan with a very little rapeseed oil. Alternatively, if you are partial to popcorn, it's worth investing in one of the excellent machines that simply pops the corn with hot air, avoiding the need to add any fat at all.

Smoked mackerel pâté is easy to prepare, rich in desirable fish oils, and always popular (see page 415). Toasted triangles of wholemeal pitta bread are a great accompaniment to this. A variety of low-fat dips (such as hummus) can also be served with toasted pitta, wholemeal rye crispbreads, matzos, low-fat crackers or raw vegetables. Be careful to read nutritional information on savoury biscuits and crackers. You may be surprised at the quantity of fat in some of them.

If you enjoy smoked salmon, why not serve it on thinly-sliced wholemeal bread with plenty of lemon juice? There's no need to muffle the flavour with butter.

**TRAMP: Would you give me twenty-five pence
for a sandwich, lady?
LADY: I don't know – let me see the sandwich.**

GYLES BRANDRETH,
1000 Jokes: The Greatest Joke Book Ever Known, **1980**

Sandwiches can be anything from banal to bizarre. What you put between two pieces of bread is limited more by your imagination than by anything else. And you can cater for every taste without including large amounts of saturated fat. Fresh salad and mixed-grain bread are always a good start. Low-fat yoghurt, virtually fat-free fromage frais, quark or cottage cheese lend themselves to a great variety of low-fat dressings. Tomato ketchup, lemon juice, Tabasco sauce, Worcestershire sauce, Hoisin sauce, Dijon mustard and curry paste are great for adding flavour. If you want to dress it with something 'off the peg', and

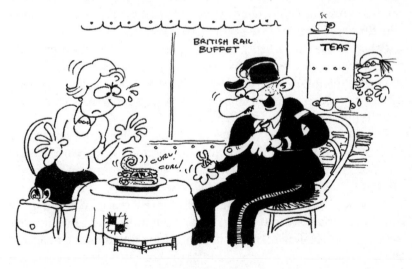

'I see your sandwich has turned up.'

I don't recommend your hat, you could try one of the commercial fat-free dressings (such as yoghurt and chive or Thousand Island style). Tinned fish and cooked chicken or turkey usually go down well.

With ingredients like these, there is no need for butter but consider Benecol or Flora pro.activ. A layer of grease will waterproof the bread. Mind you, there is nothing wrong with moist bread – as long as it's not soggy – unless you are trying to emulate British Rail. (BR earned a reputation for reliability in catering: if you ordered a sandwich, it always turned up – just round the edges.)

Mini sandwiches are ideal for parties, and you can always use shape cutters for extra fun.

Fat substitutes

'Seeing is deceiving.
It's eating that's believing.'

JAMES THURBER,
Further Fables for Our Time, 1956

The perfect fat substitute has all the feel and flavour of fat with none of the calories and is completely safe. This last point is always rather difficult to prove with a new substance, but food manufacturers know that there is a lot of money to be made from increasingly fat- and calorie-conscious consumers who won't want to change the habits of a lifetime when offered an alternative on a plate.

Polydextrose (by Pfizer) and Simplesse (by Nutrasweet) have acquired 'generally regarded as safe' (GRAS) status and are used in foods like margarine, mayonnaise, ice-cream and confectionery. They cannot be used in any foods that will be heated and a margarine made with Simplesse is no good for cooking.

Procter and Gamble developed sucrose polyesters, later called olestra (brand name Olean) by combining fatty acids with a sugar backbone in a different configuration from any natural fat molecule. Olestra is stable when heated and can even be used as a cooking oil. It behaves just like a normal fat, except for one crucial point: it is not digested. It passes right through the body unscathed by digestive enzymes. So you have double the fun: all the fun of eating it, and all the fun of excreting it. Indeed, one of the concerns about olestra has been that some people may experience the latter very rapidly after the former. Further development of olestra greatly reduced its laxative properties, but some concern remained that vital fat-soluble vitamins could go down the pan along with the unwanted calories. The product is now fortified with vitamins.

Like artificial sweeteners, good, safe fat substitutes will have their uses. The commercial potential is huge and they will be hailed as the answer to obesity and heart disease. I doubt that they will ever fulfil this hope. They will never be a satisfactory substitute for developing good food habits and enjoying the rich variety of a balanced low-fat diet.

- ◆ Fat substitutes can be useful in low-fat processed foods

- ◆ There is no substitute for learning to appreciate a balanced diet of unprocessed foods

Chapter 6

Carbohydrate

As the name suggests, carbohydrates are made of carbon and the elements in water (hydrogen and oxygen). They are an important energy source, but the proportion of dietary calories consumed as carbohydrate varies greatly across the world. The population of a developing country might obtain 85% of its calories from carbohydrate, while the diet of an industrial country contains much more fat and may provide less than 45% of the energy as carbohydrate.

The carbohydrates in our food comprise sugars, starches and fibre.

Sugar

Sugars are simple carbohydrates. In the simplest sugars, the molecule consists of only one 'building block' and these are known as the monosaccharides – glucose, galactose and fructose. When two of these are joined together, a disaccharide sugar is formed. Sucrose is a combination of glucose and fructose. Other disaccharides are maltose and lactose.

Sugars in our food can be divided into 'intrinsic sugars' and 'extrinsic sugars'. Intrinsic sugars remain where nature put them – within the cell structure of the food; they are an intrinsic part of the food. An example would be the small amount of sugar that occurs naturally within a fresh bean. Extrinsic sugars, on the other hand, have been separated from this natural structure – like table sugar and the sugar added to a can of baked beans.

Fructose (fruit sugar) is found in fruit, and lactose (milk sugar) is found in milk, but sucrose (table sugar) is found on tables.

Starch

Starches are complex carbohydrates. They are polysaccharides because they consist of many sugar units joined together. The starch in our diet is made up of lots of glucose molecules linked to one another. We get most of our starch from cereal grains and potatoes, but it is also found in peas, beans and other vegetables.

Fibre

Fibre, which used to be called 'roughage', is also in the complex carbohydrate group. In fact, nutritionists prefer to talk about non-starch polysaccharides (NSP) these days, but I suspect you will feel more comfortable if I keep calling it 'fibre'. So I will.

In westernised diets, fibre has had to play Cinderella to all those glamorous nutrients. After all, we can't digest it; it's just the dross that's left behind after the intestine has extracted all the goodness from our food. But, like Cinderella, fibre turned out to be something special and, without it, even the most princely diet would be desperately deficient.

Indeed, the relative lack of fibre in our diet may go a long way towards explaining why many medical problems (including constipation, diverticular disease, acute appendicitis, bowel cancer and gallstones) are so common here but so rare in some parts of the world (e.g. rural Africa). In addition, diets containing plenty of high-fibre foods are associated with low rates of heart disease.

There are two main types of dietary fibre.

Insoluble fibre provides bulk, which helps you to feel satisfied without devouring too many calories. It is also important for normal bowel function and helps to prevent constipation. Simply adding insoluble fibre to the diet probably doesn't lower blood cholesterol but, in practice, when people eat more high-fibre foods, they get less of their energy from saturated fat and the cholesterol level falls. Vegetables (including the skins) and cereal husks provide insoluble fibre. Good sources are: wholemeal bread, wholegrain cereals, brown rice and jacket potatoes.

Soluble fibre does have a direct cholesterol-lowering action. That means that adding enough soluble fibre to the diet, without changing anything else, causes some drop in blood cholesterol levels.

We do not fully understand the mechanisms responsible for this cholesterol reduction. It may be partly that soluble fibre clings to bile acids in the large intestine and prevents their re-absorption back into the body. These bile acids contain cholesterol that has been made in the liver. In this way soluble fibre could encourage the excretion of cholesterol produced by the liver.

Even so, the big reductions in blood cholesterol are seen in people who eat plenty of high-fibre foods *instead* of foods containing a lot of saturated fat.

We obtain soluble fibre from fruit and vegetables generally, and especially from pulses (peas, beans, lentils, chickpeas), as well as from oats. Apples, pears and citrus fruits (such as oranges) are important sources of pectin – one form of soluble fibre. Experiments have shown that adding pectin to the diet lowers cholesterol, but you would generally have to eat a big pile of fruit every day (e.g. five pounds of apples) to match the quantities of pectin given in these experiments.

Too much of a good thing?

Very high carbohydrate diets, in which more than 60% of the calories come from carbohydrate, can raise blood triglyceride levels and lower HDL-cholesterol – the 'good cholesterol' (see Chapter 4). This is a very unwelcome effect. However, people eating very high-carbohydrate diets in developing countries also eat very little saturated fat; they have low levels of LDL-cholesterol – the 'bad' cholesterol – and low rates of heart disease. Even so, you would do much better to keep up your HDL-cholesterol and avoid raising your triglycerides.

So what should I eat?

Where carbohydrate is concerned, standard advice is simple: keep it complex.

It has been generally assumed that simple carbohydrates (sugars) are bad for you because they cause a rapid rise in blood sugar, while complex carbohydrate (starch) is good for you because it releases energy slowly.

It turns out that this view is far too simple. The very fibre of this dietary doctrine has been dealt a death blow by recent research into the glycaemic index of foods.

What's the glycaemic index?

The starch in our food is broken down by digestion and absorbed into the bloodstream as glucose. It doesn't matter whether the food is bread, rice, pasta, potato or something else: the starch it contains has to be converted to simple glucose before it can be absorbed. Some foods are easily broken down causing a rapid rise in blood glucose, while others take longer to digest so that glucose is released more slowly.

Sugars, too, end up as glucose. Some foods contain glucose itself which is absorbed immediately into the bloodstream. Disaccharides are broken down within the intestine to glucose, fructose and galactose which can then pass through the wall of the intestine; fructose and galactose only get as far as the liver where they are converted to glucose.

So, sooner or later, all digestible carbohydrate becomes blood glucose. And when we talk about 'blood sugar', we always mean glucose.

Clearly, some carbohydrate foods give up their energy more quickly than others. It was back in 1981 that David Jenkins and colleagues at the University of Toronto recognised the need to quantify this. They proposed the use of a glycaemic index (GI) – a measure of the impact a food has on blood glucose levels.

How is GI measured?

Jennie Brand-Miller and her colleagues at the Human Nutrition Unit at Sydney University have played a central role in GI research. Tests on hundreds of foods gave rise to the International Tables of Glycaemic Index, published by the *American Journal of Clinical Nutrition*.

No matter how sophisticated your laboratory, you can't measure a food's GI in a test tube. It's all about the way the food is handled by the body, so you need healthy volunteers – at least ten of them. After an overnight fast, each volunteer eats a precisely measured quantity of the test food – enough to provide 50 g of available (digestible) carbohydrate; the fibre, which cannot be digested or absorbed, doesn't count.

Over the next two hours, finger-prick blood samples are taken every 15 to 30 minutes to determine capillary blood glucose levels. A graph is plotted (Figure 4) for each volunteer to show the change in blood glucose concentrations over those two hours; the area under the curve (AUC) is a measure of the total impact of the food on that volunteer's blood glucose levels. On a separate occasion, the same ten people go through exactly the same process after consuming 50 g of pure glucose instead of the test food.

GI is simply the ratio of the two glucose response curves, expressed as a percentage:

$$\text{GI of test food} = \frac{\text{AUC test food}}{\text{AUC glucose}} \times 100$$

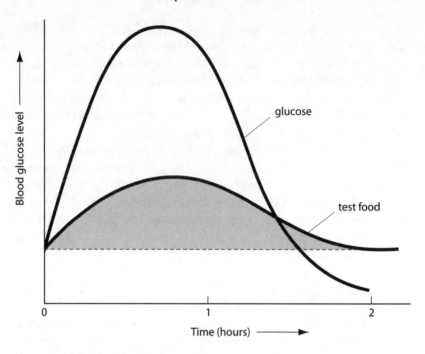

Figure 4 Calculating GI: glycaemic responses to glucose and a test food.

Naturally, glucose – the reference food – has a GI of 100; it's absorbed immediately, causing a rapid rise in blood glucose. A food producing only half this blood glucose response has a GI of 50. The more slowly glucose is released from the food, the lower the GI. The published GI is the average of the results from all ten people. Table 10 shows the GI numbers of some common foods.

Confusion has been caused by the fact that some studies have used white bread as a reference food, generating GI numbers up to 140. (It's easier to get volunteers to eat bread than to drink a sickly solution of glucose.) So it's always wise to check that you're dealing with a standard scale based on comparison with glucose. If you find yourself in bread territory, multiplying the numbers by 0.7 will make them comparable with the standard table.

You might think that if the test period were extended beyond two hours, slow-release foods would eventually catch up with glucose, producing a graph of equal area but more elongated shape. (After all, in time, all 50 g of digestible carbohydrate in the test food will be turned into glucose.) But no. Glucose, of course, is constantly being removed from the blood; it's entering cells in tissues all over the body to produce energy. That's what this is all about.

Does it matter?
Suddenly flooding the bloodstream with glucose is a bit like giving your builder five cups of tea all at once. If this is what you do, try spreading the supply more evenly through the day; you could see a marked improvement in performance.

When blood glucose shoots up after eating high-GI foods, more insulin is released to reduce it again. Raised insulin levels make you feel hungry and can lead to fat storage. It's bad news for the heart and arteries if insulin levels are persistently raised, as they are in the metabolic syndrome (see page 313) and Type 2 diabetes.

Perhaps it always was naïve to think that sugar was of the devil, and wholemeal bread a virtuous food – when the starch in bread ends up as simple blood sugar. But the big surprise has been the finding that some starchy foods, such as bread, have a higher GI than table sugar! And wholemeal bread has virtually the same GI as white bread.

More enlightened doctors have realised for some time that people with diabetes benefit from eating a low-GI diet. Conventional advice in recent years, however, has been to control blood glucose by cutting out sugary foods and eating plenty of low-fat, starchy foods, such as bread and potatoes. How much sense does this make when wholemeal bread and baked potatoes push up blood glucose faster than table sugar?

Not only that, but in the light of recent research it seems that those of us who don't have diabetes are better off on a low-GI diet as well. For a start, eating a higher proportion of low-GI foods helps to reduce fat storage and control body weight. It also seems to improve the balance of blood lipids, raising protective HDL-cholesterol and lowering triglycerides. There is now evidence that men and women who keep to a low-GI diet are less likely to develop diabetes and heart disease.

How do I follow a low-GI diet?

Have a look at Table 10 and simply replace foods that have a high number with ones that have a low GI. It is, of course, a continuous scale but foods are sometimes divided into three bands:

- low GI (less than 55)

- medium GI (55–70)

- high GI (over 70).

If you get into the habit of choosing the foods with low numbers, while cutting right down on those with a GI above 70, the overall GI of your diet will be low.

You will see that new potatoes have a lower GI than baked potatoes. Basmati rice has a lower GI than instant rice. Apples, pears and plums have lower GIs than tropical fruits such as melons and pineapples. In general, pastas and pulses (peas, beans and lentils) have low GI numbers – although broad beans are a notable exception.

How can the glycaemic index help athletes?

The slow release of energy from low-GI foods can keep you going for longer than the quick rise in blood sugar that results from eating foods with high GI numbers. Endurance will be increased by eating a low-GI meal, such as pasta, one or two hours before embarking on strenuous activity that goes on for more than 90 minutes. So whether you plan to climb a mountain or go cross-country skiing, if you're going to be at it for at least 90 minutes, stoke up with long-range (low-GI) fuel about 90 minutes beforehand.

By contrast, when athletes are training hard every day, they need to put energy (glycogen) back into their muscles quickly after each training session. Experiments have shown that foods with *high* GI numbers are better for this because they allow the body to make glycogen more rapidly.

Are low-GI foods always healthy?

No. Don't fall into the trap of thinking that all foods with a low GI are a good choice. Crisps have a GI of 54 – much lower than a baked potato; that's because the fat in crisps delays digestion. The GI only tells you about one thing – the effect on blood glucose. Low-GI foods – like crisps – can still be loaded with unhelpful fat and salt.

All-Bran has a lower GI than Shredded Wheat, but it also contains added salt while Shredded Wheat is nothing but wholewheat. Although wholegrain foods aren't guaranteed to have a low GI, they are still preferable to overprocessed products which are spoilt by having important nutrients and fibre removed, and undesirable ingredients added. A good variety of whole grains each day can help to protect you against heart disease and cancer.

Table 10 Glycaemic index and glycaemic load of common foods

Food	GI	Serving (g)	Available carbohydrate (g)	GL
BREAKFAST CEREALS				
All-Bran	39	30	18	7
Muesli (variable)	54	30	16	8.7
Porridge	56	200*	16.2	9.1
Weetabix	75	30	18.9	14.2
Special K	69	30	20.8	14.4
Shredded Wheat	67	30	21.7	14.5
Cheerios	74	30	20.4	15.1
Puffed Wheat	74	30	21.2	15.7
Cornflakes	76	30	25.2	19.2
Rice Krispies	82	30	26.3	21.6
*includes milk				
BREAD				
Mixed grain	40	30	12.8	5.1
Pumpernickel	46	30	13.4	6.2
Sourdough rye	48	30	13.5	6.5
Sourdough wheat	54	30	13.4	7.2
Wholemeal	69	30	11.4	7.9
White	70	30	13.4	9.4
Baguette	95	30	15.9	15.1
Pitta, wholemeal	56	60	27.8	15.6
Pitta, white	69	60	30.7	21.2

Table 10 Glycaemic index and glycaemic load of common foods (*cont'd*)

Food	GI	Serving (g)	Available carbohydrate (g)	GL
CRACKERS				
Rye crispbread (Ryvita™)	66	25	15.7	10.4
Water biscuits, plain	71	25	17.8	12.6
Rice cakes, white	74	25	18.5	13.7
CEREAL GRAINS, BOILED				
Barley (boiled 20 min)	25	150	31.7	7.9
Couscous (boiled 5 min)	65	150	14.3	9.3
Cracked wheat (bulgar)	46	150	25.8	11.9
Quinoa	53	150	25.5	13.5
Buckwheat	51	150	28.8	14.7
Millet	71	150	34.8	24.7
Barley (boiled 60 min)	35	150	123.3	43
RICE				
Brown	55	150	42	23.1
Wild	57	150	42	23.9
Basmati	58	150	42	24.4
White, high-amylose	58	150	42	24.4
White, low-amylose	88	150	42	37
Instant	90	150	42	37.8

Table 10 Glycaemic index and glycaemic load of common foods (*cont'd*)

Food	GI	Serving (g)	Available carbohydrate (g)	GL
		PASTA		
Spaghetti, protein enriched	27	180	44.3	12
Vermicelli, white	35	180	45.4	15.9
Spaghetti, wholewheat	42	180	44.3	18.6
Spaghetti, white	44	180	44.3	19.5
Macaroni	47	180	44.3	20.8
Udon noodles	62	180	44.3	27.5
		POTATOES		
New	57	150	19.5	11.1
Mashed	74	150	18.5	13.7
Boiled (average)	72	150	19.5	14
Baked	85	150	21.8	18.5
Instant mashed	85	150	22.8	19.4
		ROOT VEGETABLES		
Carrots, raw	16	150	7.9	1.3
Carrots, boiled	41	150	8.6	3.5
Swede (rutabaga)	72	150	6.2	4.5
Beetroot	64	150	12.6	8.1
Sweet potato	46	150	26	12
Yam	42	150	33.3	14
Parsnips	97	150	15	14.6
Cassava	46	150	45.6	21

Table 10 Glycaemic index and glycaemic load of common foods (*cont'd*)

Food	GI	Serving (g)	Available carbohydrate (g)	GL
PULSES: BEANS				
Soya	18	150	3.6	0.6
Butter	30	150	3.5	1
Kidney	29	150	24	7
Haricot	38	150	19.8	7.5
Broad (fava)	79	150	9.8	7.7
Baked	48	150	16.8	8.1
Blackeye	42	150	21.5	9
PULSES: OTHER				
Peas, dried	22	150	11.3	2.5
Split peas, yellow	32	150	11	3.5
Lentils	30	150	14.9	4.5
Chickpeas	33	150	24	7.9
FRUIT, FRESH				
Strawberries	40	120	3.2	1.3
Grapefruit	25	120	5.8	1.5
Cherries	22	120	12.5	2.8
Plum	39	120	7.8	3
Peach	42	120	7.4	3.1
Orange	42	120	9.2	3.9
Pear	38	120	11.3	4.3

Table 10 Glycaemic index and glycaemic load of common foods (*cont'd*)

Food	GI	Serving (g)	Available carbohydrate (g)	GL
FRUIT, FRESH (cont'd)				
Watermelon	72	120	6	4.3
Apple	38	120	14.6	5.5
Pineapple	59	120	9.6	5.7
Banana, unripe	30	120	23.9	7.2
Mango	51	120	15.1	7.7
Grapes	50	120	18	9
Banana, ripe	52	120	23.9	12.4
FRUIT, DRIED				
Prunes, pitted	29	60	19.5	5.7
Apricots	31	60	23.3	7.2
Figs	61	60	32.7	19.9
Dates	45	60	45	20.3
Raisins	64	60	42.7	27.3

Where a range of GI values is available for the same food, an average or a typical value has been given.
Based on data collected by Professor Jennie Brand-Miller at the Human Nutrition Unit of the University of Sydney.

So don't just look at GI. Look at how much the food has been mucked about by the manufacturer and, in particular, how much fat and salt has been added.

Do I have to remember lots of numbers?
Absolutely not. The numbers have no value apart from helping you to get into the habit of eating more of the foods with lower numbers in

place of ones with high numbers. Once mixed-grain breads and pumpernickel have ousted baguettes from your regular shopping list, the numbers are unimportant.

Remember, too, that these numbers are produced by testing foods in isolation under laboratory conditions. In real life, the foods are eaten as part of a meal – mixed with other foods which alter the speed of conversion to glucose. Fat (e.g. olive oil) and acid (e.g. lemon juice or vinegar) make the stomach empty more slowly. So vinaigrette dressing on your potato salad will reduce its impact on blood glucose (and add a lot of calories). Soluble fibre (e.g. from psyllium or beans) makes it harder for digestive enzymes to get to carbohydrate in the intestine, reducing the overall GI of the meal. Cooking makes a big difference. Overcooking your pasta increases its GI; eat it *al dente*.

You may also notice that similar foods can have significantly different GI numbers. Some varieties of potato or rice, for example, will be more rapidly digested than others. Also, the published GI relates to a particular group of volunteers; you couldn't expect an identical result on a different group. While some GI tests have used 'normal' people, others have been done on people with diabetes.

So, although the GI of a food in your meal may be quite different from its GI in the laboratory, including foods with lower numbers will reduce the impact of your meal on blood glucose levels; it's the overall effect of the meal that counts. The glycaemic impact of your meal will also be reduced by including a good portion of a high-protein food (such as tofu, fish or chicken) and plenty of vegetables (e.g. broccoli, courgettes, mangetout, peppers, spinach and tomato). These foods don't appear in GI tables because their digestible carbohydrate content is insignificant. Also, some fruits (such as berries) contain too little carbohydrate to be granted a GI number; eating the whole fruit will have little effect on your blood glucose; drinking the juice is another matter!

◆ The glycaemic index (GI) of a food tells you how fast it pushes up blood glucose and insulin levels

◆ Some foods rich in complex carbohydrate have a higher GI than table sugar

◆ Pastas and pulses have low GI numbers

What about glycaemic load?

You may be horrified to see that watermelon has a GI of 72. This sounds like something to be avoided – until you realise that you'd have to chomp your way through one whole kilogram of melon to notch up 50 g of digestible carbohydrate. Remember that GI is measured by giving the volunteers enough of the food to provide 50 g of available carbohydrate. (We can only hope they liked watermelon.)

Eating a small slice of watermelon would have much less effect on your blood glucose than you might have assumed, knowing the GI is over 70.

No matter how rapidly the carbohydrate in melon is converted to glucose, if your portion contains very little carbohydrate, it can't do a lot to disrupt your blood glucose levels. The fastest gun in the West is no threat if he's loaded with nothing but blanks. What we really need to know is the glycaemic load (GL). This was defined by Walter Willett and his associates at Harvard in 1997.

GL takes into account both the speed of conversion to glucose (GI) and the quantity of available carbohydrate:

$$GL = \frac{GI}{100} \times \text{available carbohydrate in grams}$$

You probably remember that calculating GI involved multiplying by 100 to give us a score out of 100 – a percentage. In dividing by 100 here, we are simply getting back to the original fraction expressing how rapidly the carbohydrate in this food gets into the blood (compared with pure glucose). We can now apply this factor to the quantity of digestible carbohydrate in a portion of the food to find out the true impact on blood glucose – the GL. The available carbohydrate is simply the total carbohydrate content of a portion minus the fibre – fibre being carbohydrate that passes into the large bowel undigested.

Let's find out the glycaemic impact of eating a 120 g slice of watermelon which will contain approximately 6 g of available carbohydrate:

$$GL = \frac{72}{100} \times 6g = 4.3g$$

One way of looking at the glycaemic effect of eating this slice of watermelon, then, is that it's similar to the effect of eating 4.3 g of glucose. We've taken the digestible carbohydrate content and adjusted it for 'speed' using the GI. Of course, you're much better off eating the melon than the glucose because the melon also gives you water, fibre, vitamins and minerals – not to mention taste and texture.

Like GI, we can divide GL into three bands:

- low GL (up to 10)

- medium GL (11–19)

- high GL (20 and over).

Suddenly, that watermelon looks much more innocent. Despite its high GI, a standard portion has a low GL because it's not a very carbohydrate-dense food.

Now consider those broad beans with their surprisingly high GI of 79. A normal portion of 80 g would provide 5.2 g of available carbohydrate, so the GL would be reassuringly low at 4.1.

On the other hand, when it comes to foods more densely packed with digestible carbohydrate, the GL can be surprisingly high. Take one serving (180 g) of a spaghetti with a pleasantly low GI of 41. That would give you 44.3 g of available carbohydrate and a GL of 18.2.

So GI can be misleading until you apply it to the carbohydrate content of your serving to reveal what you really want to know – the GL.

If you keep the GL down to no more than 15 for main meals and 5 for snacks, so that your total for the day is around 60, you will be doing very well. A typical high-GL diet scores over 120 in a day. But I don't want you to bother with adding numbers. It really isn't necessary. If you follow the recommendations in this book, keeping to average portions of lower-GL foods, the rest will take care of itself.

Why not just eat a low-carb diet?

You may think it's not worth bothering with all this when you could reduce the glycaemic loading of a diet simply by avoiding carbohydrate.

After all, in theory, you can limit the effect of the meal on blood glucose levels either by selecting foods with lower GI numbers or by reducing the total intake of carbohydrate. That's the theory. Some people have been suspicious of GI and GL because they are mathematically derived. But it actually works in practice too.

In a study published in *The Journal of Nutrition* in 2003, Jennie Brand-Miller and colleagues fed healthy young adults foods with different carbohydrate contents and different GI ratings. The calculated GL effectively predicted the blood glucose response. As GL went up, so did the area under the graph of blood glucose concentration over time.

So you can, indeed, reduce peaks in blood glucose by eating very little carbohydrate. But a low-carbohydrate diet is a blunt instrument. You could lance a boil with a poker but I don't advise it. You could protect yourself from damaging relationships by avoiding people altogether; alternatively, you could choose your friends carefully.

Not only does a very low-carbohydrate diet deprive you of helpful foods like whole grains and pulses, it also makes you eat more protein and fat. The high intake of saturated fat that some people have on the Atkins Diet is particularly harmful.

GL to the rescue

Carbohydrate is like sex (obviously). Speed and content both matter. The impact of carbohydrate on blood glucose levels depends on quality and quantity – and GL takes both into account. Knowing about GL allows you to select the most helpful foods and eat appropriate portions.

You now know that although pasta is digested quite slowly, it is also packed with carbohydrate, and a standard (180 g) portion is too much. Have a palmful, not a plateful. (No, I don't mean you should eat it from your hands.) Pasta should be a bit on the side, not the main attraction in a meal.

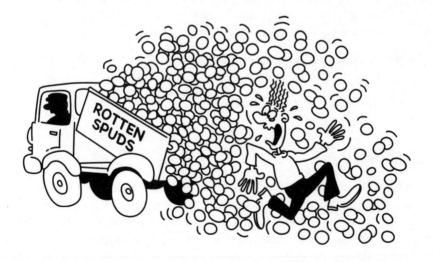

The impact of carbohydrate depends on quality and quantity.

White bread, potatoes and rice aren't much help when you're try-ing to eat a low-GL diet. Keep the portions small. Better still, use mixed-grain or rye bread, chickpeas, couscous and quinoa. Limit bread to a maximum of two slices a day; have less if you are struggling to lose weight. New potatoes have a lower GL than most others. If you particularly want to use rice, choosing a variety with a high amylose content will help to keep the GL down (because the amylose portion of starch is more slowly digested than amylopectin).

Remember that the total GL of your meal is influenced by every-thing on your plate. So if at least half of the plate is covered with vegetables (including pulses), and a quarter is taken up by a low-fat source of protein (such as skinless poultry, fish, tofu or Quorn), you're off to a very good start.

◆ Glycaemic load (GL) takes both the GI of a food and the carbohydrate content of a portion into account

◆ A normal portion of a high-GI food (such as broad beans or watermelon) can have a low GL

◆ Most pastas have a low GI, but because they are packed with carbohydrate, the GL of a normal portion is high

◆ A low-GL diet can help to control body weight, prevent diabetes and heart disease, and improve the balance of blood fats (raising HDL and lowering triglycerides)

◆ Choosing mixed-grain bread, chickpeas, couscous and quinoa in place of white bread, potatoes and rice helps to lower GL

Less simple

Discoveries about the glycaemic index of different foods have revolu-tionary implications, but advice to have less simple carbohydrate (sugar) is still valid. When sugar is added to your food, it gives you calories without nourishment (so-called 'empty calories').

Don't worry about the intrinsic sugar in fruit and vegetables, but try to cut down the extrinsic sugar that is added to so many foods and drinks. The table sugar added to a bowl of cereal or to a cup of tea is obvious, but so much extrinsic sugar is hidden – in breakfast cereals, soft drinks, and many different processed foods, both sweet and savoury. Check food labels to spot the hidden sugar, remembering that ingredients are listed in order of quantity present (by weight). Sugar will probably be the first ingredient listed on a jar of jam. This simply means there is more sugar than anything else in the jam.

Sugar appears in many guises. Honey, molasses, sucrose, maltose, lactose, fructose, glucose, glucose syrup, dextrose, invert sugar and caramel are all variations on the same theme – sugar.

Sugar is bad for the teeth (especially when eaten frequently throughout the day) and may contribute to obesity. It often comes with fat in factory-made cakes, biscuits and other snacks.

Here are a few practical tips for cutting down unnecessary sugar.

- If you are still adding sugar to tea and coffee, why not join the millions who now find that drinks taste better without?

- Most of us would benefit from drinking more water. Carbonated drinks like cola and lemonade conceal an awful lot of extrinsic sugar, so the low-calorie varieties are better from that point of view. (A can of soft drink might contain seven teaspoons of sugar.)

- Artificial sweeteners have their place but, if you use them routinely instead of adjusting your palate (or your 'tooth'), you end up having sweeteners in addition to too much sugar.

- Many recipes, including those for jams and marmalades, can stand a big reduction in sugar. Reduced-sugar jams or pure fruit spreads are best kept in the fridge once opened.

- Dried fruits – such as dates, raisins, sultanas, apricots, figs and prunes – can be used to sweeten cakes and biscuits. The sugar is intrinsic and they are also high in fibre.

- Select low-sugar breakfast cereals (less than 10% sugar) and enhance them with chopped bananas and dried fruit.

- Get into the habit of finishing meals with fruit. Save traditional puddings for special occasions.

- Buy tinned fruit in natural juice, not syrup.

> JACKIE: Pity there's no such thing as Sugar Replacement Therapy.
> VICTORIA: There is. It's called chocolate.
>
> ────────────
>
> **VICTORIA WOOD,**
> *Mens Sana in Thingummy Doodah*, 1990

More complex

In the light of recent research, the simple recommendation to eat more complex carbohydrate is not very helpful; choosing the best high-carbohydrate foods is a little more complex than it first appeared.

Knowing about GI and GL (see Table 10) can help you make the very best choices. You can see that a baguette will send your insulin levels soaring almost as much as pure glucose, while a mixed-grain loaf – especially one containing barley and rye – would be a particularly good option.

Regular **pulses** are good for your heart: peas, beans (including baked beans, kidney beans, soya beans, borlotti beans, butter beans) lentils and chickpeas are great sources of soluble fibre that can help lower cholesterol. Beans also provide quality protein reducing the need for meat; replacing animal protein in the diet with vegetable protein reduces both total and LDL-cholesterol. On top of all this, we now know that pulses help to keep down the total GL of your diet, so give them leading roles in your cuisine.

> **'Bread that must be sliced with an axe
> is bread that is too nourishing.'**
>
> ────────────
>
> **FRAN LEBOWITZ,** *Metropolitan Life*, 1978

Cereal grains give you starch and fibre (as well as protein). Many breakfast cereals contain a lot of added sugar. This is quite obvious if the product is advertised as honey- or sugar-coated, but with other cereals you will often find that sugar is still the second ingredient listed. Shredded Wheat (including 'Bitesize') and Puffed Wheat are remarkable for having only one ingredient – wheat – with no added sugar or salt. Even so, the GL is medium, not low.

A bowl of Shredded Wheat and skimmed milk needs no extra sugar if topped with sliced bananas and raisins or other dried fruit. Soft fruits (like raspberries, strawberries and blackberries) and stewed fruits

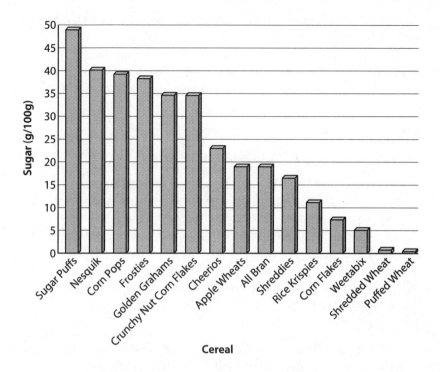

Figure 5 Sugar content of some common breakfast cereals.

also make lovely accompaniments to breakfast cereals. If you feast frequently on very sugary cereals, consider mixing them with less sugary ones (see Figure 5). Mix your Sugar Puffs with a good helping of Puffed Wheat and you'll munch through much less sugar. Don't bother with this advice if you need to gain weight and you've already lost all your teeth.

**'Breakfast cereals that come in the same colors
as polyester leisure suits make oversleeping a virtue.'**

FRAN LEBOWITZ,
Metropolitan Life, **1978**

Oats and **oat bran** are useful sources of soluble fibre – not to mention taste and texture. A bowl of porridge oats with skimmed milk or water takes a few minutes to cook in the microwave, and there's no dirty saucepan! Try topping this with sliced banana or berries instead of golden syrup.

Why not make your own muesli with a mixture of cereal grains and dried fruit? If you are buying ready-made muesli, it's worth avoiding brands with a very high sugar content and those with coconut.

ADAPTING TO CHANGE

We are creatures of habit. Don't forget that you've been eating food for longer than you can remember. It's a habit. If you've been having porridge with cream for 20 years, don't expect to be ecstatic the first time you try it with skimmed milk. Don't chuck it away in disgust and conclude that healthy eating's not for you. Give yourself a chance. You've spent years getting used to a high-fat, high-salt diet; you can learn to enjoy a low-fat, low-salt diet much quicker than that. But don't give up on day one because it's not what you're used to.

I'm not suggesting you should force yourself to eat porridge made with water every day until you feel grateful! For a start, you can make changes gradually. You could change from cream to skimmed milk via whole milk and semi-skimmed milk – or any blend of these – if you wanted. It may be that porridge is not for you at all. A recipe that I enjoy may not appeal to you. Don't let that put you off. There are countless other possibilities.

You are embarking on a voyage of discovery. Don't turn back at your own front gate.

'The critical period in matrimony is breakfast-time.'

A P HERBERT,
Uncommon Law, 1935

The average intake of fibre in Britain would need to be increased by 50% to reach the recommended level.

Of course, you can boost fibre intake by adding wheat bran to porridge or any other moist food, but overdoing this may reduce absorption of certain minerals, and not everybody's intestine takes kindly to having large quantities of wheat bran dumped in it. It is better generally to eat plenty of foods (pulses, fruit and vegetables, starchy foods and cereal grains) that have not had their natural fibre removed.

There is an important principle here: try to eat as much of your food as possible in its natural, whole, unprocessed form. A whole apple gives you starch, fibre, intrinsic sugar, vitamins, minerals and water. If it's a good apple, you may eat a second one, but you are unlikely to eat more than two in one go. Now, if you convert apples into apple juice, most of the sugar becomes extrinsic and you lose the fibre. You can gulp down the juice of a dozen apples without a second thought – all those calories without the fibre. I'm sure that new juicer will be a godsend on occasions, but perhaps it should go to the back of the cupboard. Smoothies made from whole fruit – with nothing added or taken out – are a huge improvement. But the process of turning the fruit into a drink could raise the GL, and it is still better to eat most of your fruit uncrushed.

ACTION POINTS

◆ Eat less sugar. Watch out for hidden sugar in processed foods

◆ Choose wholegrain cereals, bread, pasta and rice when possible

◆ Fruits and vegetables provide fibre and starch – eat plenty

◆ Large amounts of soluble fibre (from beans, oats and fruit) help to lower cholesterol

◆ Eat most of your food whole/unprocessed (apples rather than apple juice)

Chapter 7

Salt

We all need just a little salt (not a Lot). You are probably consuming at least six times as much common salt, or sodium chloride, as you need. Yes, even if you don't add any salt to your food, you will be eating several times the amount your body requires.

So what? The problem is that there is a link between eating excessive salt and having raised blood pressure – hypertension. If your blood pressure is high, you are more likely to have a stroke or heart attack.

◆ Our high-salt diet is linked with high blood pressure which leads to strokes and heart attacks

◆ On very low-salt diets, blood pressure doesn't rise with age

◆ Up to 85% of our salt comes from processed foods

◆ Reducing average UK salt intake by a third would dramatically cut strokes and heart attacks

◆ The palate adjusts to salt reduction, but do it gradually or food will taste bland

◆ Potassium helps to lower blood pressure; you get it from fruit and vegetables

---

The salt of the earth

Although salt is abundant on the surface of the earth, many folk around the world eat much less of it than we do.

In 1988 the *British Medical Journal* published the findings of the Intersalt study. This huge research project (on 10 079 men and women from 52 population samples in 32 different countries across the world) investigated the relationship between salt consumption and blood pressure. The researchers measured the quantity of sodium excreted in the urine over a 24-hour period as an indicator of salt intake.

The conclusions were inescapable. People with very low salt intakes had low blood pressures; high average salt consumption was linked with high average blood pressure.

And that wasn't all. We are so used to blood pressure rising as we get older that it is commonly considered a normal part of the ageing process. It isn't. The Intersalt study showed that it didn't happen in the groups of people with very low salt intakes. And the higher the average salt intake of a population, the more pronounced the age-related rise in pressure.

Inescapable conclusions? Yes, but, predictably, the Salt Institute (the salt producers' trade organisation) has made every attempt to escape them. The Institute criticised the statistical method that the Intersalt team had used to reveal the link between salt intake and the rise in blood pressure with advancing age. The Intersalt researchers responded with a complete re-analysis of their data – published in the *British Medical Journal* in 1996. In fact, *four* different methods of analysis all confirmed the link between bigger salt consumption and higher blood pressure in middle age.

The great salt scandal

You might think that a few grains of salt are neither here nor there but, of course, the salt producers are in business to shift mountains of salt from their mines to our meals. They have fought fiercely to undermine the evidence and obscure the facts. The Salt Institute pooh-poohed the statistical method of the Intersalt team, then ignored their new analyses that used methods suggested by the Institute itself, and rubbed salt into the wound by producing its own analysis of Intersalt data, riddled with statistical and biological flaws. The *British Medical Journal* was good enough to publish this; it shows the contortions of a group with a commercial interest. The Institute's analysis involved fictional figures such as the estimated blood pressure at birth (based on data about ages 20–59). This is nonsense! But it is symbolic of the salt producers' strategy.

To be fair, the salt producers are not the only ones to have expressed doubts about the implications of Intersalt. Notably, Professor John Swales urged caution before applying the results of a population study to individual people. Mind you, further analysis of the Intersalt data has strengthened the evidence that, *within* populations, salt consumption of the individual is linked with blood pressure. Apart from Intersalt, there is a lot of other experimental evidence that the blood pressure of individuals is influenced by salt intake.

Evidence comes from several types of study.

- Clinical trials on people with raised blood pressure have shown a reduction in blood pressure when salt is restricted; in some cases this has avoided the need to take drugs to treat raised blood pressure.

- Migration studies on people who move from rural areas to towns have shown that when salt intake goes up, so does blood pressure.

- Animal studies have confirmed that blood pressure can be pushed up and down by varying the salt content of the diet. (I know chimpanzees aren't people but they are certainly individuals.)

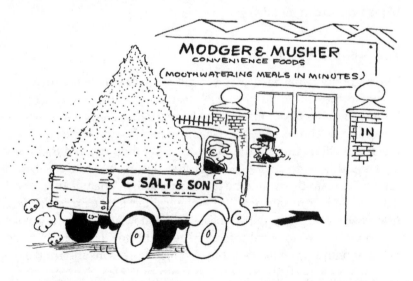

They take a grain of truth and make a mine of misinformation.

There's no doubt that some people are more sensitive than others to the effects of salt on blood pressure. And there is still a debate about the value of restricting salt intake in people with normal blood pressures. Indeed, you may even have been told by a doctor that you needn't bother about salt because your blood pressure's OK. But what will your blood pressure be like in five or ten years' time? The crucial point that is so often overlooked is that blood pressure tends to rise with age – except in communities with very low salt intakes. Anyway, although your blood pressure is 'OK' now, you would probably be better off if it were lower still. Besides, a high-salt diet may raise the risk of other problems such as osteoporosis (weak bones) and cancer of the stomach.

Although some independent scientific voices have posed proper questions about the significance of salt, many of the salt cynics turn out to be driven by the food industry. Adding salt is a cheap way of making processed foods palatable – to palates that have adapted to salt concentrations similar to that of sea water. Unfortunately, our physiology is not well adapted to marine life. To improve flavour by increasing the content of real food, such as fruit and vegetables, would be expensive. It is far cheaper to feed the consumer if you feed the controversy too. Fortunately, consumers are becoming more aware of the dangers of excess salt. There's a lot at stake. In fact, the evidence suggests that merely reducing the average salt intake of our population by one-third would prevent more deaths from strokes and heart attacks than all the current treatment for high blood pressure!

In 1994 the British government's committee of experts recommended that the average daily salt intake of the population should be reduced from its present level of 9 g to 6 g. Note that we are talking about salt here – sodium chloride – and not sodium. Six grams of salt contains a little less than 2.4 g of sodium (see Table 11). The recommended reduction in salt of 3 g is roughly half a teaspoonful. It was recognised that this would not be achieved without reducing the salt content of processed foods. The government endorsed the committee's recommendations on other aspects of food policy, but not this. It turned out that the food industry had lobbied ferociously against action on salt. Seven years later, in 2001, the Department of Health officially backed the recommendation that the average salt consumption of adults should be reduced to 6 g a day.

Frustrated by the lack of government action, a number of eminent medical scientists formed a group for Consensus Action on Salt and

Health (CASH). Their aim is to work with the food industry to reach a consensus on salt and blood pressure and then to find ways of reducing the amount of salt in food. This approach seems to be working. Over recent years, the quantity of salt added to some foods has been reduced significantly. This is very good news, but a lot more needs to be done.

Won't salt restriction cramp my style?

You can get cramps due to salt depletion, can't you? Well, this can happen to people labouring in tropical conditions, but it need not concern you in our climate.

Eating foods (such as fruit, vegetables, meat and fish) in their 'natural' state gives you all the sodium you need. Unfortunately, eating processed foods adds large quantities of superfluous salt to your intake. Using a saltcellar adds insult to injury. (Which is more insulting to the cook: to add salt to a meal before even tasting it, or to taste it first and then add salt? I'm not sure.)

Table 11 Typical salt content of foods

Food	Sodium content (g/100 g)	Salt content (g/100 g)
Cornflakes	0.7	1.8
All-Bran	0.6	1.5
Bran flakes	0.5	1.3
Rice Krispies	0.65	1.7
Special K	0.45	1.1
Frosties	0.55	1.4
Shredded Wheat	trace	trace
Shreddies	0.3	0.7
Weetabix	0.3	0.7

Table 11 Typical salt content of foods (*cont'd*)

Food	Sodium content (g/100 g)	Salt content (g/100 g)
White bread	0.53	1.4
Brown bread	0.54	1.4
Wholemeal bread	0.55	1.4
Wholemeal flour	trace	trace
White flour	trace	trace
Self-raising flour	0.36	0.9
Cream cracker	0.61	1.6
Rye crispbread	0.22	0.6
Digestive biscuit	0.6	1.5
Spaghetti (boiled)	trace	trace
Spaghetti (in tomato sauce)	0.42	1.1
Rice (boiled)	trace	trace
Salted butter	0.75	1.9
Margarine	0.8	2.0
Cheddar cheese	0.67	1.7
Edam cheese	1.02	2.6
Processed cheese	1.32	3.4
Cottage cheese	0.38	1.0

Increasingly, nutritional labels provide information on salt content, not just sodium. There are 393 mg of sodium in every 1 g (1000 mg) of sodium chloride (salt). So, to convert grams of sodium into grams of salt, you would divide by 0.393 – or simply multiply by 2.5.

The figures given here for cereals reflect the welcome reduction in salt added to some products. Note that the salt content of cereal brands can differ from one country to another.

Assault on the taste buds

If you stop adding salt in the kitchen and at the table, you'll be surprised at how quickly your palate adjusts. Cut down gradually and you will avoid the initial shock. Before long you will begin to appreciate natural food flavours, which once you would have overpowered with salt, and heavily salted food will taste unpleasant.

This is a change worth making. Unfortunately, though, most of the salt in the UK diet (65%–85% of it) comes from processed foods (Figure 6). It's already in the food before it reaches your kitchen. Salt, like fat, is a cheap ingredient and you'll get a good helping of both in sausages, pâtés, pies, crisps and a host of other manufactured savoury foods. I'm sure these fatty foods won't be top of your shopping list any more.

Here is a shocking fact: the biggest single source of salt in the British diet is factory-made bread! Fortunately, since the first edition

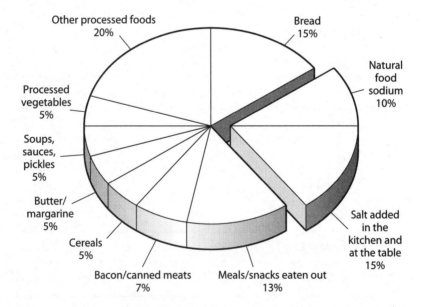

Figure 6 The contribution of various foods to the sodium intake of the population will be something like this. The picture will be quite different in some individual people. For example, bacon or canned soup will account for higher proportions in those who eat a lot of these foods. The natural sodium in food makes up no more than 10% of the intake; 15–25% is added during cooking or eating; 75% comes from food processing.

of *Stop That Heart Attack!* was published, it has become easier to find reduced-sodium loaves in the shops. Still, the best way to get the bread you really want is to make it yourself. Wait! Don't hold your hands up in horror. This has never been easier. With an automatic bread maker, just a few minutes of your time to throw in the ingredients is all it takes to have a fresh loaf whenever you want. And there's no need to add salt. Admittedly, if you are on the breadline, a machine like this seems expensive, but it can soon pay for itself if you eat a lot of bread.

Alternatively, join with friends and neighbours and ask a local baker to make a batch of bread without salt. You can keep extra loaves in the freezer. Of course, if you're eating less than a slice of bread a day to reduce GL, it won't seem worth it (unless you have 16 people in your family).

Some savoury foods, such as crisps, are very obviously salty. But it probably wouldn't occur to you that the concentration of salt in your breakfast cereal may be similar to that in sea water. In 2005, Kellogg announced a 25% salt reduction in some cereals; this was a welcome step in the right direction. When the label tells you about sodium, **you must multiply by 2.5** to convert it to salt.

Lots of good products are spoiled by their high salt content. Why buy a can of sweetcorn with added sugar and salt when there are excellent brands without? So check those labels for sodium content. Any supermarket worth its salt will offer reduced-sodium alternatives. You will find some tinned soups with 0.3 g/100 g sodium or less, and other varieties with three times that quantity. (Even the lower-salt brands will give you about a gram of sodium per can; a really low-salt home-made soup would be better.)

A tin of tuna in water (not brine) might contain only 0.1 g/100 g sodium, while a tin of anchovies in olive oil would have about 6 g/100 g – yes, sixty times the concentration. Of course, you may well eat the whole tin of tuna in one meal, but the thing to do with the anchovies is to scatter a few finely cut shreds on your pizza topping.

Apart from sodium chloride, common salt, various other compounds can bump up the sodium content of manufactured foods. The most notable example is monosodium glutamate, which is frequently used as a flavour enhancer.

Keeping your sodium intake down is a wise move. A small reduction in blood pressure could make all the difference – the difference between having a stroke or heart attack and not having one. Sadly, there will always be those who take this kind of advice with a pinch of salt. It's not just a question of lowering your blood pressure now: a reduced-sodium diet helps to prevent blood pressure rising with age.

Potassium, on the other hand, helps to lower blood pressure. We all get too much sodium but many of us could do with more potassium. Don't worry. You don't have to go round checking food labels for potassium content. This is another problem which is solved by eating enough fruit and vegetables.

What about salt substitutes?

It is far better to re-educate your taste buds than simply to load your saltcellar with a salt substitute, but on those occasions when you really feel a little salt makes all the difference, you could use a tiny amount of 'LoSalt' or 'Solo'; these are low-sodium products containing a mixture of potassium chloride and sodium chloride. You can use them in home-made bread. One container should last for ages. If it doesn't, you're using too much.

There are other salt substitutes consisting entirely of potassium salts. These are useful for people on very low sodium diets for specific medical reasons, but they are less palatable than products containing some sodium.

If you are taking a potassium-retaining drug (such as an ACE inhibitor) or have kidney disease, it is generally unwise to add potassium to your diet. Discuss this with your doctor who will be checking your potassium levels from time to time.

There's always pepper, I suppose

True. We still haven't discovered anything terrible about pepper. And freshly ground black pepper can do a lot for a meal. But seasoning doesn't end there. Reducing salt opens the way to an exciting exploration of herbs and spices. Get fresh herbs whenever you can. Why not grow some in your garden (or window box)? Don't forget garlic, mustard powder, lemon juice and vinegar (including wine vinegars and balsamic vinegar). It's no surprise that celery salt is mostly salt, but beware other ready-made seasonings: you may find salt is the main ingredient.

So, should I rid my larder of salt? No. It would be wise to be well stocked – or you'll regret it when the path freezes over.

ACTION POINTS

◆ Eat as much of your food as possible whole/unprocessed

◆ Don't add salt when cooking or eating

◆ If you feel added salt is essential, consider 'LoSalt' and 'Solo'

◆ When buying processed foods, go for lower-sodium products

◆ Season skilfully with: pepper, garlic, herbs, spices, mustard, lemon, wine, sherry, vermouth, vinegar, etc.

◆ Take care with ready-made flavourings such as stock cubes, soy sauce, etc.

◆ Season for a reason. Halt! That's salt!

Chapter 8

Fish

A fishy theory

It is often said that Inuit people, eating their traditional diet which was very rich in fish oils, had low rates of coronary heart disease. This may be true but there must be some doubt about the causes of death as they were not determined by post-mortem examination. As Professor Durrington has pointed out, we cannot be certain that some of the deaths put down to 'hypothermia' or 'drowning' were not, in fact, caused by heart attacks. So could the oily fish turn out to be a red herring?

Inuits aside, we do have good evidence of the beneficial effects of eating fish, including oily fish. In the Zutphen Study, the dietary habits of 852 Dutch men were examined and these men were followed up for 20 years. During this time, 78 men died from coronary heart disease, but the death rate from heart disease was more than 50% lower in the men who ate at least 30 g (1 oz) of fish a day than in those who did not eat fish. About one-third of the fish consumed was of the oily type.

The Japanese generally eat lots of fish and have low rates of heart disease. Japanese fishermen eat more fish than the general population and have even lower rates of heart disease.

In 1989, the DART study on men who had recently suffered a heart attack found that those advised to eat oily fish (at least two portions a week) were significantly less likely to die (during a follow-up period of two years) than those who were not given this advice.

What do you mean by oily fish?

This does not refer to tinned tuna in vegetable oil! Fish contain the special polyunsaturated fatty acids, eicosapentaenoic acid (EPA) and docosahexaenoic acid (DHA). These are also known as omega-3 fatty acids. You may remember that polyunsaturated fatty acids have more than one area of the molecule with room for extra hydrogen. Well, 'omega-3' simply means that the last position on the molecule that is not saturated with hydrogen is the third carbon atom from the end of the chain. This chemical structure makes these omega-3 fishy fatty acids behave quite differently from the omega-6 polyunsaturates like linoleic acid found in vegetable oils.

The quantity of EPA and DHA present in a fish depends particularly on the species of fish, but also on factors like the season and whether the fish is wild or farmed. Fish with high levels of these omega-3 fatty acids are often called 'oily fish'. They live in cold water. Common examples are mackerel, salmon, herring, sardines and pilchards. You will sometimes find tuna listed as an oily fish and, indeed, fresh tuna can be a good source of omega-3 fatty acids, but the tinned tuna you are likely to find in the supermarket will probably have a very low fat content (e.g. 0.5 g/100 g) – provided you don't buy it in vegetable oil!

The total fat content of oily fish is very variable (see Table 13) and only a small proportion of this is made up of omega-3 fatty acids, but in every case the saturated fatty acid content is low.

One way of ensuring a regular intake of fish oils is to take a concentrated supplement. The GISSI-Prevenzione trial published in *The Lancet* in 1999 recruited 11 324 people who had recently survived a heart attack. Adding 1 g/day of omega-3 fatty acids (one Omacor™ capsule daily) to the standard treatment reduced the overall death rate by an extra 20% and the risk of sudden death by 45%.

◆ High fish diets are linked with low rates of heart disease

◆ Fish oils (EPA and DHA) reduce the risk of thrombosis and abnormal heart rhythms

◆ All fish are helpful to your heart – especially oily fish (e.g. sardines, mackerel, salmon)

What's so special about these omega-3 fatty acids?

Consumption of fish oils has several significant effects on the circulation.

First, the blood doesn't clot as easily. Tiny cells in the blood called platelets have to stick together before a blood clot can form in the circulation. EPA gets into the platelets and makes them less 'sticky'. 'Coronary thrombosis', which means the formation of a blood clot in one of the coronary arteries supplying the heart, is another name for a heart attack. We saw in Chapter 5 that saturated fats can make thrombosis more likely, increasing the risk of a heart attack. Fish oils make thrombosis less likely.

Secondly, large amounts of fish oil can reduce the level of triglycerides in the blood. Permanently raised triglyceride levels do seem to increase the risk of heart disease. Fish oils do not normally make a significant difference to the blood cholesterol level.

There is some evidence that large doses of EPA and DHA can slightly reduce raised blood pressure. The effect on people with normal blood pressure seems less consistent. One study in older people found that fish oils were better at lowering blood pressure if salt intake was reduced as well.

More fish in the sea

Other sea fish (such as cod, haddock, bass, flatfish, red snapper and dogfish) contain some EPA and DHA even if it's not enough for them to be classed as oily fish. And fish don't have to come from the sea to contain useful amounts of oil: trout and carp have enough to qualify as oily fish.

There's more to fish than omega-3 fatty acids. All fish from sprats to sharks will do you good (as long as it's *you* eating *them*). They make an excellent, low-saturated fat replacement for meat. As well as protein, they provide important vitamins, minerals and trace elements. Fish are good suppliers of various B vitamins (e.g. niacin, vitamin B_6, vitamin B_{12}) and oily fish contain vitamin D. They will top you up with iron and potassium; sea fish will give you iodine and the important antioxidant, selenium. Canned sardines and pilchards are excellent sources of calcium. And, of course, fish is delicious as well as nutritious.

I know some people say they don't like fish; they are missing so much and I do hope you're not one of them. If you are, perhaps I could ask you just to consider the possibility that you have been put off by some ill-chosen or badly presented fish. Smelly fish and slimy fillets are excellent bait for crab fishing, but they are not fit for your

Table 12 Fat content of white fish

Fish	Total fat (g/100 g)	Saturates (g/100 g)	Mono-unsaturates g/100 g)	Poly-unsaturates (g/100 g)
Bass, sea (raw)	2.5	0.4	0.6	0.6
Cod (raw)	0.7	0.1	0.1	0.3
Cod (steamed)	0.9	0.2	0.1	0.4
Cod (fried in sunflower oil)	15.4	1.8	3.1	9.7
Coley (raw)	1.0	0.1	0.3	0.3
Haddock (raw)	0.6	0.1	0.1	0.2
Halibut (raw)	1.9	0.3	0.6	0.4
Monkfish (raw)	0.4	0.1	0.1	0.1
Mullet, grey (raw)	4.0	1.1	0.9	0.5
Plaice (raw)	1.4	0.2	0.4	0.3
Rock salmon/Dogfish (raw)	9.7	1.4	2.6	2.7
Shark (raw)	1.1	0.2	0.2	0.4
Skate (raw)	0.4	Trace	0.1	0.2
Turbot (raw)	2.7	0.7	0.6	0.6
Whiting (raw)	0.7	0.1	0.2	0.2

Fatty acids do not account for 100% of the weight of fat, which also contains substances such as phospholipids and sterols.

table, however well seasoned or cooked. Fish should be fresh – firm and bright-eyed (but not bushy-tailed). And overcooking is a common mistake.

Table 13 Fat content of oily fish

Fish	Total fat (g/100 g)	Saturates (g/100 g)	Mono-unsaturates g/100 g)	Poly-unsaturates (g/100 g)
Herring (raw)	13.2	3.3	5.5	2.7
Kipper (raw)	17.7	2.8	9.3	3.9
Mackerel (raw)	16.1	3.3	7.9	3.3
Pilchards (canned in tomato sauce)	8.1	1.7	2.2	3.4
Salmon (raw)	11.0	1.9	4.4	3.1
Salmon, pink (canned in brine, flesh only)	6.6	1.3	2.4	1.9
Salmon, red (canned in brine, flesh only)	9.0	1.7	3.7	2.4
Sardines (raw)	9.2	2.7	2.5	2.7
Sardines (canned in oil, drained)	14.1	2.9	4.8	5.0
Swordfish (raw)	4.1	0.9	1.6	1.1
Trout, rainbow (raw)	5.2	1.1	1.8	1.7
Tuna (raw)	4.6	1.2	1.2	1.6
Tuna (canned in brine, drained)	0.6	0.2	0.1	0.2

Fatty acids do not account for 100% of the weight of fat, which also contains substances such as phospholipids and sterols.

NOTE: the fat content of fish varies with the season and the maturity of the fish. Oily fish caught in British waters (such as mackerel and herring) contain more fat in winter. Herring, for example, might contain 5 g/100 g in spring and 20 g/100 g in winter.

Data from *Fish and Fish products*, the 3rd supplement to McCance and Widdowson's *The Composition of Foods*, Holland, Brown and Buss, 1993, © Crown copyright.

ACTION POINTS

◆ Eat fish at least twice a week

◆ Avoid fish canned in 'vegetable oil'; choose those in olive oil or water

◆ If you're not a fish fan, disguise fish in casseroles, etc.

◆ Grill, bake or microwave; avoid deep-fried fish; shallow frying in a little rapeseed or olive oil is OK

Fish come in so many forms, and can be prepared in such a variety of ways, that most people can find something acceptable. If grilled plaice doesn't appeal, a tuna salad might be more to your liking. If you are put off by a whole trout staring you in the face, you may feel at ease with a fillet. Or perhaps you'd prefer your fish disguised in a casserole or pasta sauce. Most of us can appreciate any of these but, if

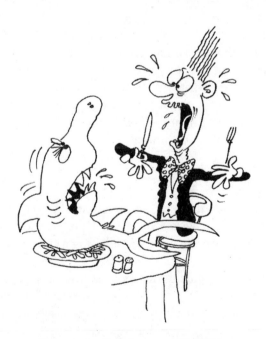

You may be more at ease with a fillet.

you're not a fish lover, it's well worth finding one or two fish dishes you can enjoy. To start you off, an outing to a first-class fish restaurant might be a good investment.

I'm not talking about fish and chips, of course. The problem with traditional fish and chips is that two excellent ingredients (fish and potato) have been drenched in fat. It wouldn't be so bad if you could be sure that a good quality oil, rich in mono-unsaturates or poly-unsaturates, had been used. Even if it started that way, reheating may have caused oxidation, making the oil much less friendly to your arteries. Oven chips have a much lower fat content (e.g. 5%) than those cooked in deep fat (e.g. 15%). Thin chips, such as french fries, are more fatty than fat chips.

All fins bright and beautiful . . .

The magnificent sight of a gleaming salmon or bass, dorsal fin erect, delights the fish enthusiast. All the better if he or she has hunted the creature in its habitat, cleaned it, prepared it and brought it to the table. What better way to procure fresh fish?

If you are the non-enthusiast, already squirming at my description, get your fishmonger to do as much of the preparation as possible. Gutting and filleting are not for you. Neatly packaged fillets, frozen or fresh (as long as they are), make a convenient option. Tinned fish is a good standby. Don't buy it in unspecified 'vegetable oil'. Sardines in olive oil, drained, are great with salad or on toast.

Despite all the salt in the sea, fish are naturally low in sodium but variable quantities of salt are added to tinned fish and it's as well to keep an eye on the sodium content.

How often?

When it comes to sex, it's pointless recommending a frequency. Some people are happy with twice a year; others prefer twice a day. As long as both parties are content, it's futile advising a change. Fish is different.

I recommend that you have fish at least twice a week. One of these meals should include oily fish (two or three portions of oily fish a week are recommended for those who have already had a heart attack). This is a minimum and, if you want to eat fish every day, so much the better.

Table 14 Fat and cholesterol content of shellfish

	Total fat (g/100 g)	Saturates (g/100 g)	Mono-unsaturates (g/100 g)	Poly-unsaturates (g/100 g)	Cholesterol (mg/100 g)
CRUSTACEA					
Crab (boiled)	5.5	0.7	1.5	1.6	72
Crayfish (raw)	0.8	0.1	0.2	0.3	105
Lobster (boiled)	1.6	0.2	0.3	0.6	110
Prawns (raw)	0.6	0.1	0.2	0.1	(195)*
Prawns (boiled)	0.9	0.2	0.2	0.2	(280)
Scampi, in bread-crumbs (fried in sunflower oil)	13.6	1.6	3.1	8.2	110
Shrimps (boiled)	2.4	0.4	0.5	0.8	130
MOLLUSCS					
Clams, canned in brine (drained)	0.6	0.2	0.1	0.1	(67)
Cockles (boiled)	0.6	0.2	0.1	0.2	53
Cuttlefish (raw)	0.7	0.2	0.1	0.2	110
Mussels (boiled)	2.7	0.5	0.4	1.0	58
Octopus (raw)	1.3	0.3	0.2	0.5	48
Oysters (raw)	1.3	(0.2)	(0.2)	(0.4)	(57)
Scallops (steamed)	1.4	0.4	0.1	0.4	47
Squid (raw)	1.7	0.4	0.2	0.6	225
Whelks (boiled)	1.2	0.2	0.2	0.3	125
Winkles (boiled)	1.2	0.2	0.2	0.4	105

*Figures in brackets are estimated.

Fatty acids do not account for 100% of the weight of fat, which also contains substances such as phospholipids and sterols.

Data from *Fish and Fish products*, the 3rd supplement to McCance and Widdowson's *The Composition of Foods*, Holland, Brown and Buss, 1993, © Crown copyright.

Of course, oily fish contain a lot more calories than white fish. And there is some concern that the traces of toxic pollutants (dioxins, PCBs and mercury) found in some oily fish could build up to significant levels if you over-indulge.

For many of us, the benefits of eating up to four portions of oily fish a week will outweigh any risk from pollutants (a portion being about 140 g). Girls and women who may become pregnant at some point in the future should have up to two portions a week. During pregnancy, avoid swordfish, marlin and shark altogether as they build up higher levels of mercury. Those of us who are not pregnant would be wise to eat these big predators no more than once a week; I have them only occasionally.

With all this talk of toxins, you may choose to keep oily fish down to once a week and eat other varieties the rest of the time. That's fine. It's worth noting that recent studies have found significant levels of PCBs and dioxins (similar to the levels in oily fish) in sea bream, sea bass, turbot, halibut, dogfish and crab.

If you are looking for alternative sources of omega-3 fatty acids, see the box in Chapter 19 on *Fishing for alternatives.*

What about fish oil supplements?

One way to obtain omega-3 fatty acids without the worry about pollution is to take a capsule of purified fish oil. Each capsule of Omacor contains 460 mg EPA and 380 mg DHA, strictly purified to remove cholesterol, pesticides, heavy metals and other impurities. If you read the labels, you will notice that many other supplements contain much smaller amounts of EPA and DHA. Omacor is available on prescription for people who have had a heart attack (or those with very high triglyceride levels); you can also buy it from a pharmacist without a prescription.

In 2007, the National Institute for Health and Clinical Excellence (NICE) advised that prescription of Omacor should be considered for people who had suffered a heart attack within the last three months if they were not managing to eat the recommended two to four portions of oily fish a week. NICE indicated that prescription of the supplement could be continued for up to four years after the heart attack, but that doctors should not normally *start* prescribing it more than three months after a heart attack.

Benefits of fish oil in doubt

In 2006, the *British Medical Journal* published a paper which pooled the results of lots of studies investigating the impact of fish oil on heart disease. The results sent shock waves through the fishing community and the medical profession. The analysis failed to confirm any effects of omega-3 fatty acids on total mortality, strokes, heart attacks or cancer!

When you look closely at this analysis, you find it is mainly one study that is rocking the boat. In 2003, Burr and colleagues published an investigation (DART-2) into the effect of omega-3 consumption in 3114 men with stable angina. Surprisingly, the men taking more omega-3 had more heart attacks – especially those taking fish oil capsules rather than eating oily fish.

Interestingly, it was Burr and colleagues who carried out the original DART study in 1989 which showed the benefit of eating oily fish after a heart attack.

Well, if you remove the DART-2 study from the 2006 analysis, it totally changes the outcome to show a benefit from higher omega-3 intake. Fishy, eh?

So what should we do? I'm certainly not suggesting that we ignore the shocking results of DART-2. Clearly, more research is needed. In the meantime, here are some thoughts:

- One study does not overturn the accumulated evidence for the benefits of eating fish, including oily fish;

- Omega-3 fatty acids are essential (the body can't make them or do without them) so deficiency is bad – bad for the brain apart from anything else;

- Pending further evidence, if you have not had a heart attack but have angina, you should be wary of taking fish oil supplements. Omega-3 capsules can help to prevent abnormal heart rhythms after a heart attack, but they may have unwanted effects in stable angina;

- You can't go wrong with two portions of fish a week – one of them oily fish;

- If you have had a heart attack within the last two years, there is a good case for eating two to four portions of oily fish a week.

Shellfish indulgence?

Shellfish are sometimes depicted as forbidden fruit for the cholesterol conscious on account of their reputation for being rich sources of cholesterol. In fact, if you have a passion for shellfish, there is no reason why it should not be indulged.

The term 'shellfish' covers crustaceans like crabs, lobsters, shrimps and prawns as well as molluscs such as clams, mussels, oysters, scallops, squid and octopus. All have a very low total and saturated fat content. In addition, they contain useful quantities of the omega-3 fatty acids EPA and DHA – generally comparable with the quantities in non-oily fish (see Table 14).

The reputation for being loaded with cholesterol probably comes partly from old figures which, for technical reasons, were too high. Also, it may be that two or three higher-cholesterol members of the group have tarnished the reputation of others. There are always a few shellfish individuals that get others into trouble.

Shrimps, prawns, lobsters and squid have high cholesterol levels (but I don't know how often they get heart attacks). Even so, there is the question of portion size, and you needn't worry about the number of prawns in a prawn cocktail (unless you've discovered a generous restaurant); I'd be more concerned about whether it was a low-saturated fat seafood sauce. When it comes to controlling your blood cholesterol level, the cholesterol in your food is much less important than the saturated fat. A lot of the cholesterol we eat passes through the intestine without being absorbed – although some people are genetically programmed to absorb more.

Make sure your shellfish is fresh and properly cooked, or your intestine won't be absorbing anything much for a while.

◆ Shellfish (such as mussels, oysters, prawns, crabs) are low in fat

◆ Have shellfish if you want to

◆ Use low-fat seafood sauces

◆ Shrimps, prawns, lobsters and squid are low in fat but not in cholesterol: keep to moderate portion sizes

Chapter 9

Antioxidants

A few years ago, antioxidants were stuck in the pages of scientific journals, but now they have hit the big time. Everybody's talking about them. You can't even buy a simple moisturiser these days without being told you need one with antioxidants to mop up the free radicals in your skin.

What are free radicals?

This has nothing to do with the release of political prisoners. Free radicals are unstable molecules which are formed as by-products of the body's normal metabolism. If you were being rude about a free radical, you might say it was 'one electron short of a pair' (and, indeed, the chemical definition is: 'having one or more unpaired electrons'). They are, in chemical terms, highly active and, just like an unstable political activist, they are always trying to provoke a reaction – and they can cause a lot of damage in the process.

> 'A conservative is a man with two perfectly good legs
> who, however, has never learned to walk forwards . . .
> A reactionary is a somnambulist walking backwards . . .
> A radical is a man with both feet firmly planted – in the air.'
>
> FRANKLIN D ROOSEVELT, 'Fireside Chat', 1939

Oxidation

When chemists refer to 'oxidation' of a substance, they are talking about a chemical reaction in which electrons are removed from the substance. ('Reduction' is the opposite process in which electrons are added.) Now free radicals are short of electrons and they will seize any opportunity to steal them. This is what makes them unstable, provoking the reaction of oxidation whenever they can.

The oxidative damage that free radicals cause to the body's fats, proteins and DNA plays an important part in the development of heart disease, ageing processes and cancer.

Normal body chemistry produces some free radicals, but they are also generated by pollutants, including cigarette smoke.

'I simply can't believe nice communities release effluents.'

WILLIAM HAMILTON,
William Hamilton's Anti-Social Register, **cartoon, 1974**

- ◆ Free radicals are unstable molecules that cause damage

- ◆ The damage done by free radicals leads to heart disease, ageing and cancer

- ◆ Smoking produces extra free radicals

- ◆ The antioxidant vitamins (A, C and E) mop up free radicals

- ◆ Antioxidants can block the free-radical attack on arteries

- ◆ Too much polyunsaturated fat without antioxidants could cause atherosclerosis

Where do antioxidants come in?

Antioxidants are substances that stop these free radicals from acting and prevent them from causing damaging chemical reactions. You can think of an antioxidant as a 'scavenger' that goes round 'gobbling up' harmful free radicals. The best known antioxidants are beta-carotene (which is related to vitamin A), vitamin C and vitamin E; they are often called the 'ACE vitamins'.

Apart from these vitamins, we get several other important antioxidants from our diet (see Table 15). The chemicals that give vegetables their colour are called carotenes and flavonoids. By having vegetables of three different colours on your plate, you will be covering a good range of antioxidants. Selenium is a chemical element found in small quantities in certain foods.

Table 15 Antioxidants

Antioxidant	Common sources
Vitamin E	Vegetable oils, whole grains, nuts, dark green vegetables
Vitamin C	Fresh fruit and vegetables
Carotenes	Yellow/orange fruit and vegetables (e.g. carrots, apricots, peppers) and green vegetables (e.g. broccoli, spinach)
Flavonoids	Apples, onions, red wine, tea, skins of fruits and vegetables
Selenium	Brazil nuts, cashew nuts, walnuts, bread, cereals, poultry, sea fish

Selenium

Concern has been expressed recently about the falling levels of the antioxidant selenium in British and other European diets. This is largely because we import less wheat from North America nowadays. The British and European varieties used for making bread have a lower selenium content. Selenium is one of the antioxidants that helps to prevent atherosclerosis (furring and hardening of arteries) but also has important roles in thyroid balance and sperm production.

You could certainly correct any selenium deficiency by eating brazil nuts, which are a very rich source of selenium. Just three brazil nuts contain all the selenium you need for a day, and only about 1.6 g of saturated fat. Lots of other foods (such as cashew nuts, walnuts, sea fish and cereals) contain useful amounts of selenium, although not in the concentration supplied by brazil nuts. Of course, if you can't stop at three brazil nuts, the dose of saturated fat will start to mount up.

What's the benefit?

This raises a useful point: don't just get carried away with the antioxidant content of a food; consider whether it is helpful in other ways. I am reminded of that newspaper article claiming that chocolate protects against heart disease – a claim which was based on the fact that chocolate contains flavonoid antioxidants. Regrettably, any beneficial effect of the antioxidants obtained from a chocolate binge would be overshadowed by the large intake of fat and sugar.

Measuring antioxidant power

Scientists have come up with various laboratory tests to measure the antioxidant power of different foods. One system that has gained popularity in recent years rates foods according to their *oxygen radical absorbance capacity* (ORAC).

Comparing ORAC ratings for different foods can be misleading. Some ORAC values relate to a typical serving of the food; others to a given dry weight or wet weight.

Most of us are interested in blocking damaging oxidation that causes ageing and disease. ORAC research has been followed by a lot of hype about superfoods, and the inevitable appearance of 'concentrated ORAC' products in pots.

Here are some of the foods with high ORAC scores: kidney beans, pinto beans, blueberries, blackberries, raspberries, strawberries, spinach, kale, broccoli, cauliflower, peppers, beetroot, onion and garlic.

These are all really useful foods which should be prominent in your diet – and not just because of their high ORAC ratings. Apart from being delicious, they deliver vitamins, minerals and fibre with a very low GL. It's not an exhaustive list: other fruits and vegetables (as well as nuts and whole grains) make an important contribution to your battle against destructive free radicals. Variety is essential. No single superfood can fight the battle on its own. (I'm getting a picture of a cartoon character – ORAC the Superberry. You read it here first.)

How could antioxidants protect against heart disease?

It is likely that antioxidants are involved in a range of biochemical processes that help to prevent heart disease. Probably one of the most important of these is protection of LDL (low density lipoprotein) from oxidation by free radicals. A simple illustration of the way in which free radical attack on LDL can lead to fatty deposits in arteries is given in Figure 7.

Fat in LDL particles is attacked by free radicals producing oxidised LDL. Along come macrophages, which are special scavenging white cells, to engulf the oxidised LDL. Once the macrophages are laden with cholesterol droplets they are known as foam cells. These foam cells can deposit fat on the artery lining causing 'fatty streaks' and eventually atherosclerosis.

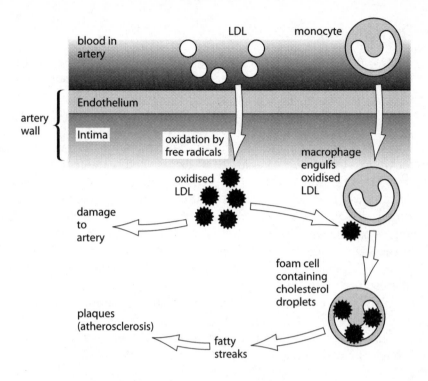

Figure 7 Free radical attack leads to fatty deposits in arteries.

Antioxidants block this chain of events by protecting the LDL from attack by free radicals. We have seen that polyunsaturated fatty acids in the diet can help to lower LDL-cholesterol – the 'bad' cholesterol – but they are not helpful unless there are enough antioxidants around. Too many polyunsaturates without enough antioxidants can increase this LDL oxidation by free radicals and lead to more atherosclerosis.

Vitamins C and E work together. As vitamin E gets used up in the battle against free radicals, vitamin C restores it and gets it fit to fight another day.

One of the damaging effects of smoking is to use up antioxidants, and smokers need more antioxidants than non-smokers. Unfortunately, you cannot reverse *all* the harmful effects of smoking by supplementing antioxidants.

The irony in store

There is now some evidence that iron stored in the body can lead to the formation of free radicals; more free radicals could mean more atherosclerosis. Before the menopause, women usually store much less iron than men do because they lose iron every month with their periods. In fact, young women can easily become anaemic if there is not enough iron in the diet to replace this menstrual loss. It is very rare for women to develop coronary heart disease before the menopause (but, after the menopause, they start catching up with men; see Chapter 24). It is widely assumed that oestrogen is protecting them. Perhaps it is, but it's possible that lack of iron is another factor reducing the risk of heart disease in young women. (You have to be very bad at shaving to match a woman's menstrual blood loss; this could be a powerful argument for a man to become a blood donor – out of self-interest if nothing else.) It's quite reasonable for a young woman to supplement her diet with multivitamin tablets containing iron. Men may be better off taking preparations without iron.

What an irony if it transpires that being fortified with iron has brought some down, while others have been shielded by deficiency!

◆ High levels of stored iron in the body could produce more free radicals

◆ Before the menopause, women have low iron levels and this could help protect arteries

◆ Men should avoid iron supplements unless a blood test shows they're needed

◆ Being a blood donor may reduce a man's coronary risk

Homocysteine

Everyone's heard of Homer Simpson. Many people still haven't heard of homocysteine and yet this substance may play an important role in the development of free radicals, foam cells and atherosclerosis.

Homocysteine is produced when protein is digested; it results from the breakdown of an amino acid called methionine – one of the building blocks of protein. The body can also convert homocysteine back to harmless methionine.

Studies show that persistently raised blood levels of homocysteine are linked with an increased risk of coronary heart disease and stroke; the higher the level of homocysteine, the greater the risk.

But this doesn't prove that homocysteine causes heart disease and strokes. If there are high rates of excessive beer drinking among men with tattoos, you cannot assume that the tattoos cause the beer drinking. Even if you discover that excessive beer drinking is more common in men with big tattoos than in men with small tattoos, you still shouldn't assume that the tattoos are to blame.

In the same way, if people with damaged arteries (which may become blocked causing a stroke or heart attack) tend to have higher levels of homocysteine, it doesn't prove that the homocysteine causes the damage. Mind you, evidence from laboratory experiments gives us every reason to think that homocysteine is bad for arteries. Research indicates that homocysteine can damage the smooth lining of arteries (endothelium) and trigger formation of blood clots in the circulation (thrombosis). It seems that homocysteine may also reduce the availability of nitric oxide – a very important substance that helps arteries to relax and widen.

Raised blood levels of homocysteine are very common, especially in older people. Your homocysteine level is influenced by your genes and your diet. To convert homocysteine back to methionine, your body needs a good supply of the B vitamin folic acid (also known as folate, folacin, and pteroylglutamic acid); vitamins B_{12} and B_6 play a minor role.

A lot of people are not getting enough folic acid from food to bring their homocysteine level down to the ideal range. Taking a supplement of 0.4 mg daily is usually effective. (This is the dose that women are advised to take before conceiving and in the first 12 weeks of pregnancy.) For a long time there has been a debate in scientific and government circles about whether folic acid should be added to foods such as bread (as it is in the USA).

So what are we waiting for?

High blood levels of homocysteine are linked with an increased risk of strokes and heart attacks. These high homocysteine levels are common. Laboratory evidence confirms that homocysteine is bad for arteries. Supplementing the diet with extra folic acid reduces blood homocysteine levels. So why on earth don't we just put extra folic acid in staple foods, as they do in America?

Frankly, we've been waiting for that final piece of evidence – the evidence that when you give groups of people folic acid and reduce their homocysteine levels, they have fewer heart attacks and strokes.

A Scandinavian scandal

NORVIT, the Norwegian Vitamin Trial, recruited 3749 men and women who had suffered a heart attack within the previous week. They were divided at random into four groups, each receiving one of the following daily treatments:

1 0.8 mg of folic acid plus 0.4 mg of vitamin B_{12} plus 40 mg of vitamin B_6

2 0.8 mg of folic acid plus 0.4 mg of vitamin B_{12}

3 40 mg of vitamin B_6

4 placebo – a capsule containing no B vitamins

All the treatments were taken as a single daily capsule for over three years, in addition to standard treatment after a heart attack. The outcome was published in the *New England Journal of Medicine* in 2006.

The results were shocking. The group with the lowest risk of suffering a stroke or heart attack was the placebo group! And the risk appeared to be 22% higher for those taking all three vitamins. Although the two groups taking folic acid had a 27% reduction in homocysteine levels, it didn't seem to be doing them any good. I certainly couldn't recommend taking high doses of B vitamins after a heart attack on this basis.

◆ High blood levels of homocysteine are linked with heart disease

◆ Homocysteine can damage arteries and trigger thrombosis

◆ Folic acid reduces homocysteine levels

◆ In clinical trials, folic acid supplements did not reduce the risk of having a heart attack or stroke

◆ Green vegetables and blackeye beans are rich in folic acid

◆ Folic acid is lost when greens are cooked, but can be recovered by using the cooking water to make gravy

Several other large trials (HOPE-2, VISP and WAFACS) have reported that lowering homocysteine with folic acid, vitamin B_{12} and vitamin B_6 failed to prevent strokes and heart attacks. These trials, like NORVIT, were properly randomised and controlled; they all recruited people who already had coronary heart disease, or had suffered a stroke, or were at very high risk (through diabetes or a combination of risk factors). The possibility raised by NORVIT, that treatment with B vitamins might be positively harmful, has not been confirmed by other studies.

An analysis of 12 controlled trials was published in the *Journal of the American Medical Association* in December 2006: there was no evidence that people with diseases of the heart and circulation could reduce their risk by taking folic acid supplements.

What now?

Remember that a stroke or heart attack usually follows decades of silent damage to arteries. Clearly, taking high doses of B vitamins is not a remedy for diseased arteries. It is still likely that avoiding deficiency of folic acid (and high blood levels of homocysteine) over the years – along with all the other strategies in this book – helps to prevent arteries becoming diseased in the first place.

Good sources of folic acid include green vegetables (especially Brussels sprouts, broccoli, spinach and kale), blackeye beans, chick-peas, peas and fortified breakfast cereals.

A lot of folic acid is lost when vegetables are cooked; much of it, rather than being destroyed, escapes in the water the vegetables were cooked in. If you make gravy or sauce with your spinach water, you'll recapture a lot of the folic acid.

It is always far better to ensure you are having enough of the right foods than to put your faith in concentrated nutrients in a pill. Grandma was right: you should eat up your greens.

Do antioxidants really prevent heart disease?

We know from laboratory work that antioxidants can block the damaging effects of free radicals. How does this work out in real life? Do they really protect us from disease?

A lot of evidence has been gathered from animal work. For example, the arteries of rabbits or hens with high cholesterol levels will fur up quickly with fatty deposits, but this can be prevented by giving vitamin E to the animals. What about people?

In the United States Nurses' Health Study involving 87 000 women, low intakes of vitamin E and beta-carotene were linked with an increased risk of coronary heart disease. Women with the highest antioxidant intakes had a 30–40% lower risk of heart disease. Research on 1605 men from Eastern Finland found that men with vitamin C deficiency were more likely to have a heart attack.

Investigations like these – so-called observational studies – generally report a link between higher antioxidant intakes and low rates of heart disease or cancer. So far, so good.

There is every reason, then, to expect that giving people antioxidants such as vitamins C or E will reduce their risk of having a heart attack or getting cancer. We have to look to well designed controlled trials to put this to the test.

The Heart Protection Study published in 2002 (see page 329) failed to show any additional benefit or risk when 600 mg of vitamin E and 250 mg of vitamin C were added to treatment. Some controlled trials have suggested that taking antioxidant supplements is beneficial, and some have suggested it's risky; most of the bigger trials show neither benefit nor risk.

Should I take vitamin supplements?

Having analysed all the evidence from controlled trials, we cannot recommend taking antioxidant supplements to treat or prevent heart disease or cancer.

On the other hand, there is strong evidence for the benefit of regularly eating foods rich in antioxidants – fruit and vegetables, whole grains and nuts.

No doubt, the antioxidants in these foods play a vital part in protecting us against heart disease and cancer, but we know that fibre, starch and minerals are important as well. If you extract 'pure nutrients' from whole foods because you think they are the most important, you may leave something even more important behind.

Observational studies have suggested that eating foods high in beta-carotene is beneficial. Unfortunately, beta-carotene supplements have not proved beneficial in trials, and there is strong evidence that they increase the risk of lung cancer and death in smokers. Perhaps it was something else in the beta-carotene-containing foods that was doing the good.

And there is really no evidence that you are better off taking much bigger doses of vitamins (antioxidant or otherwise) than you can obtain from your food.

The biggest mistake is to think you can make up for a poor diet, lacking in a balanced variety of helpful foods, by taking a vitamin pill. Supplements aren't substitutes.

By all means take a multivitamin pill, if you wish – in addition to eating a good diet. Avoid megadoses of one favoured vitamin. If you want to take a folic acid supplement, I would stick to 0.4 mg daily, especially if you have just had a heart attack, unless advised by your doctor to take more. Similarly, don't take more than 10 mg of vitamin B_6 in a pill, except on medical advice.

ACTION POINTS

◆ Eat at least five portions of fruit and vegetables a day

◆ Have whole grains every day

◆ Enjoy up to 28 g (1 oz) of nuts (e.g. almonds, walnuts) most days

Chapter 10

Garlic

It is, of course, an old wives' tale that garlic is good for you. It seems that this may be one of those occasions when old wives know best.

The medicinal powers of the garlic plant (*Allium sativum*) were proclaimed by the ancient Egyptians and by Hippocrates. Respiratory infections, boils, fungal infections and infestations with worms and other parasites are among the many conditions that have been treated with garlic over the ages. In recent times, science has provided some evidence that garlic can have remarkable effects on the cardiovascular system.

There must be something in it

Actually lots of different substances have been identified in garlic cloves, but the main ingredient responsible for its medicinal properties is a sulphur-containing compound called allicin. Unfortunately, this is also the stuff that stinks. Attempts to extract a garlic essence with all the medicinal zest of fresh garlic and none of the odour have failed: you can't have the ping without the pong! Some odourless garlic preparations contain no active ingredients.

> **'I did not realize what it had done to my breath – one doesn't with garlic – until this afternoon when I stood waiting for somebody to open a door for me and suddenly noticed that the varnish on the door was bubbling.'**
>
> **FRANK MUIR,**
> *You Can't Have Your Kayak and Heat It,* 1973

The quantity of allicin present in fresh garlic varies greatly and is influenced by agricultural conditions, as well as the origin of the garlic. When fresh garlic is stored at room temperature, the amount of allicin that can be obtained from it decreases substantially over a few weeks.

However, when garlic powder preparations have been carefully dried and stored, they can retain up to 90% of available allicin over five years; those derived from the best Chinese garlic are good sources of allicin.

Allicin itself would be difficult to preserve as it is chemically unstable. Fresh whole garlic cloves contain the inactive, odourless amino acid called alliin. Crushing the garlic sets the enzyme allinase to work on alliin, releasing allicin and its familiar odour.

Of course, for most people, the aroma of garlic is a delight in the kitchen and at the dinner table – but not on the breath of your colleague the next morning. It is claimed that you can neutralise the odour of allicin by eating parsley. There may be something in this but I'm sure that there are many people blissfully believing that they are enjoying all the benefits of garlic without the social consequences; their friends don't like to tell them that they are living in a fantasy world – allicin Wonderland.

The best solution is for all of us to eat lots of garlic every day, so that we cannot detect it on anyone else's breath; then only the occasional alien will be offended. Of course, this is not such a fantastic idea. In some countries they have been doing it for centuries. It would be rather hard, I suppose, on that small minority of people who genuinely cannot tolerate garlic.

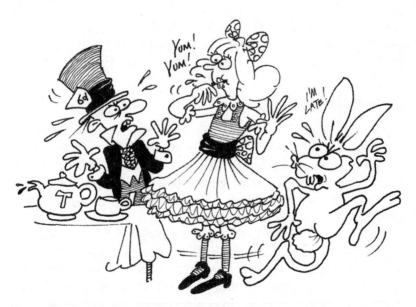

'I'd be a social outcast if it weren't for parsley.'

Kwai tablets contain garlic powder prepared by drying good quality Chinese garlic cloves. The special coating prevents the release of any allicin until the tablet reaches the digestive system. The tablets certainly are odour-free, but the people who take them may not be. In one large study, a garlic odour was reported (usually by the spouse) in 21% of those taking the tablets but also in 9% of the placebo group whose tablets contained no garlic!

Garlic and cholesterol

Various animal experiments, in which animals were fed diets that cause fatty deposits in arteries, have shown that garlic can protect the arteries against these changes. The studies have generally found a fall in the undesirable LDL-cholesterol together with a rise in the protective HDL-cholesterol in subjects treated with garlic.

In a large German study published in 1990, Dr Mader examined the effects of garlic in 261 people whose cholesterol and triglyceride readings were above the recommended levels. This was a randomised, double-blind, placebo-controlled trial: people were either given Kwai tablets or 'dummy' tablets, which looked the same, and neither the people nor researchers knew who was getting what until the code was cracked at the end. Reduction in cholesterol was significantly greater in those receiving garlic (12% at 16 weeks compared with 3% in the placebo group). Triglyceride levels dropped too (17% in the garlic group and only 2% in those receiving placebo tablets).

Garlic and thrombosis

If our blood didn't clot, we would bleed to death. On the other hand, if the blood clots too easily, thrombosis (the formation of a clot in the circulation) can cause a heart attack or stroke. The body is constantly keeping a balance between these extremes. Eating saturated fat increases the risk of thrombosis; several studies have shown that both garlic and onion can help protect against it.

The body's system for reversing the chain of events that leads to thrombosis is called 'fibrinolysis'. In one study there was a 70% increase in fibrinolysis within a few hours of eating fried or raw garlic and this increase continued during a month of eating garlic. Onions contain a substance called cycloalliin (and you will notice the similarity to alliin in garlic). Cycloalliin significantly increased fibrinolysis 1½ hours after it was given to people who had suffered a heart attack.

Platelets (also known as thrombocytes) are the smallest blood cells but they are a vital part of the blood-clotting system. By sticking to each other or to the walls of a damaged artery they can help to bring bleeding under control. If platelets become too 'sticky', they can add to the plaques that cause narrowing of arteries and they can provoke thrombosis leading to a heart attack or stroke.

Various experiments in animals and humans have indicated that garlic can stop platelets clumping together too easily. This action of garlic is similar to the effect of aspirin; low-dose aspirin is prescribed for some people who are at increased risk of thrombosis (e.g. people who have had a heart attack or suffer from angina). We do not yet have enough information about the effect of garlic on platelet function to recommend it as an alternative to aspirin for people at high risk of thrombosis.

Garlic and blood pressure

More relevant is the work done on humans. Auer and colleagues published a study in 1990 in which 600 mg a day of dried garlic powder (Kwai tablets) was given to people with raised blood pressure in a controlled trial. Very satisfactory reductions in blood pressure were observed in those taking garlic. Several other studies have also reported that blood pressure was reduced by garlic consumption, but others have found no change.

Survival in stink?

Maybe garlic does fight infection and protect against heart disease. You could propose that its widespread use around the world is explained by natural selection – that more garlic eaters have survived. Perhaps we too should become a nation of garlic eaters before we are wiped out by heart disease. I wouldn't go that far myself, but it is intriguing that this traditional, natural food flavouring could turn out to have so many beneficial effects.

The combination of actions on blood fats, cholesterol, blood pressure and thrombosis could make garlic a powerful protector against heart disease, but the evidence for this is incomplete.

Ideally we would have confirmation from carefully controlled trials that eating garlic results in fewer heart attacks. The trial design must ensure that the only difference between the groups under comparison is in their garlic consumption. As it is, a handful of experiments show that garlic reduces some important risk factors and we can point to groups of people that eat a lot of garlic and have low rates of heart disease (but also differ in other ways from groups of people with high rates).

If you enjoy garlic in your food, perhaps you will enjoy it all the more now. Unfortunately, it is likely that daily consumption of large quantities of good quality fresh garlic would be required to obtain maximum benefit, but nature has the last laugh and even tiny amounts can wreak havoc in your social life.

A practical way of eating the quantities of active garlic used in clinical trials is to take Kwai tablets, provided you are one of the eight out of ten who can do so without smelling of garlic, and you don't mind swallowing six to eight tablets a day. There is certainly not enough evidence for me to recommend this; more research is needed. It could never make up for an unhealthy diet or lifestyle, but at least you would have the assurance that you were simply taking a dried preparation of something that has been safety-tested on millions across the globe. It would also remove any pressure to add garlic to your food as if it were a medicine, leaving you free to delight in its flavour whenever it suits you and your diary.

GARLIC FACTS

◆ Lowers cholesterol and triglyceride levels

◆ Reduces platelet stickiness and the risk of thrombosis

◆ Lowered blood pressure in some trials but not in others

◆ The active ingredient, allicin, is the stuff that stinks

◆ Clinical trials used large amounts of allicin

◆ More research is needed

◆ Garlic is lovely. Enjoy it!

Chapter 11

Alcohol

'We drink one another's healths,
and spoil our own.'

JEROME K JEROME,
Idle Thoughts of an Idle Fellow, 1886

To your health!

Is that glass of wine a further step towards health and happiness or another nail in the coffin? It really depends whether it's the first drink of the evening or the fifth. A lot of research has been done on this subject and it is quite clear that light to moderate drinking can help to protect you against heart disease but heavier drinking will damage your health.

The J-shaped curve

A graph showing the link between death rate (from all causes) in an industrialised population and alcohol consumption is a J-shaped curve (Figure 8).

This means that the risk of death is higher for people who drink no alcohol at all than for those who drink a little. (Yes, I know 100% of us die eventually but when we talk about death rate or 'mortality' we are referring to the proportion of a population that dies in a specified period.) The lowest risk, the lowest part of the J, is at one to two units a day and the risk shoots up after four units a day.

This reduction in death rate among light and moderate drinkers results from reduced coronary heart disease (which is such a common killer that it has a big influence on total mortality figures). Heavier drinking increases the risk of having a stroke or developing liver cirrhosis, pancreatitis or certain cancers, or even damaging the heart

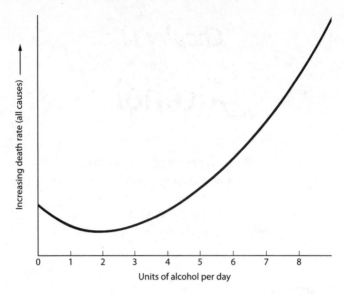

Figure 8 The J-shaped curve. This shows the link between alcohol consumption and death rate. The lowest risk, the lowest part of the J, is at one or two units a day.

muscle (cardiomyopathy) – not to mention road accidents or falling off a cliff.

This J-shaped curve hides differences within the population. Alcohol is not politically correct. It is ageist and sexist.

Young adults (under 40) are more likely to die in an accident or as a result of violence than from a heart attack. The relationship between drinking and death rates in this age group is not a J-shaped curve. It's a straight line. The more you drink, the more likely you are to die. This is not surprising as alcohol is often involved in accidents and violent deaths. Older people are more likely to die from heart disease and less likely to die as a result of an accident or violence, so the protective effect of alcohol becomes significant.

An interesting footnote for older people is that French researchers published an investigation in 1997 which concluded that older people who drink wine moderately are less prone to develop senile dementia and Alzheimer's disease than non-drinkers. Perhaps this is a J-shaped curve as well. In 2004, the *British Medical Journal* published a study showing that the risk of dementia in old age was increased by drinking either no alcohol or too much alcohol in middle age.

For women, the risk of heart disease rises after the menopause and the risk is higher for teetotallers than for light drinkers, but the recom-

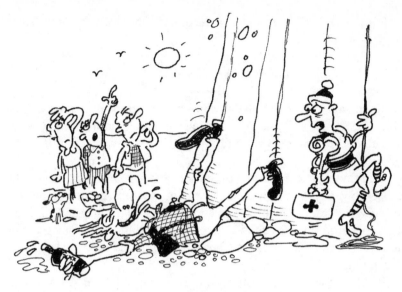

'At least he died with a healthy heart.'

mended safe drinking limit is lower for women than men. This is not because the limits are set by a committee of men. In general, a woman's body contains less water than a man's and it takes less alcohol to reach a harmful concentration. There is some evidence that even modest consumption of alcohol can increase the risk of breast cancer.

What's the limit?

Adding up your alcohol intake is made easier by referring to units. One unit of alcohol is 8 g or 10 ml of ethanol. Traditional advice states that the following drinks give you one unit of alcohol:

- 1 half pint of normal strength lager or beer;

- 1 small (125 ml) glass of wine;

- 1 measure (25 ml) spirits;

- 1 measure (50 ml) fortified wine, e.g. sherry, Martini.

This is very misleading now. Some drinks have become stronger and pubs often give larger measures. (Of course, home measures are usually doubles anyway!)

To work out the number of units in a drink, just multiply the volume of the drink (ml) by the percent alcohol by volume (% ABV) and divide by 1000:

$$number\ of\ units = \frac{volume\ (ml) \times \%\ ABV}{1000}$$

You need to divide by 1000 to convert the volume into litres; a drink that is 13% ABV will have 13 units in every litre. Simple! If the volume is stated in centilitres (cl), multiply by ten to convert it to ml: 75 cl is 750 ml.

Traditional advice is based on the assumption that your wine is 8% ABV. Nowadays you're more likely to find it's 13%. So that small (125 ml) glass contains 1.63 units. And if your glass is actually 250 ml, you'll be knocking back 3.25 units! A large glass of wine can easily give you four units of alcohol – enough, perhaps, to put you over the legal limit for driving.

In 2007, the government announced that labels on all alcoholic drinks would include sensible drinking advice by the end of 2008. Labels should state how many units of alcohol are in the drink and include the government's guidelines on safe limits (including advice to avoid alcohol if pregnant or trying to conceive).

Current guidelines recommend that men should not drink more than three to four units a day and women should not go above two to three units a day. Drinking the maximum allowance every day is not recommended as this can damage health.

I have something very important to explain to you. These are the official limits because the really damaging effects of alcohol become apparent when people drink more than this. You'll be better off drinking less. You will get most of the protection that alcohol can give you against heart disease by drinking as little as one unit a day on five days of the week. For the under 50s, the risks of drinking up to the limit outweigh any benefits.

An important improvement in the revised guidelines was the emphasis on daily rather than weekly limits. Previously, the safe limits were said to be up to 21 units a week for a man and up to 14 units a week for a woman. So a man drinking 10 pints of beer a week would be meeting the guidelines, but if he drinks it all at the weekend it's a very unsafe pattern of drinking. Binge drinking is bad for you. Apart from the risk of accidents and the social problems that come with alcoholic intoxication, it pushes up the blood pressure and does not protect the heart like moderate drinking spread throughout the week.

In fact, a bout of heavy drinking can bring on a heart attack even when the coronary arteries are normal!

◆ Light drinking helps protect against heart disease

◆ Heavier drinking damages health, risking strokes, cirrhosis and cancers

◆ In the under 40s, the benefits of alcohol are outweighed by the risks

◆ 1 unit of alcohol a day, 5 days a week is enough to help your heart

◆ Binge drinking is dangerous and can even cause heart attacks

How can alcohol protect against coronary heart disease?

It has often been pointed out that the higher rate of heart disease among non-drinkers does not prove that alcohol protects against heart disease. Perhaps this odd group of people who drink no alcohol at all is at higher risk because it includes those who have had to give up alcohol for health reasons. This is a very important point but researchers have now shown that the difference cannot be explained by ex-drinkers among the non-drinkers. After many studies on the subject, it is widely accepted that a modest alcohol consumption reduces the risk of coronary heart disease. But how?

An interesting case report published in 1984 by Breier and Lisch concerned a 69-year-old man with a condition known as familial hypercholesterolaemia. Sufferers from this inherited problem have very high cholesterol levels and, unless treatment is given to lower the cholesterol, arteries become clogged causing early heart disease. You may remember the actor Richard Beckinsale who died tragically young as a result of this condition. Well, the remarkable thing about the man studied was that he had reached the age of 69 without any evidence of narrowed arteries.

It seemed that, although he had a very high cholesterol level, his arteries were being protected by an unusually high concentration of HDL_2-cholesterol (a sub-fraction of the beneficial HDL-cholesterol). The other thing the doctors noticed was that this man drank 375 ml (three glasses) of red wine daily.

They decided to test whether the red wine was causing the high level of protective HDL_2-cholesterol. The man went through a cycle of drinking no alcohol for 21 days, followed by 21 days of drinking his usual three glasses of red wine a day. During the time without alcohol, the concentration of HDL_2 in his blood fell to about one-quarter of the original level. After 21 days back on the red wine, the HDL_2 level had returned to its original value.

It is important to understand that this was a study on one particular man, and not everybody will have the same response. (Otherwise, we should adopt this dose of red wine as a standard treatment for familial hypercholesterolaemia for a start.) Nevertheless, several other studies have shown that drinking alcohol generally raises HDL-cholesterol levels. No doubt this is one of the ways in which alcohol can protect us against coronary heart disease. In fact, statistically, you could explain about half the extra heart disease occurring in non-drinkers in terms of lower HDL-cholesterol levels.

Raising HDL-cholesterol levels will help to stop arteries furring up over the years. Another very important way of reducing heart disease risk is to reduce the chance of a thrombosis – a blood clot in the circulation. Alcohol is known to make the blood platelets less active and to decrease fibrinogen levels; both of these actions will lower the risk of thrombosis.

Red wine contains antioxidants. The actual substances are polyphenols (notably flavonoids such as quercetin and epicatechin) but that shouldn't put you off your wine. On the contrary, their discovery is a cause for celebration because, like other antioxidants, they have been shown to reduce oxidation of LDL (see Chapter 9). So, theoretically at least, the antioxidants in red wine could help to stop fatty plaques forming in arteries. These antioxidants come from the grape skin and can also be found, in lower concentrations, in red (but not white) grape juice.

What's your poison?

Should you choose beer, wine or spirits to give your heart the best protection?

Much publicity has been given to 'the French paradox'. This has nothing to do with French paramedics treating heart attack victims. The point is that the French suffer fewer heart attacks than you would expect from the amount of saturated fat in their diet; it has been

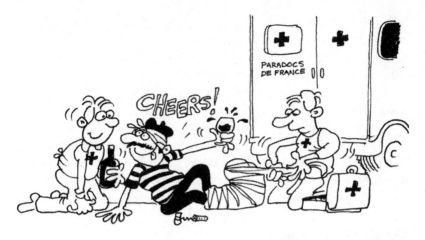

Nothing to do with French paramedics.

suggested that all the red wine they drink is protecting their hearts. The cynic might say that they die of alcoholic cirrhosis before they get a chance to have a heart attack. Certainly there are many factors apart from wine consumption that may contribute to this paradox (see page 162).

Over 60 studies have found lower rates of heart disease among light and moderate drinkers compared with non-drinkers. Some of these investigations have, indeed, concluded that wine offers better protection than other beverages but some studies have found in favour of spirits or beer. One of the problems is that one type of drink may be associated with a different drinking pattern from another type, according to the social customs of the community studied. If wine is normally consumed in moderation with meals, the effect will be very beneficial compared with binge drinking of spirits. A study on health professionals found spirits to be the most protective; spirits were the most commonly consumed type of drink and were generally taken in moderation throughout the week rather than in binges at the weekend.

Many studies on this subject were collected and analysed by Rimm and colleagues in 1996. They concluded that there was strong evidence linking all alcoholic drinks, when consumed in moderation, with a lower risk of heart disease, but not that one type of drink gives better protection than another.

It may be that the antioxidants in red wine offer additional benefits but, clearly, most of the protection against heart disease comes from the alcohol. On current evidence, then, despite what you may have heard about the health benefits of drinking red wine, it is pointless to take it like a medicine if you prefer to drink white. Personally, there is nothing I would rather drink with my evening meal than a glass of red wine, even if I am eating fish or poultry.

So, the important question is not so much 'What's your poison?' as 'How do you take it?' The beverage you choose is less critical than your pattern of drinking. This was borne out by an Australian study published in 1997 by McElduff and Dobson. They found the risk of having a heart attack was lowest in men who reported having one to four drinks a day – and in women who reported one or two drinks a day – on five or six days a week.

Should I start drinking?

If you do not drink any alcohol, you may be thinking by now that you should start. I would rather encourage you to concentrate on all the other strategies in this book for reducing your risk of heart disease than to start drinking. And, if you are a young person, don't forget that the health hazards of drinking alcohol may outweigh the benefits. Obviously, nobody should mix drinking with driving.

◆ Alcohol can increase HDL-cholesterol and reduce thrombosis risk

◆ The pattern of drinking is more important than the type of drink:

- 10 glasses of red wine on Friday night increases risk

- ½ pint beer 5 times a week helps the heart

◆ Antioxidants in red wine may give added protection but this is not proven

◆ When society increases average alcohol intake, the number of heavy drinkers rises

---

Doctors have a problem when it comes to advising people about the benefits of light drinking. I don't mean that old saying about an alcoholic being defined as someone who drinks more than his doctor. Though it is true that heavy drinkers tend to underestimate how much they are drinking. Indeed, Dylan Thomas apparently said 'An alcoholic is someone you don't like who drinks as much as you do'. True alcoholics, of course, are one group of people who should not attempt light drinking. The only path for them is to avoid alcohol completely. No, the problem doctors have when advising about the benefits of light drinking is that there will always be those who say to themselves, 'If a little will do me good, then a lot will do me more good.' I hope you understand by now that nothing could be further from the truth. It is also a sad fact that the percentage of heavy drinkers in any group of people is related to the average alcohol consumption of that group. Encouraging more people to drink, however well-intentioned, is likely to result in more people drinking heavily. Our objective to convert the majority of people into light drinkers seems impossible to achieve.

Drinking to your heart's content

Alcohol is one of God's good gifts. It is there to be enjoyed but, tragically, is often abused. Savouring a glass of wine, five days a week is quite enough to help your heart; you can get most of the health benefit from a glass every other day.

Cheers!

ACTION POINT

◆ Enjoy up to 1 or 2 units of alcohol a day – not more!

Chapter 12

Coffee or tea?

**'Look here, Steward, if this is coffee, I want tea;
but if this is tea, then I wish for coffee.'**

Punch (1841–1992) Vol. 123, 1902

You can often divide a roomful of people into coffee- and tea-drinkers. Some people are coffee potty, while others are total-teaers. Is there any evidence that our choice of beverage influences our risk of getting heart disease?

Both coffee and tea contain caffeine, of course. Caffeine can stimulate the heart, provoking palpitations, and the brain, causing insomnia. It is also a diuretic: drinking a cup of strong coffee stimulates more urine production than drinking the same volume of water. Caffeine addicts will know the withdrawal headaches that occur if they abstain for a time. For all this, there is no consistent evidence that caffeine is linked with coronary heart disease and I see no reason for moderate coffee- or tea-drinkers to be concerned about their caffeine intake (as long as they are not suffering palpitations or insomnia).

The mystery ingredient

For years it has been suspected that drinking a lot of coffee might contribute to the development of heart disease. It has been established by several research teams that drinking Scandinavian boiled coffee causes a rise in blood cholesterol levels. If it isn't the caffeine in this boiled coffee that raises cholesterol, what is it? It was discovered that the mystery ingredient is removed by passing the coffee through filter paper; filtered coffee doesn't increase blood cholesterol.

We now know that two lipids, or fatty substances, called cafestol and kahweol are to blame. They seem to be unique to the coffee bean.

- ◆ Coffee beans contain lipids that raise LDL-cholesterol
- ◆ 6 cups of cafetière coffee a day could raise cholesterol by 10%
- ◆ Filtered coffee (paper filter) does not raise cholesterol

But we don't boil our coffee like the Scandinavians

It has long been known that the Scandinavians' coffee-boiling habit is disastrous for cholesterol levels, but, if cafestol and kahweol are present in the coffee bean, what about the types of coffee that we normally drink?

A Dutch group of researchers, Urgert and colleagues, published an interesting study in the *British Medical Journal* in November 1996. In this randomised controlled trial, half the subjects drank five to six cups (0.9 litres) a day of strong cafetière coffee and the other half drank the same amount of strong filtered coffee. The two types of coffee contained the same amount of caffeine. They kept this up for six months and repeated blood samples were taken before, during and after the six-month period.

Cafetière coffee raised the total cholesterol level by 6–10%. Worse still, most of that rise was due to increased LDL-cholesterol (the damaging one), which went up by 9–14%. These changes continued for the six months of coffee drinking. Every one percentage rise in total cholesterol results in a two percentage rise in risk of coronary heart disease. So, drinking five to six cups of cafetière coffee a day produced a 12–20% rise in coronary risk!

There was also a 26% rise in triglyceride levels in the cafetière drinkers but this had settled to 7% by the end of the six months. In addition, the researchers found that cafetière coffee raised the level of a liver enzyme (alanine aminotransferase) but there was no evidence of liver damage and the significance of this is unclear.

So, cafetière coffee can push up cholesterol levels just like boiled Scandinavian coffee but filtration removes the problem. A word of warning: the researchers used paper filters and you could not expect filtration through a metallic mesh to have the same effect.

What about other types of coffee?

Turkish coffee, although served in small cups, is very concentrated stuff. (I think it must have been the origin of that old joke. You know. Man: 'Waiter, waiter, this coffee tastes like mud.' Waiter: 'It was only ground this morning, sir.') It contains similar quantities of cafestol and kahweol per cup to cafetière and boiled coffee.

Italian espresso coffee is also served in small cups and is a less concentrated source of cafestol and kahweol. It is estimated that about 25 cups of espresso would be equivalent to five or six of cafetière in this regard.

Instant and percolated coffee have low concentrations of the problem substances and their effect on cholesterol will be minimal.

Having filtered the evidence, what does it all boil down to? Remember: these alarming effects were produced by five or six cups of cafetière a day. If you are a frequent coffee drinker, you would be better off with instant, percolated or (paper) filtered. If cafetière coffee is an occasional indulgence, there is no need to lose any sleep over it (but you may do if you have it late at night). Confirmation that you can confidently carry on enjoying your coffee came from a large study published in *Circulation* in 2006. The risk of heart disease was not increased by coffee drinking in the 44 000 men and 84 000 women who were followed for up to 20 years. Most of them drank filtered coffee.

What about tea?

'English cuisine is generally so threadbare that for years there has been a gentlemen's agreement in the civilized world to allow the Brits pre-eminence in the matter of tea – which, after all, comes down to little more than the ability to boil water.'

WILFRID SHEED,
'Taking Pride in Prejudice', *GQ*, 1984

The good old English cuppa (of Asian tea) appears to be completely innocent as far as coronary heart disease is concerned. In fact, because tea contains flavonoid antioxidants, it may offer some protection against heart disease.

Several observational studies have found that tea drinking is linked with a lower risk of heart disease. Other studies have failed to confirm this. These observations are always difficult to interpret because of 'confounding factors': in one culture, tea drinking may be associated with poverty and smoking; in another, the tea drinkers may have relatively healthy lifestyles.

In the laboratory, tea consumption has been shown to have positive effects on the circulation. Research published in the *American Journal of Cardiology* in 2004 showed that drinking black tea improved blood flow in the coronary arteries supplying the heart. It seems that tea enhances performance of the artery lining (endothelium), improving production of nitric oxide which helps arteries to relax. And, in case you're thinking it's all down to the caffeine or hot water, researchers have tested both – and it's not.

Isn't herbal tea more healthy?

Well, what is normal tea if it isn't a herbal tea made from the dried leaves of the shrub *Camellia sinensis*? Of course, there is a wide variety of other plant extracts sold under the label 'herbal tea' and sometimes people imagine that they must be better for you than traditional tea. Indeed, some people think that anything 'herbal' or 'natural' must be quite safe and will probably do you a power of good. They overlook the fact that some of our most toxic drugs and poisons are simply plant extracts.

I'm not suggesting that any of the herbal teas in your local health food store are toxic. Some of them contain very familiar ingredients and offer a good caffeine-free alternative to tea. None of them will have been tried and tested and researched on anything like the scale of our traditional cuppa.

Hard to beat

Talking of making tea, isn't it a nuisance when the kettle element scales up in hard water areas? Before you rush to soften your drinking water, you may like to reflect on the fact that studies have repeatedly shown lower death rates from cardiovascular disease in hard water areas. The mortality difference is small, and you certainly shouldn't worry about it if you happen to live in a soft water area, but it has been a consistent finding. A water hardness level of 170 mg/l of calcium carbonate is fine and there is no apparent advantage in having it any harder than that.

**ERIC: I always take my wife morning tea in my pyjamas.
But is she grateful? No – she says she'd rather have it in a cup.**

ERIC MORECAMBE and ERNIE WISE,
The Morecambe and Wise Joke Book, 1979

◆ Tea appears safe and its antioxidants might even help your heart

◆ Some studies link tea drinking with lower rates of heart disease

◆ In laboratory tests, tea improves blood flow through arteries

◆ 'Herbal' teas are probably OK but have not been researched like tea and coffee

◆ Hard water areas have lower rates of heart disease; the difference is small

Chapter 13

Getting your balance

*'When Marilyn Monroe was married to Arthur Miller,
his mother always made matzo ball soup. After the tenth time,
Marilyn said, "Gee Arthur, these matzo balls are pretty nice,
but isn't there any other part of the matzo you can eat?" '*

ANN BARR and PAUL LEVY,
The Foodie Handbook, 1984

Variety is vital. How can we be sure our choice of foods is giving us all the nutrients we need and in the right balance?

To make a detailed analysis of your diet, a dietitian would use food composition tables or a computer to calculate your intake of various nutrients. Don't even attempt this. There is quite enough to contend with in the supermarket without taking a laptop computer.

A simple, practical method of making sure we keep the right balance is to use food groups. Table 17 (page 140) shows the five main food groups:

- Cereals and starchy foods;

- Fruit and vegetables;

- Milk and dairy products;

- Meat and high-protein foods;

- Fatty and sugary foods.

The eatwell plate

Use the eatwell plate to help you get the balance right. It shows how much of what you eat should come from each food group.

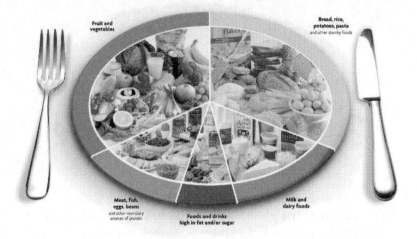

Figure 9 The eatwell plate.

Crown copyright 2007, Food Standards Agency

Every day you should eat a variety of different foods from each of the first four groups.

The fifth group is foods containing lots of fat, lots of sugar or both. You don't need to select any items from this group for a healthy, balanced diet; if you do, keep the quantity right down. Yes, some of these foods (such as the cooking oils) are sources of essential fatty acids, but you can get these in adequate quantities from foods in the other four groups. This is not a completely comprehensive list of foods; the examples given will enable you to put other foods in the correct category (Figure 9).

Most of your food should come from the first two groups – the starchy foods and the fruit and vegetable group. Have several different foods from the starch group each day. Examples are porridge, muesli, rye bread, mixed-grain bread, barley, wholemeal pasta and couscous. Always choose wholegrain varieties where possible and try to avoid sugary breakfast cereals, biscuits and cakes.

Most people in the UK are not eating the recommended five portions of fruit and vegetables a day. Eat **at least** two portions of fruit and three of vegetables every day. More would be better. Theoretically, a portion is 80 g (and you don't count the bits you don't eat, such as stones and cores). In practice, a portion could be a piece of fruit the size of an apple, two plums or apricots, or three heaped tablespoons of vegetables, chopped fruit or berries. Just one heaped tablespoon of dried fruit (e.g. raisins) makes a portion; without the bulk and weight of water, it's concentrated stuff (see Table 16).

Table 16 Examples of one portion (80 g) of fruit or vegetable

---

1 apple, pear, orange, peach, or banana

2 plums or apricots

1 slice of melon

Half a grapefruit

1 heaped tablespoon of raisins or other dried fruit

1 bowl of salad (the size of a cereal bowl)

3 heaped tablespoons of vegetables/pulses

3 heaped tablespoons of chopped fruit, cherries, grapes or berries

---

Milk and dairy products are a very important source of calcium. They provide protein too. If you stick to skimmed milk and very low-fat dairy products, you can use them freely. Aim for three servings a day from this group. Examples of a serving would be the milk taken in tea throughout the day, or a carton of yoghurt, or quark added to a pasta dish.

Most people in the developed world are eating enough protein to meet their 'nutritional requirements', i.e. to replace nitrogen lost from the body. This is calculated as 0.75 g of protein a day for every kg of body weight. So typical daily requirements are 55 g for a man and 45 g for a woman. This is easily covered by two servings from the protein group. But you may benefit from more, especially if you are finding it difficult to lose weight or trim your tummy (see Chapter 18).

The trouble is that so much of the protein people eat comes with a good helping of saturated fat in meat and dairy products. Use pulses and fish in abundance; use red meat sparingly. Pulses, of course, as well as providing protein, give you starch and soluble fibre.

Variety is the key. Five apples do not count as five portions.

Table 17 The five main food groups

---

1. CEREALS AND STARCHY FOODS

Bread, including wholemeal, mixed-grain, granary loaves, rye bread, pumpernickel, white bread, French bread, pitta bread, rolls, baps

Crumpets, crispbreads, matzos

Breakfast cereals, muesli

Oats (including porridge), barley, rye, wheat, bulgar, buckwheat, millet, maize, polenta, semolina, couscous, tapioca, quinoa

Rice, including brown rice and wild rice

Pasta: spaghetti, lasagne, tagliatelle, macaroni, noodles, etc.

Potatoes, including sweet potato, cassava, yam, taro

---

2. FRUIT AND VEGETABLES

Salad vegetables, including lettuce, cucumber, tomatoes, peppers, etc.

All vegetables (not potatoes) – fresh, frozen or canned

All fruit – fresh, frozen or canned (in fruit juice)

Dried fruit e.g. prunes, figs, apricots, raisins, sultanas

Unsweetened fruit juice

---

3. MILK AND DAIRY PRODUCTS

Milk, skimmed recommended for most adults

Cheese: most have a high fat content

Cottage cheese, quark, and a little Parmesan/pecorino recommended

Yoghurt, especially very low-fat varieties

Fromage frais, particularly virtually fat-free

Buttermilk

Table 17 The five main food groups (*cont'd*)

---

4. MEAT AND HIGH-PROTEIN FOODS

Meat: beef, pork, lamb (lean cuts, remove fat), lean bacon (or smoked turkey rashers), ham, rabbit, venison, ostrich, kangaroo

Meat products: reduced-fat sausages/burgers (still not very low-fat)
Poultry: chicken, turkey

Fish: white fish – cod, haddock, plaice, sole, etc.

Oily fish – mackerel, herring, sardines, pilchards, salmon

Shellfish – scallops, oysters, cockles etc.

Nuts: hazelnuts, almonds, walnuts, peanuts

Seeds: sunflower, sesame

Eggs

Pulses: lentils, chickpeas, beans (e.g. baked beans, kidney beans, broad beans, mung beans, blackeye beans, pinto beans, soya beans), peas, split peas

Dhal, hummus, tofu, textured vegetable protein (TVP)

Quorn

---

5. FATTY/SUGARY FOODS

Fatty foods (some also have high sugar content):

Fat spreads, margarine, butter

Olive oil, rapeseed oil, corn oil, sunflower oil, safflower oil, soya oil, sesame seed oil, grapeseed oil, walnut oil, groundnut (peanut) oil, palm oil, coconut oil, 'vegetable oil'

Suet, lard, dripping

Oil-based dressings, fatty sauces, mayonnaise

Cream, ice-cream

Cakes, biscuits, puddings, pastries, crisps

Chocolate, chocolate spread, toffee/butterscotch sauces

Coconut bars

Sugary foods (some also have high fat content):

Sweets

Sweet snacks

Sweetened drinks, squashes

Sugar, jams

ACTION POINTS

◆ Have wholegrain foods every day (e.g. porridge, muesli, pasta)

◆ Eat *at least* 5 portions of fruit and vegetables a day

◆ Use skimmed milk, low-fat yoghurt, fromage frais, buttermilk, quark

◆ Have lots of pulses (peas, beans, lentils, chickpeas)

◆ Use fish, lean poultry (skinned), egg white, tofu, TVP, Quorn

◆ Avoid meat products (sausages, burgers, pies, etc.) and fatty red meat

◆ Fill most of your menu with the first two food groups and beware the fifth

On balance

The food group principle can help people of all ages to achieve a balanced diet. Obviously, portion sizes and energy requirements vary from individual to individual. Some people have food allergies, or intolerances, or special dietary needs requiring professional advice, but everyone should get the best balance that they can.

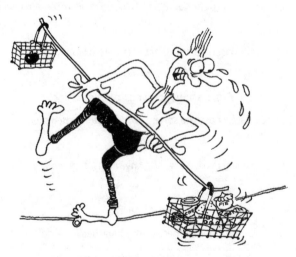

Getting your balance needn't be so difficult.

When you're getting on

It's a bit irrelevant at 80, isn't it? Not at all. Eating well and exercising are extremely important at any age. After the age of 65, there is a sharp rise in the rates of stroke and heart disease. You cannot avoid death – although you may postpone it – but this is particularly about life. It's about living it to the full, in the best health possible. 'I will never be an old man. To me, old age is always fifteen years older than I am,' is what the American statesman Bernard Baruch had to say about it. On the other hand, as Bob Hope said, 'You know you're getting old when the candles cost more than the cake.'

By all means enjoy your birthday cake but, as you get older, please don't neglect vegetables, fruit and fish.

This book says more about eating than about not eating. If you are frail and have a poor appetite, it is all the more important that you get the right balance of nutrients. Misguided dietary restriction must be avoided; energy intake is crucial. You may need advice from your doctor or a dietitian.

When you're expecting

If you are pregnant, and here I am no longer addressing older readers, balanced nutrition based on the first four food groups is very important for you. There is no special pregnancy diet but there are a few important precautions.

To reduce the risk of a neural tube defect in the baby (such as spina bifida), you should take a folic acid supplement (0.4 mg daily); this should have been started before pregnancy, from the time of stopping contraception, and should be continued for the first 12 weeks of pregnancy. If you are less than 12 weeks pregnant and not taking folic acid, simply start now. The supplement should be taken in addition to eating foods containing folic acid (e.g. Brussels sprouts, spinach, cooked blackeye beans and fortified cereals).

Liver should be avoided during pregnancy as the high levels of vitamin A could harm your baby. Eat up to two portions of oily fish a week, but not swordfish, marlin or shark (as they contain more mercury).

Toxoplasmosis is one of those infections which is not normally serious but in pregnancy it can be catastrophic. You can catch it from undercooked meat (and from handling cat litter).

Listeriosis (caused by the bacterium *Listeria monocytogenes*) is another infection to avoid in pregnancy. It can cause miscarriage, stillbirth or an ill baby. Some foods can be heavily contaminated with Listeria, which thrives at fridge temperatures but is killed by cooking. Foods to avoid are: soft cheeses like Camembert, Brie, goats' and ewes' milk cheeses; pâté and non-canned meat products like sausage rolls and pies; ready-made salads and coleslaw. Cottage cheese is fine.

Of course, pregnancy brings bizarre changes in appetite for some women. Cravings for certain foods (or even non-foods like clay or matchboxes) and aversion to others can temporarily threaten the balance of nutrition. All the more reason to get nutritionally fit well before getting pregnant.

> ◆ Balance is important at all ages
>
> ◆ Fish and fruit are often neglected
>
> ◆ In pregnancy, avoid toxoplasma, listeria, liver, swordfish, marlin and shark; take folic acid in the first three months

The balanced shopper

Help! The supermarket closes in half an hour and you have a family of four to feed. Don't panic. You've done it before. You know the layout of the supermarket. You collect a trolley and set off. Ah, the shopping list – it must be by the kitchen sink. How could you forget it? Are you finally going off your trolley? You dash up and down the aisles, hoping you'll remember what you need when you see it. Ugh! You're certainly going off this trolley; one wheel keeps making for the check-out and you're nowhere near finished. Oh, what are those? They look interesting. No time to check prices, let alone food labels. Sling them in the trolley. Was that your tummy rumbling? Those cakes would fill the gap.

All right. It's a good description of someone else – not you. That's good. Because, if you go to the supermarket hungry, hurried and harassed, there's no hope of the family eating a good and balanced diet for the rest of the week. What you put in that trolley ends up in their bodies (OK, not the toilet rolls, but the food). You cannot escape that consequence, but you can easily lose sight of it.

Healthy shopping means healthy eating. And vice versa. Plan the shop, eat first, give yourself time, and take a list. The shopping list should be based on the first four food groups (Table 17) because, if you have an unbalanced larder, you'll have an unbalanced diet.

At the end of the shop, you should be able to see at a glance that you have a balanced trolley – mainly full of fruit and vegetables, cereal and starchy foods, pulses and fish. No doubt you will also have a range of very low-fat dairy products and perhaps some skinless chicken or turkey breast or some game. Yes, you may have a little red meat or higher fat cheese, but these should be difficult to spot – swamped by other foods.

You have only to glance at the trolleys of some shoppers to see why heart disease is claiming people by the thousand – trolleys laden with fatty meat pies and sausages, fatty red meat and full-fat cheeses, whole milk, fat spreads, and manufactured cakes and biscuits. Two or three small bags containing fruits or vegetables have a tiny space at one end.

I realise that you may not buy all your food from a supermarket. Perhaps, for example, you get your fruits and vegetables from a market (or grow some yourself) and your fish from a fishmonger. If you favour organic fruits and vegetables, it's well worth finding out if there is a local, weekly delivery service. This is a good way of ensuring that you never run out of fresh produce, provided you order enough. It's usually a matter of pot luck which particular items turn up each week and you may need to buy more with your weekly shop.

Why not make a shopping checklist based on Table 17? Of course, there are additional food items that are sometimes needed such as herbs, spices and seasonings.

Give yourself time to read food labels. Take a magnifying glass if you need one. In due course you will need less and less time to do this as you become familiar with more products.

As a general rule, reject processed foods with more than four grams of fat per 100 grams – especially when most of the fat is in the form of saturates. Remember to avoid unspecified 'vegetable oil' and hydrogenated vegetable oil unless the quantities are tiny. Don't worry: even if you don't add fat to your food, you can get all the fatty acids you need from the first four food groups. Certainly, if you use a little olive oil or rapeseed oil in your cuisine, and keep up a good intake of oily fish, there is no fear of lacking any fatty acids or fat-soluble vitamins; you simply have more control over the quantity and type of fat that you are eating.

Some items will be labelled as having no added salt or sugar. Anything approaching one gram of sodium per 100 grams is an awful lot when you are trying to limit your salt intake. Check how much of the total carbohydrate content is in the form of sugars. Table 18 gives you some help on food labelling.

Table 18 Guide to food labelling.

Quantities per 100 g	
This is a lot	**This is a little**
10 g sugars	2 g sugars
20 g fat	3 g fat
5 g saturates	1 g saturates
3 g fibre	0.5 g fibre
0.5 g sodium	0.1 g sodium

Source: Adapted from *Eating for Your Heart*, published by the British Heart Foundation, March 1999, with permission. For many meals and foods you eat in large amounts, look at the amount per serving. For snacks and foods you eat in small amounts, look at the 'per 100 g' information. Work out from the table whether there is a lot or a little of each nutrient in the food. Remember – the most important nutrient to look for is FAT.

ACTION POINTS

◆ Make a shopping list from the 4 important food groups

◆ Don't go shopping on an empty stomach

◆ Take a magnifying glass if you need one to read food labels

◆ Reject processed foods with:

- more than 4 g fat/100 g (especially saturates)

- 'vegetable oil'/hydrogenated vegetable oil

- high sodium content (e.g. 0.9 g/100 g)

◆ Before you go to the check-out, make sure you have a balanced trolley

What about the bank balance?

'There are several ways in which to apportion the family income, all of them unsatisfactory.'

ROBERT BENCHLEY

I'd love to eat a healthy diet, but how can I afford it? Food is expensive. This is a real problem for some people. Poverty has been defined as the need to spend more than 30% of available income on food. Certain foods mentioned in this book will be beyond the reach of some readers or could be an occasional luxury for others, but a healthier diet need not be a more expensive one.

Here are a few tips on eating well but keeping down the cost. For a start, eating more foods from the high-starch group (like bread, potatoes, pasta and rice), and less meat, is good for your heart and your budget.

There is a wide variety to choose from in the way of peas, beans and lentils, which are good sources of protein and cost less than meat. If you use them with foods from the cereal group, all your essential amino acids are provided. It's very convenient to buy them in tins, ready-cooked. Add them to casseroles, or any meat dish, and you'll need far less meat.

Buy foods on special offer. Cash flow permitting, stock up on canned foods or skimmed milk powder when the offer is good (as long as you know the brand, so there's no risk of being disappointed).

A freezer allows bulk-buying of many other foods when the price is low. Salmon steaks would be an extravagant luxury for many people but the price varies enormously. If you can afford it, stock the freezer (or freezer compartment of your fridge) when they are half-price.

Fruit and vegetable prices fluctuate with changes in season and agricultural conditions. Buy whatever is cheap at the time. You will often find much better prices on a market stall than in the supermarket. But beware: it's no economy if it goes bad before you can eat it. Be choosy. Get to know the good market stalls, and avoid the bad ones. Even better, grow your own fruits and vegetables. If you don't have a garden, consider an allotment. Sharing with another family can make this easier.

The same is true of shopping expeditions; if you don't have a car, sharing the cost of transport to a supermarket may be more economical than relying on local shops.

And finally, if worry about your budget is driving you to spend lots of money on cigarettes, you should read Chapter 21.

TIPS TO SAVE MONEY AND STAY HEALTHY

◆ Eat more starchy foods and pulses, but less meat

◆ Buy foods on special offer

◆ For fruit and vegetables, use a good market stall and buy cheap

◆ Grow your own produce; consider a shared allotment

Chapter 14

Eating in – eating out

Eating in

'Kissing don't last: cookery do!'

GEORGE MEREDITH (1828–1909)

Well done! A successful shopping trip has stocked your cupboards, fridge and freezer. A large basket of fruit; a full rack of vegetables; a shelf of cereal grains, rice and pasta; a fridge replete with fish, chicken breasts, low-fat dairy products and salad vegetables; and a full rack of spices: this sounds like a very good start. Of course, the fresh herbs, onion and garlic, and the sun-dried tomatoes (dry-packed) will help things along. And you can never have too many cans of pulses, tomatoes, pimentos and sweetcorn. The frozen peas, beans and spinach are an excellent standby.

So you're all ready to cook. Here are a few hints on doing it the healthy way.

For a start, like any job, food preparation is a lot easier with the right tools. A good set of knives is a sound investment (and with blunt ones you'll make a meal of it – eventually). You need at least two chopping boards so a separate one can be used for raw meat. Those made of soft white plastic are excellent: they won't blunt your knife and they can be washed with piping hot water or in a dishwasher. A food processor speeds up many recipes and, again, thorough cleaning is made easier if you have the luxury of a dishwasher.

The importance of scrupulous hygiene cannot be overstated. Like all family doctors, I frequently attend people with gastroenteritis, and many of these cases are avoidable. Raw meat must be treated like poison. Anything – whether a hand, a worktop or a cloth – that comes into contact with it must be properly cleaned before contamination is spread to something that will be eaten uncooked. Meat must be stored at the bottom of the fridge so that no drips can land on other food. Check the fridge temperature; it should be 4°C. Uncooked meat, even if pre-packed, should be placed immediately into a separate bag at the time of purchase to avoid contaminating other products. Assume all poultry has salmonella; if properly handled and cooked, this is no threat. If you are unfortunate enough to purchase a piece of beef contaminated with *E. coli* 0157, nothing short of the best kitchen practice will save you from disaster as so few organisms are required to cause catastrophic infection. Thorough cooking will kill bacteria in the meat, but woe betide you if the tiniest drop of uncooked meat juice ends up on your salad. (This is a good argument against buying cooked meats from someone who handles raw meat as well.)

Wash all fruits and vegetables carefully. A soft brush, such as a washing-up brush, is useful for fruit but a hard brush is good for root vegetables. Then there's no need to remove those potato skins: whether boiling, baking or roasting, they add to the flavour and nourishment.

ACTION POINTS

◆ Keep shelves stocked with fruits, vegetables, grains, pasta, pulses, etc.

◆ Use good knives and chopping boards

◆ Handle raw meat like poison

◆ Store meat at the bottom of the fridge

◆ Check that your fridge temperature is 4°C

◆ Wash fruit and vegetables carefully with a brush

You may have heard that you should chuck out the frying pan. I wouldn't – unless it's of poor quality. You'll need a good, heavy-bottomed pan, not so much to fry as to sauté – that is, to toss in the minimum of oil (*sauter* means 'to leap' in French). Or try sautéing in vegetable stock, perhaps with added wine or sherry, for a lower-fat dish. If using oil to fry or sauté, the oil must be hot enough to crisp the food quickly otherwise much more fat is taken up. You can now purchase an olive oil spray (one calorie per spray) which makes it easier to add tiny amounts of oil.

Another good way to move food quickly in a small amount of hot oil is to stir-fry in a wok. The trick is to have all the ingredients prepared and cut to similar sizes before starting and, working quickly, to add them to the hot oil – ending with those that need least time to cook.

Steaming is also an oriental method of cooking and a bamboo steamer that fits over a wok is not expensive. It's a particularly good way of cooking vegetables but can be used for rice, fish, or even chicken breasts.

If you boil vegetables, keep it short and shallow: use a short cooking time and shallow, boiling water. Put the lid on the pan, cook over high heat and serve immediately. How many children have been put off vegetables by limp and colourless specimens? Overcooking spoils nutrients. You can always use the water for stock.

- ◆ A heavy-bottomed pan is good for sautéing in very little oil and for 'dry-frying'

- ◆ To stir-fry, cut ingredients to similar sizes; move them quickly in the minimum amount of hot oil until cooked

- ◆ The microwave oven is ideal for vegetables, jacket potatoes and fish

- ◆ Vegetables are good steamed or boiled quickly in shallow water

---

A microwave oven is great for vegetables. They can be cooked in a covered serving dish and you generally need only a tablespoon or two of water – just enough to wet the bottom really. Not only is this a very convenient method, but it's also good at preserving the colour and texture of vegetables.

The microwave oven is ideal for cooking fish such as whole trout or salmon steaks. And jacket potatoes can be turned out in a fraction of the time needed in a conventional oven. It's a good idea to wrap them in foil after cooking, to keep them hot until you are ready to serve.

No kitchen is complete without a grill. Unlike frying, grilling allows fat to run away from the food. Oily fish do well under the grill; great care is needed to avoid overcooking white fish. Make sure meat is cooked right through: a fierce heat will burn the outside before the inside is cooked. A good marinade adds flavour and helps to stop the meat drying out. A charcoal barbecue is ideal for grilling – as long as you cook over hot charcoal and not in fierce flames. You don't have to opt for the traditional beefburgers and sausages; chicken kebabs and fish go down very well.

Even if you are a microwave enthusiast, you will probably do much of your roasting and baking in the main oven. Traditional recipes can often be made much healthier with a little modification.

EGGS IN PERSPECTIVE

Many recipes call for eggs. They're highly nutritious. Egg white is just protein (albumen) and water. But the yolk contains a fair amount of fat and a lot of cholesterol. An egg yolk contains about 6.5 g of fat and almost 2 g of this is saturated. (Don't forget that nutritional information gives quantities per 100 g and one egg weighs about 60 g.) The amount of cholesterol in one egg yolk is spectacular – about 230 mg. We've seen that, when it comes to controlling blood cholesterol, the fat in food is more important than the amount of cholesterol. Even so, if you are struggling to get your blood cholesterol down, one egg yolk gives you enough cholesterol for the whole day.

An egg a day is a sensible limit and you could choose to have no more than three yolks a week. You can leave egg yolk out of most recipes. Simply use two egg whites for every whole egg demanded by the recipe. An alternative is to use an 'egg replacer' (sold by health food shops). This is a powder containing no animal products; it's particularly useful for vegans and those with an allergy to eggs. In baked recipes, people aren't going to notice that you've used egg replacer instead of eggs, but you wouldn't use it to replace a fried egg, of course!

But do keep eggs in perspective. They won't bite (until well after they've hatched) and there's no need to be afraid of them (unless you suffer from egg allergy). Eating a couple of boiled eggs will give you a massive dose of cholesterol, but for most people, one whole egg a day will supply useful nutrients without raising blood cholesterol.

The Sunday roast need not be steeped in saturated fat. Remember, the rule with meat is: SLIM, TRIM and SKIM (see page 47). Roast potatoes and parsnips are excellent if prepared by tossing the par-boiled (i.e. briefly boiled) vegetables in a tiny amount of hot olive oil or rapeseed oil. Drain off the meat fat before making gravy.

When baking, remember that hard fats can often be replaced with rapeseed oil or lightly-flavoured olive oil (see page 53) or with prune purée. Many recipes call for eggs. As egg yolk has a high fat and cholesterol content, you could restrict yourself to three eggs a week. Columbus eggs supply omega-3 fat but are still full of cholesterol. To avoid egg yolk, you can simply use two egg whites for every whole egg demanded by the recipe. It is often convenient to use dried egg white, which can be bought as a powder in sachets (made by Supercook). Alternatively, 'egg replacer' can be purchased in health food shops. But, in most people, eating one whole egg a day has no significant effect on blood cholesterol levels.

Make sauces with skimmed milk and cornflour. Forget the roux. It'll taste just as good without the added fat. You can always add extra skimmed milk powder to make it more 'creamy'.

Whatever you're cooking, consider doubling the quantity and freezing some. Ready-made meals in the freezer can save you from resorting to fatty takeaways when you haven't got time to cook.

ACTION POINTS

◆ Grill instead of frying

◆ Roast vegetables in a tiny amount of hot olive or rapeseed oil

◆ Replace hard fats with rapeseed or lightly-flavoured olive oil

◆ Use prune purée instead of fat for cakes and/or puddings

◆ Eat no more than 1 whole egg a day; you can replace 1 egg with 2 whites

◆ For sauces, use skimmed milk with cornflour instead of a roux; or use quark with skimmed milk for savoury sauces

◆ Cook and freeze big batches to avoid takeaways and convenience foods

Eating in – South Asian style

'The art of cooking is simple and needs to be so.'

DAS SREEDHARAN,
The New Tastes of India

If you are South Asian (having roots in India, Bangladesh, Pakistan or Sri Lanka), the information in this book is especially relevant to you. The statistics for heart disease in South Asians are shocking. In the UK, the rate of premature death (i.e. before the age of 75) from heart disease is about 50% higher for South Asians than for white people. This epidemic affects both men and women, and risk factors for heart disease can even be found in South Asian children.

The explanation for this has a great deal to do with the metabolic syndrome (see page 313), which is so common in South Asians. And the answer to it is to take enough exercise (see Chapter 20) and eat a protective diet; an unhealthy diet, full of fat and sugar, merely 'feeds' the metabolic syndrome and accelerates the decline into diabetes and heart disease.

Some simple changes to traditional methods of cooking can make all the difference. Here are a few tips.

- Don't use ghee, coconut oil, coconut cream or butter for cooking.

- Choose olive oil or rapeseed oil and measure it instead of pouring it directly into the pan; one tablespoon of oil is usually enough to make curry for four to six people, although it will seem too little if you're in the habit of using more; you'll soon adjust.

- Avoid deep frying. Foods such as chips, bajhias, sev, chevra/chevda, and samosas take up huge quantities of fat. Items like samosas can simply be brushed with a little oil and baked or grilled.

- Don't re-use cooking oils as some of the unsaturated fats become saturated.

- There is no need to add oil or ghee to chapati dough.

- Some dishes such as keema and dhal can be made very successfully without any added fat or oil.

- Avoid adding butter to cooked dhals and vegetables.

- Use a little water to replace some of the oil when cooking subjhis with more absorbent vegetables like methi (fenugreek), brinjals (aubergines) and karela (a bitter gourd).

- Choose lean meat and trim off all visible fat. If you use red meat such as beef, pork, lamb or mutton, keep to small portions.

- Use lots of high-fibre foods such as fruit, vegetables, dhals, chickpeas, beans (e.g. soya, red kidney and blackeye beans) and oatbran. Select wholegrain versions of chapati, bread and rice.

- Avoid full-fat dairy products and use very low-fat yoghurt, skimmed milk and cottage cheese. You can produce home-made yoghurt from skimmed milk. Remember that reduced-fat cheeses may still be very high-fat foods.

- Gradually reduce added salt, allowing all members of the family to adjust their palates. If you think a little salt is essential, use LoSalt or Solo.

- Avoid sweets such as jalebi and halva which are full of fat and sugar. A plate of chopped fresh fruit makes a refreshing end to a meal!

- ◆ High rates of heart disease among South Asians living in the West are linked with the metabolic syndrome

- ◆ Regular exercise and simple changes in cooking methods can help to protect against diabetes and heart disease

- ◆ Cutting down fat (especially saturated), sugar and salt can make a huge difference to health without spoiling your food

Eating out

**'The best number for a dinner party is two –
myself and a damn good head waiter.'**

NUBAR GULBENKIAN,
quoted in the *Observer*, 1965

For most of us, eating out with friends is a great social pleasure. With good food and good company you can't go wrong. But restaurant food is loaded with fat, isn't it? How can you eat out without damaging your coronary arteries? Watching your friends tuck into steak and chips while you pick at your lettuce and cucumber is not such a pleasure.

Certainly some restaurants have very little to offer the health-conscious customer. Traditional French establishments use lots of butter and cream; burger bars serving nothing but grease and chips are no help either. Study the menu before selecting your restaurant. There are plenty that offer enough variety to meet your needs.

While awaiting your meal, eat bread, if it is offered, but without the butter or spread.

You will want to choose a starter such as melon or other fruit or fruit juice. Seafood is fine if it isn't swimming in a high-fat sauce (although if it is swimming at least you know it's fresh). Perhaps you could have the sauce served separately and use it very sparingly. A deep-fried appetiser will get you off to a fatty start.

For the main course you could select grilled fish, chicken or turkey. These can be absolutely delicious if they've been skilfully seasoned, marinated and char-grilled. Beware any dishes covered with sauce because sauces in restaurants usually have a very high fat content – even though it's quite possible to make lovely low-fat sauces.

At a carvery you might choose lean turkey breast. Have plenty of vegetables but avoid those smothered in butter or cheese sauce. Go easy on the gravy.

It's a mistake to assume that vegetarian dishes are necessarily low in fat. They could even be made with palm oil or coconut oil, which would bump up the saturated fatty acid content.

Of course, you can always ask about the ingredients of a dish. Don't be shy. You're paying. If the waiter or waitress doesn't know, ask to see the manager or the chef. There's no reason why you shouldn't request simple changes such as having your potatoes sautéed in olive oil instead of butter. If the staff can't cope with such requests, it doesn't say much for the restaurant.

Boiled new potatoes or jacket potato would be wise choices in preference to sautéed potatoes, roast potatoes or chips. You won't want to top your jacket potato with sour cream or butter, but you could ask for some chutney or pickle instead.

You can never be quite sure what's in a creamy salad dressing; at least with vinegar and a little olive oil you know what you're getting.

The sweet trolley usually confronts you with cheesecakes, gateaux, pastries and lashings of cream. Wise options may be limited to fresh fruit, fruit salad or sorbet.

No doubt many different parts of the world are represented by the restaurants in your local town. Although the native cuisine of some Mediterranean and oriental countries is ideal, you cannot rely on the anglicised version being equally healthy. Again, you should ask how a dish has been prepared and which oil has been used.

From the orient, Chinese restaurants are the most familiar but Japanese and Thai restaurants are also worth exploring. Dishes that are stir-fried in a small amount of hot oil don't take up too much fat; deep-fried items, such as spring rolls, will generally take up more. Enjoy the variety of vegetables and have plenty of plain rice. Chicken and seafood are good choices; lamb and pork will be higher in fat. Unfortunately, Peking Duck is a very high-fat dish.

There's nothing quite like a curry. Sadly, much Indian cuisine involves the use of ghee (clarified butter) which has a very high saturated fat content. We have a local Indian restaurant that guarantees to use rapeseed oil – or to leave the oil out altogether if you prefer. In general, dishes without a sauce will be lower in fat. For example, chicken tikka would be less fatty than chicken tikka masala. At least the sauce in chicken jalfrezi is based on tomatoes and it should be a reasonable choice. It's better to have enough rice and naan bread than to fill up with lots of high-fat dishes, but remember that naan bread contains about six times as much fat as ordinary brown or white bread. Enjoy side dishes such as raita (cucumber, yoghurt and spices).

Restaurants of a Mediterranean tradition, such as Greek and Spanish, usually have something acceptable on the menu, whether it's chicken kebab or grilled fish. Beware the pasta sauces in Italian restaurants: they are usually loaded with fat. Some pizza houses have excellent salad bars these days – enticing rows of wholesome ingredients. If you've paid for unlimited visits, you'll sample most of them. If it's one visit only, the bowl is too small. The secret here is to part-fill the bowl and then arrange cucumber slices vertically around the rim, secured with a ring of rice. The extra height greatly increases the capacity of the bowl. Watch the croutons (which are deep fried), salads in mayonnaise (e.g. coleslaw, vegetable salad) and oily dressings. Some outlets do serve fat-free or yoghurt-based dressings.

Eating out gives you far less control over your diet than eating in. If this is something you only do occasionally, the most important rule is this: relax and enjoy it!

ACTION POINTS

When eating out:

◆ Avoid restaurants with unsuitable menus

◆ Eat bread without butter or spread

◆ Select fruit, fruit juice or seafood (not covered in sauce) for starters

◆ Order grilled fish, chicken or turkey (without skin)

◆ Avoid sauces (or have them served separately and use very little)

◆ Choose boiled or jacket potatoes; or specify sauté in olive oil

◆ Request a low-fat topping for jacket potatoes (e.g. chutney or pickle) and avoid butter/sour cream

◆ Ask about salt and fat used; request olive oil rather than butter

Chapter 15

Foreign food

Nobody wants a heart attack, but eating a typical British diet is a good way to go about having one. It wasn't always so. The vast increase in heart disease throughout the UK over the past century has gone hand in hand with a huge change in our diet. Responding to this, a Welsh researcher conducted an odd experiment, which was discussed in the *British Medical Journal* in 1979.

He reconstructed a typical Welsh labourer's diet, as recorded in 1863, consisting mainly of potatoes, oatmeal and wholemeal bread. There was also a little cheese and milk but this diet was far lower in fat and higher in carbohydrate than a diet based on the Department of Health's current recommendations. The researchers didn't eat this diet themselves. They converted it into pellets, which they fed to a group of rats. An identical group of rats was fed pellets made from a contemporary Welsh diet. Rats on the 1863 diet lived far longer than rats on the modern diet.

I know you're not a rat. And I'm sure you are not attracted to the diet of a nineteenth-century Welsh labourer. However, there is a great deal for us to learn from interesting, contemporary diets around the world that are not linked with coronary heart disease. Nations with Northern European traditions have high cholesterols and high rates of heart disease, while people of Southern Europe, rural Africa and the Orient have low cholesterols and low rates of heart disease. Many of the low-risk people are eating delicious diets.

The Japanese diet

'You do not sew with a fork, and I see no reason why you should eat with knitting needles.'

MISS PIGGY

The Japanese have the lowest average cholesterol level and the lowest rates of heart disease in the developed world. Perhaps this is a genetic characteristic of Japanese people? Not so. The Japanese who settled in San Francisco adopted the American diet. As their saturated fat intake rose to mirror that of the Californians, so did their blood cholesterol levels and rates of heart disease. On the other hand, the Japanese who moved only as far as Hawaii took on a diet that was somewhere between the Japanese and American diets with an intermediate saturated fat intake. They developed more heart disease than the Japanese who had stayed in Japan, but not as much as the mainland Americans. Perhaps the Japanese would agree with Fred Allen's alleged remark: 'California is a great place – if you happen to be an orange'.

Japanese cuisine features:

- plenty of cereals (especially rice);

- fresh fruit and vegetables (which are not overcooked);

- lots of fish;

- soya beans including tofu (soya bean curd);

- very little red meat or saturated fat.

No doubt all these features play a part in reducing Japanese rates of heart disease. Evidence for the role of soya protein in lowering cholesterol and protecting arteries has been building up in recent years. The interesting thing is that this diet protects them from heart disease even though smoking and raised blood pressure are common in Japan. The one thing that stands out as being unsatisfactory in the Japanese diet is its high salt content. Since making a big reduction in their sodium intake, the Japanese have seen the prevalence of raised blood pressure decline dramatically and the figures for heart disease have become even lower!

Sadly, many young Japanese are now picking up some Western eating habits and we may see rising levels of heart disease as they reach middle age.

The least we can do is to return the compliment and pick up some oriental eating habits.

The Mediterranean diet

'In Rome people spend most of their time having lunch.
And they do it very well – Rome is unquestionably
the lunch capital of the world.'

FRAN LEBOWITZ, *Metropolitan Life*, 1978

The people of Mediterranean countries such as Italy and Greece suffer much less heart disease than Northern Europeans. This may well have something to do with the olive oil that plays such an important part in their cuisine. Olive oil is a rich source of the mono-unsaturated fatty acid, oleic acid. We know that using olive oil instead of more saturated fats helps to lower the harmful LDL-cholesterol without reducing the level of protective HDL-cholesterol. Olive oil also provides antioxidants.

But it must be remembered that there are lots of other good things about the diet of Mediterranean countries apart from olive oil. Compared with a typical British diet, there is much greater emphasis on fruit and vegetables; evidence for their vital role in maintaining health has mounted. Seafood is given due prominence and use of garlic is the norm.

The Lyon Diet Heart Study was published in the *The Lancet* in 1994. (This is the correct spelling and it was nothing to do with eating, or being eaten by, big cats.) It was a controlled trial involving people who had already had one heart attack.

The control group was given routine advice about a 'prudent diet', while the experimental group was put on a Mediterranean diet that was rich in oleic acid and alpha-linolenic acid (related to fish oils). They were advised to eat more bread, fruit, root vegetables, green vegetables and fish, but less meat – beef, lamb and pork being replaced by poultry. A special margarine based on rapeseed oil was supplied free to those in the experimental group and their families. They were allowed to use olive oil or rapeseed oil, but no other fats, for cooking and dressing salads. A moderate amount of wine was permitted with meals.

In just 27 months, there was a marked reduction in heart attacks among those on the Mediterranean diet.

'The French paradox'

'France is the largest country in Europe,
a great boon for drunks, who need room to fall . . .'

ALAN COREN, *The Sanity Inspector*, 1974

The French appear to get off lightly. They put the pâté and profiteroles on our menus but seem to have low rates of heart disease themselves. This disparity between their saturated fat intake and their statistics for coronary deaths is known as 'the French paradox'. (See also Chapter 11.)

Red wine has largely been given the credit for this. Certainly the French drink a lot of it – too much, in fact. No doubt it reduces their level of coronary heart disease but they pay for this with higher rates of liver cirrhosis, cancer of the mouth and gullet, suicide and violent death.

Apart from alcohol, there are other factors in the French diet that would be expected to lower the risk of heart disease, including the generous use of fruit, vegetables, onions and garlic and the tradition of eating plenty of unbuttered bread with meals. Also, France is a big place and in parts the diet is more Mediterranean with less saturated fat and more olive oil.

Bon appetit!

◆ Oriental, Southern European, and rural African diets are linked with low rates of heart disease

◆ The Japanese diet is high in cereals (rice), vegetables, soya and fish but low in red meat and saturated fat

◆ Mediterranean cuisine includes fruit and vegetables, bread, pasta, fish, olive oil, garlic, wine

◆ Rapeseed oil and nuts (e.g. walnuts) supply alpha-linolenic acid which is related to fish oil and helps to protect against heart disease

◆ There's more to the French paradox than red wine

Chapter 16

Feeding children

'Maybe you know why a child can reject a hot dog
with mustard served on a soft bun at home,
yet eat six of them two hours later at fifty cents each.'

ERMA BOMBECK,
If Life is a Bowl of Cherries –
What am I doing in the Pits? **1978**

We all want our children to get off to a good start but how much of
the dietary advice in this book is relevant to young children? This
chapter explains easy ways to introduce healthy eating to children, so
that they learn to make heart-safe choices.

Feeding children can be a source of anxiety and frustration. If you
never have to do it, you may want to skip this chapter.

An early start

Research suggests that there is a link between the size of a baby at
birth, and death of the adult from heart disease or stroke in later life.
Professor Barker and his team followed the fortunes of 1586 men who
were born in a Sheffield maternity hospital between 1907 and 1924.
They found that the bigger the baby (birth weight, head circumference
and weight/length[3]) the lower the death rate.

The weight of an infant at the age of one year is an even better
guide to his risk of coronary heart disease in adult life. Professor
Barker's team published findings on about 8000 men who were born
before 1931 in Hertfordshire. The results were striking. The death rate
from coronary heart disease was three times higher among those who
had weighed only 17 pounds at one year than among those who had
weighed 28 pounds. A study on women published in the *British
Medical Journal* in 2005 found that the risk of heart disease was highest in the overweight women who had been small at birth.

In fact, the risk of having high blood pressure, diabetes or heart disease as an adult is increased by being too small at birth and in the first two years of life – but also by gaining too much fat after the age of two. Fat children often become fat adults.

So it's never too early to start considering the child's adult health (before conception is ideal) but misguided attempts to impose a healthy diet on young children can be very damaging.

◆ It's never too early to bother about healthy eating

◆ Nutrition, even before birth, can affect heart health in adult life

◆ Breast milk is the ideal food in the first few months

◆ Baby cereal fortified with iron is helpful from 4 months

◆ Giving fruit with a meal helps absorption of iron

Feeding an infant – the first two years

Infants are growing rapidly. They are not miniature adults. Unlike older children and adults, they need to take in about 50% of their energy as fat. Breast milk is the ideal food in the first few months of life. Either breast milk or infant formula should be continued during the first year but neither can supply all the nutritional needs of a baby in the second six months of life. Weaning foods add important nutrients and introduce a wide variety of tastes and textures. Food is fun (but it doesn't always seem that way when you find it behind a radiator several months later).

The commonest nutritional problem in infancy (in the developed world) is iron deficiency anaemia, which affects about 12% of 1- and 2-year-old children. It is even commoner in some Asian groups. We know that anaemia in early childhood can interfere with mental development so it is very important to avoid it. Although breast milk does not have a high iron content, the iron that is present is easily absorbed and utilised by the infant; it is helpful to introduce a baby cereal fortified with iron from about four months of age. Cows' milk is a poor source of iron and is unsuitable as a drink in the first year. Indeed, cows' milk, tea and wholemeal cereal foods can reduce the absorption of iron from food. The iron in red meat and offal such as liver is in a form (called 'haem iron') which is better absorbed than iron from plant sources. Vitamin C increases iron absorption, so giving fruit with a meal will help. Infant formula milks and certain foods (such as cereals and white bread) are fortified with iron.

Don't overdo the wholemeal and high-fibre foods at this age. Applying adult guidelines to infants is the origin of so-called 'muesli belt malnutrition'. Bulking out a meal with plenty of high-fibre foods is very helpful for adults, but infants have small stomachs and big energy requirements. They need a higher proportion of energy-dense foods or they can feel full before taking in enough calories.

Reduced-fat milk and low-fat dairy products are not suitable for children under two years.

Salt intake should be restricted, just as in adults, by choosing low-salt foods and by avoiding the addition of salt during food preparation.

The main reason why nuts are not recommended at this age is that they can cause choking. There is also concern that nut allergies, which can be life-threatening, are on the increase. It is possible that avoiding exposure to nut products during the first three years reduces the risk of developing this sensitivity.

Vitamin drops (such as those containing vitamins A, D, and C, which may be available from your health visitor) are a good idea from 6 months to 5 years. They are not a substitute for a balanced and varied diet.

ACTION POINTS

- Breast feed for as long as you can, but start solids by six months

- Don't give cows' milk as a drink in the first year

- Don't give low-fat dairy products to the under 2s

- Choose from the 4 important food groups to get the best balance you can

From two to five years

Changing from an infant into a schoolchild isn't easy: it presents a host of developmental challenges; it has its ups and its downs – not only emotionally, but also nutritionally. It is futile to try to impose any rigid dietary dogma on the pre-school child, and adult guidelines are still inappropriate at this age.

Semi-skimmed milk can be introduced as a drink from the age of two years. I didn't do this with my children and, on current evidence, I can't see a lot of point in most cases. One argument for semi-skimmed milk is that it is a step towards the grown-up diet of the schoolchild for, one way or another, this adaptation should be made by the age of five.

She hardly eats a thing!

'How to eat like a child.
Spinach: divide into little piles. Rearrange again into new piles.
After five or six maneuvers, sit back and say you are full.'

***

DELIA EPHRON, *New York Times*, 1983

You are bound to be anxious when your child appears to be starving or, at least, heading for severe nutritional deficiency. This is an extremely common anxiety in parents of pre-school children. Even the child who normally tucks in will lose his appetite for a few days with a bad cold. Toddlers rapidly sense their parents' concern and food becomes a powerful weapon in the battle for independence.

In the great majority of cases, plotting the height and weight on a chart confirms a completely normal growth pattern. Parents are sometimes puzzled that their child's negligible intake is enough to sustain normal growth. An interesting experiment was published by Birch and colleagues in the *New England Journal of Medicine* in 1991. They presented 15 pre-school children with a range of familiar foods and the children were allowed to have whatever they liked for a meal or snack. Their calorie intake varied greatly from meal to meal but the daily intake of each child remained fairly constant. The message is: healthy children don't starve themselves; they regulate intake to meet their nutritional needs.

A toddler is quick to realise that it doesn't much matter about eating at mealtimes if an anxious mother is only too glad to supply milk, biscuits or crisps to 'get something into him' (or her) at any other time of day. On the other hand, if a child discovers that no amount of lying on the floor and screaming will procure any nourishment until the appointed hour, mealtimes will soon be taken more seriously. Either way, the child will meet his or her nutritional needs.

This does not mean that, if you establish regular mealtimes, your child will always clear the plate! A child's requirements vary and you might have overloaded the plate. There will be passing food fads. The important thing is to relax in the knowledge that your child's appetite is a good guide to his needs. When you're hungry, eating is fun. It's important not to turn it into a deadly task. Once you are relaxed enough to show no concern about the unfinished meal, children work out that it's their loss, and not yours, if they don't eat when food is available.

Nor does establishing a routine imply three square meals a day. It is a very good thing for the family to sit down together for main meals whenever possible but small children have small stomachs and may need snacks. Crisps and biscuits are not the only possible snacks: some children enjoy sugarsnap peas or raw carrot or bread sticks.

While toddlers are very good at getting what they need as long as food is available, it is possible for parents to jeopardise their child's nutrition by restricting foods that are considered to be unhealthy or too fatty.

Aim to give your child something from each of the first four main food groups:

- Cereals and starchy foods: bread, breakfast cereals, rice, pasta, potatoes;

- Fruit and vegetables: fresh, frozen or canned are all excellent. Dried fruits (e.g. raisins);

- Milk and dairy products: milk, yoghurt, cheese;

- 'Meat' or high-protein group: meat, fish, poultry, pulses (peas, beans, lentils), eggs.

Chips, baked beans and banana custard (made with real banana) might not have been your first choice but you've covered the four important food groups.

Young children don't demand a starter, a savoury course and a sweet. Small pieces of fruit, such as satsuma (seedless), banana, apple, pear or kiwi fruit, often slip down better nestling between pieces of meat, cheese or bread.

Children are often put off by the texture of food as much as the taste. Stewed fruit or vegetable purée (which can be added to other foods) will often go down better than lumps, and flaked fish can be smuggled in mashed potato.

You want your child to meet a wide range of tastes and textures but a new food is best introduced, just a little at first, alongside an old friend. Be prepared for rejection and conceal your disappointment; try again after a decent interval (several weeks).

When children are involved in choosing and preparing food, they are more likely to want to eat it. Another useful tip is to find out which of your child's playmates have good appetites, especially for foods your child rejects, and invite them round for meals. Example can be inspiring. Be less hospitable to the fussy ones.

Remember: food fads, awkwardness and manipulative behaviour are very common in pre-school children whereas failure to thrive is not. Of course, if there is any doubt about your child's growth or development you should discuss it with your health visitor or doctor.

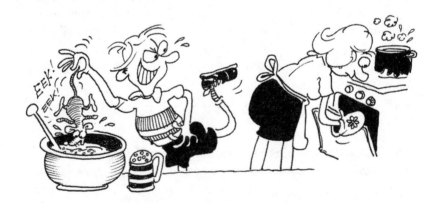

**When children are involved in the preparation of food,
they are more likely to eat it.**

◆ When food is available, healthy children make sure they get enough

◆ Food is fun! Don't turn eating into a deadly task

◆ Raw vegetables such as sugarsnap peas and carrot sticks make good snacks

◆ When children help to choose and/or prepare food, they're more likely to eat it

From five years

When a child reaches five, a diet based on the Department of Health's recommended averages for the general population is suitable – 35% of the calories coming from fat and 10% of them from saturated fat.

Ideally, a family with children of school age will sit at the table together, sharing a menu based on these guidelines. The recommended diet is significantly lower in fat than the current UK average diet. Achieving it will mean selecting some of the lower-fat options detailed in this book. A good variety of foods should be taken from each of the four main food groups, being sure to include enough fruit and vegetables as well as plenty of cereal and starchy foods.

From the age of five, fully skimmed milk can be used, not only in food but also as a drink. Of course, if you simply switch from whole milk one day to fully skimmed the next, we can predict the reaction. When the time came for our daughters to make the change, we started adding skimmed milk to their whole milk (out of their view, of course) – gradually increasing the proportion of skimmed milk. They were soon drinking fully skimmed milk quite happily.

For many adults, especially those at high risk of coronary heart disease, I would recommend a more radical diet than one based on the Government's targets for population averages (see Chapter 17). For children, who need plenty of energy for growth and to fuel the energetic lifestyle that should be encouraged, this moderate diet is sensible. It's still worth pointing out that the rapeseed oil in home-made flapjack is just as good at giving a child energy as the hydrogenated vegetable oil in a chocolate bar.

Why start so young?

If coronary heart disease is an adult problem, why bother about it in childhood?

Well, leaving aside the fact that eating well brings a whole range of health benefits apart from protecting the heart, it must be remembered that the foundations of coronary heart disease are laid in childhood.

Professor Barker's work suggests that nutritional factors in the womb and in infancy can influence adult heart disease. Other work has shown that risk factors for heart disease, such as raised cholesterol, can often be tracked from around two years of age into adult life. About 90% of the young adults with a cholesterol level of 6.2 mmol/l or above could probably be identified in childhood – either by the presence of obesity or by a raised cholesterol level (although the range is different in childhood).

Not only this, but the process of artery-clogging can actually begin in childhood! The formation of fatty plaques of atheroma in arteries begins with fatty streaks on the inside of the artery walls. Fatty streaks occur in tiny children. These streaks do not always go on to form plaques and in some cases they will be temporary. In some children, real artery-clogging plaques of atheroma appear around the time of puberty.

Isn't it worth stopping this process before it becomes established in the young adult?

Education, too, must be considered. Why should you suddenly start eating well at the age of 21 if you have never learnt how? You wouldn't leave piano playing or speaking French until then. You might be surprised at the healthy choices children can make when given the right opportunities from an early age.

◆ Adult guidelines (including fully skimmed milk) apply from age 5

◆ Children need energy-dense foods, but rapeseed oil is better than hydrogenated vegetable oil

◆ Clogging up of arteries starts in childhood!

Chapter 17

Moderation in all things?

'Moderation is a fatal thing. Nothing succeeds like excess.'

OSCAR WILDE, *A Woman of No Importance*, **1893**

Many books and articles on the subject of healthy eating will tell you that moderation is the key. At the same time, medical journals have frequently published articles lamenting the fact that giving people dietary advice has had very little impact on their raised cholesterol levels. I can tell you from my years of clinical experience that moderation is indeed the key – the key to failure in many cases.

Charts similar to that shown in Table 19 are often given out by practice nurses and doctors when they are advising people how to change their diets to lower cholesterol levels. You may have been given one yourself. These charts can be very useful. They tell you which things you can eat and drink regularly and which things to avoid altogether. The middle column shows which things you can eat and drink in moderation. Moderation is the downfall of many.

I recall a patient of mine called John. John was disappointed that after changing his diet for three months his cholesterol level had hardly altered. I asked him to keep a record of everything he ate and drank for one week. There was the roast lamb with roast potatoes and gravy, but he explained that he would only have roast lunch once a week, on a Sunday. His wife prepared this in the traditional way, using lard for the potatoes and meat fat for the gravy, but it was only once a week. Then there was the fish and chips (from the local shop) but that was only once a week, on a Wednesday, after his late shift. And by the time we had added up all the exceptions to his otherwise healthy diet, there wasn't a lot of room left for really helpful foods.

Table 19 Extract from a chart used by some advisers

Eat regularly	Eat in moderation	Avoid
	DAIRY FOODS	
Skimmed milk, low-fat yoghurt, skimmed milk soft cheese, cottage cheese, low-fat fromage frais	Semi-skimmed milk, medium-fat cheeses (e.g. Brie, Edam), reduced-fat cheeses, cheese spreads	Whole milk, cream, full-fat yoghurt, full-fat cheese (e.g. cheddar, Stilton), imitation cream
	MEAT	
Chicken, turkey (skinless), veal, rabbit, game, meat substitutes (e.g. Quorn, soya)	Beef, pork, lamb, ham, gammon (visible fat removed), very lean minced meat, duck (skinless), grilled lean bacon, liver, kidney, low-fat pâté	Sausages, pâté, salami, streaky bacon, corned beef, luncheon meats, burgers, meat pies, sausage rolls, goose

If you eat enough different foods that are moderately bad for you in moderation, there won't be much space on your menu for foods that are really good for you. Such a diet has very little impact on cholesterol levels or the risk of heart disease.

Some years ago, my own cholesterol level was over 7 mmol/l. I changed my diet and my cholesterol has been 5 mmol/l or below ever since; it's come down from a high reading to well below the population average (see Chapter 19). My 30% drop in cholesterol level amounts to a reduction in the risk of coronary heart disease by at least 60%! (A 2% reduction in risk for every 1% drop in cholesterol is a conservative estimate; in many cases, a risk reduction of 3% would be nearer the mark.)

I have found it is far easier simply to exclude unhelpful foods from my routine diet than to try eating them in moderation. Cheese is an example: I don't think about it because I'm too busy eating other things instead. And have you tried eating chocolate in moderation? Once you've started, it's difficult to stop. But if I went to a dinner party, which is something I do only occasionally, I would have no compunction about tucking into a piece of Camembert and some chocolate mints; it wouldn't matter at all because my routine diet is sound. After all, if you make a rule, you need the odd exception to prove it. Now if your social life is far more exciting than mine, and you're always off to dinner parties, you would need to take a different view.

Do you remember that advertisement for an anti-dandruff shampoo? Someone says to the shampoo user 'I didn't know you had dandruff'. The reply, of course, is 'I don't'. And when someone, seeing that I am careful about my diet, says to me, 'I didn't know you had a cholesterol problem', my reply, of course, is 'I don't'.

Perhaps you have been told that your cholesterol is normal and you are thinking that all this discussion about eating a better diet doesn't concern you. It may be that you haven't had your cholesterol measured yet; when you do, Chapter 19 will help you to interpret the result. One of the most unhelpful things that health professionals can do is to give people the impression that because their cholesterol level is 'normal' they needn't bother about their diet! That's nonsense. If you've come away with this idea, your visit to the 'health promotion clinic' may have increased your risk instead of reducing it.

The average cholesterol level in our population is too high and lots of people have heart attacks with average and even below average cholesterols.

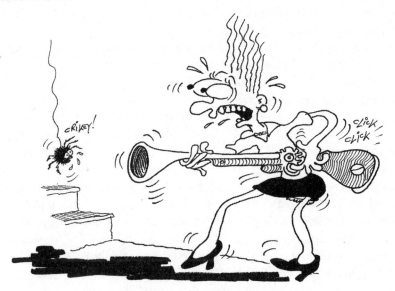

Nothing succeeds like excess.

◆ Advice about diet often fails to lower cholesterol

◆ Moderation is the downfall of many

◆ Excluding unhelpful foods from your routine diet is easier than trying to eat them in moderation

◆ If your cholesterol is 'normal', healthy eating is still essential

If you think about earlier chapters in this book, you will realise that a good diet protects your heart and arteries in lots of ways that have nothing to do with lowering cholesterol. Reducing sodium intake helps to control blood pressure; cutting down saturated fat reduces thrombosis risk; fish oils make platelets less 'sticky'; and antioxidants in fruit and vegetables help to prevent fatty deposits forming in arteries. You need all this protection even if your cholesterol reading was 'normal'.

At the other end of the scale, there are people who have an inherited disorder of cholesterol metabolism resulting in a very raised cholesterol that cannot be brought down to normal by diet. They may need drug treatment, but, even if drugs control their cholesterol, a healthy diet is still vital to protect their heart and arteries in other ways.

Apart from avoiding heart disease, the diet recommended in this book reduces the risk of cancer as well.

What about the idea that giving people dietary advice doesn't make much difference to their cholesterol levels? It's often true. And why? In most cases it's because only moderate changes have been made to a basically unhealthy diet. The quality of dietary advice is often poor. People come away from it confused and poorly motivated. To give effective dietary education is very time-consuming. Doctors and nurses may conclude that their patient's raised cholesterol is 'metabolically resistant' – in other words, that it will not respond to a change in diet – when the real problem is that the diet hasn't changed enough. Certainly, as I have said, there are cases of metabolic resistance, but these are less common than the resistance of people to dietary change.

How do I know this? Studies carried out in metabolic wards or laboratories – where changes in diet are carefully controlled – show that big reductions in cholesterol levels can normally be achieved if the diet is altered enough.

Can this be achieved outside the laboratory? Yes. The Lifestyle Heart Trial published in *The Lancet* in 1990 was a properly constructed controlled trial on 48 people with coronary heart disease. The narrowing of their coronary arteries was carefully measured by a special investigation known as coronary angiography. Each person was then randomly allocated to either the experimental group or the control group. The 28 people in the experimental group were given a lifestyle programme that involved: a very low-fat vegetarian diet; help with giving up smoking; stress management and moderate exercise. The 20 people in the control group were given routine care. Those in the experimental group changed their diet so much that, after one year, their fat intake had dropped from 31.5% of total calories to just 6.8%. There was no significant change in the diet of the control group. Cholesterol levels fell significantly in the experimental group, but not in the control group.

After one year on the programme, all the people had their coronary arteries re-examined by angiography. The results were striking. In the control group receiving routine care, the coronary arteries had become narrower – the heart disease had progressed. This progression of heart disease had been prevented in the experimental group. Not only that, their coronary arteries were actually wider than they had been at the start of the experiment – their heart disease had gone into reverse!

And let's debunk the myth, once and for all, that a really healthy low-fat diet is boring, limited and unappetising. It may be radically different from the average British diet, but it can be more varied and interesting. Many people are stuck in a rut with their diet and don't know how to get out of it. They haven't begun to explore the range of cereal grains, pastas, fruits and vegetables, low-fat dairy products, pulses and fish available to them. Tastes vary but the choice is so wide that everyone can be satisfied without compromising the quality of the diet.

If you are attached to traditional British cuisine, most recipes can be adapted to use more desirable oils and low-fat cooking methods. My patient, John, could have continued his Sunday roast and his fish and chips with impunity if they had been prepared in the right way. Those who are fortunate enough not to have any problem keeping their weight down can be less stingy with the olive oil or rapeseed oil (or even sunflower, safflower, soya or sesame seed oils). Don't overdo it; high-fat diets influence clotting factors, increasing the risk of thrombosis.

The information in this book will allow you to discover for yourself that meals containing very little fat can be every bit as delicious and satisfying as fatty ones. You may have already been advised by your doctor or practice nurse to adopt a low-fat diet and found it difficult to make the change. It would be impossible for a health professional to convey to you all the information contained in these pages. In this way the book can complement the efforts of your health advisers.

'The trouble with facts is that there are so many of them.'
***

SAMUEL MCCHORD CROTHERS,
The Gentle Reader

What's the point in changing my diet and lifestyle, you may ask, when I don't know whether my risk of getting heart disease is high or not? Perhaps I will live to 99 and die of cancer with a healthy heart. True, and Chapter 25 will help you to assess your risk. Whether the risk appears to be high or low, anyone living in a country where heart disease is epidemic would do well to reduce his or her risk. In any case the lifestyle that protects against heart disease also protects against cancer.

Now I have something very important to explain to you. We saw in Chapter 5 that the 1994 COMA report recommended that no more than 35% of calories should come from fat. The Government's expert committee was not making recommendations for the individual but for the population average. This is frequently misunderstood.

What's more, the committee set this target for the population – to reduce its fat intake from an average 40% of calories to 35% – because it was realistic and **not** because they believed it would result in the lowest possible risk.

In fact, I can reveal to you that some experts would have preferred a target of 20%! You may find that hard to believe, but it's true. The 1994 committee recognised that'. . . levels less than 10% have been achieved in some circumstances with evidence of benefit'. My advice is to reduce radically your intake of saturated and trans fats, while making sure you get some friendly fats from nuts, seeds and oily fish.

The fact is that the committee's moderate target of 35% was a political compromise. It was reckoned that people weren't ready to make a bigger change. Even more to the point: the food industry just wouldn't stomach it.

That's the startling truth behind the recommendations of the 1994 COMA report. And yet I come across health professionals who have picked up the idea that COMA recommendations for the population average are the ideal target for an individual person!

If your cholesterol has been measured and found to be high, you may need to make much bigger changes than this to bring it down to the ideal level.

If you have never had your cholesterol checked, consider arranging this through your doctor as part of an overall risk assessment (see Chapter 19).

Someone with a very low risk of heart disease would be well advised to maintain a healthy diet and lifestyle but can afford to relax: no drastic changes are needed. For those at high risk, moderation may be fatal.

Mind you, many people who are at high risk – especially those who have already developed heart disease – will, quite rightly, be offered drugs to control their cholesterol level. There is good evidence now that this can improve survival. The tragedy is that many people could avoid the need for lifelong treatment with cholesterol-lowering drugs if only they would change their diet substantially. But no. They scratch the surface. They make moderate adjustments. Their intake of saturated fat remains far higher – and their consumption of fruit, vegetables, starch, fibre and fish far lower – than that of many populations around the world that are not plagued by heart disease.

I can hear the voices of my critics saying that it's quite unreasonable and unrealistic of me to expect people to make radical changes to their diet. But it's not. Many have done it. I'm not actually asking you to adopt the diet of a Japanese fisherman. His tastes and preferences may be quite different from yours. With enough information, you, like many others, can discover that radically improving your diet need not mean deprivation; the great variety of helpful foods means you can satisfy all your needs without jeopardising your health. And with the right know-how, many of your family's favourite recipes can be adapted to slash the saturated fat but not the flavour. That's the purpose of this book: to give you the information and the know-how.

Current nutritional wisdom holds that there is no such thing as a 'good food' or a 'bad food' or a 'healthy food' or an 'unhealthy food' but there are good and bad diets because it's all a question of balance. OK, but I put it to you that foods with a high content of saturated or trans fatty acids are certainly very unhelpful to someone who is trying to reduce his heart disease risk – however unfashionable it may be to label them as 'unhealthy'.

◆ Big changes in diet and lifestyle can reverse heart disease!

◆ A radically different diet could be more interesting than the one you're eating now

◆ Modifying traditional recipes can make them much 'healthier'

◆ The COMA report recommended averages for the population

◆ Some people need to make much bigger changes than COMA advised

But we all need some fat, don't we?

Yes, some fat is essential – but not saturated fat. None of the saturated fatty acids is essential; we can make them for ourselves. Even if they were essential, you wouldn't have to worry: you can't avoid them altogether. Even olive oil is about 14% saturates. My advice is to avoid as much saturated fat as you can.

Surely there are dangers in making radical dietary changes?

Yes, just as there are dangers in continuing an unhealthy diet, making inappropriate changes can be damaging. I have argued that for those at high risk of heart disease on poor diets, moderate changes are inadequate, but, although moderation is no answer, balance is essential. Never forget the five food groups (see Chapter 13). The radical change required means redressing the balance; it means enjoying enough of the helpful foods as well as avoiding unhelpful ones.

It is just possible that you are losing more weight than you want to on a very low-fat diet, especially if you are young, slim and active. (Others wish they had your problem.) As well as monstrous portions of starchy foods (like bread, rice, pasta and potatoes) and enough low-fat, high-protein foods (such as turkey breast, skimmed milk and pulses) perhaps you should eat a little more fat. I'm not suggesting a high-fat diet as that would raise the risk of thrombosis, but there's no reason to stay on a **very** low-fat diet if you can't maintain your weight. Have a few almonds, hazelnuts and walnuts; use avocados if you enjoy them; dress your salads with olive oil; feast on oily fish from sardines to salmon; treat yourself to home-baked cakes and biscuits made with rapeseed oil. Enjoy it while you can: no doubt your weight will rise as you get older.

Is there a risk of vitamin deficiency on a low-fat diet? If you avoid high-fat and high-sugar foods, you have to get your energy from other foods – foods that will give you a good supply of vitamins and minerals. Fat contains the fat-soluble vitamins (A, D, E and K). Vitamin K is made in your intestine, and you won't miss out on vitamins A, D and E on the kind of diet I'm recommending which includes some nuts, oils and oily fish.

If you adopt a very low-fat diet to control your weight, make sure you include plenty of skimmed milk powder fortified with vitamins A and D. And the last thing you want to do if you are trying to reduce your risk of heart disease is to go short of essential fatty acids and the vital antioxidant vitamin E; it's wise to allow yourself some nuts and seeds. By all means take a multivitamin too.

When we talk about changing dietary habits, a very real danger for some people is the development of unhealthy attitudes to food or even eating disorders such as bulimia and anorexia nervosa. No doubt the diet and fashion industries do a great deal to foster these unhealthy attitudes; it is certainly not my intention to do the same.

It is my hope that the information in this book will set you free – free to enjoy good food without harbouring feelings of guilt or worries about your health. Food should be delicious and satisfying, but the notion that it won't be unless it's loaded with saturated fat or hydrogenated vegetable oil is absurd. Food is all the more enjoyable if you know it's doing you good instead of fearing that it's doing you in.

If you are British, your risk of getting heart disease is vastly greater than it would be if you were Japanese. The difference comes down to lifestyle – mainly diet. You could make some minor changes and marginally reduce your risk. After all, you might get away with it. On the other hand, you could cut your risk dramatically to Japanese proportions. The choice is yours.

◆ Proper balance means eating enough helpful foods as well as avoiding unhelpful ones

◆ If you are losing too much weight on a very low-fat diet, include more oily fish, nuts, rapeseed and/or olive oil (as well as starchy foods)

◆ On a very low-fat diet, don't forget essential fatty acids and vitamins A, D, and E

◆ You could cut your risk a little, or a lot. The choice is yours

Chapter 18

Weight –
dump your toxic waist!

**'I've been on a constant diet for the last two decades.
I've lost a total of 789 pounds. By all accounts,
I should be hanging from a charm bracelet.'**

ERMA BOMBECK

Mass hysteria?

Everybody's at it. The diet industry is booming. Millions of pounds are spent on books telling you foolproof ways to lose weight and on miraculous remedies like 'fat-burning pills'. And yet, the nation is getting fatter! OK, there are the tragic anorexic exceptions but, if you travel on the tube in the rush hour, you won't need any statistics on body mass index to convince you that we are expanding.

What is body mass index?

You know the one about the man whose doctor told him he wasn't too heavy – just too short. Your ideal weight range, of course, depends on your height, so doctors use the body mass index (BMI). It's a simple way to check whether you're overweight. To calculate your BMI, you take your weight in kilograms and divide it by your height in metres squared:

$$\text{BMI} = \frac{\text{Weight in kilograms}}{(\text{height in metres})^2}$$

If your BMI is 20–24.9, congratulations. This is the 'normal' or desirable range. In fact, the World Health Organization now accepts anything down to 18.5 as normal. Of course, it is important to measure your height accurately – not wearing platform shoes. And bathroom scales are notoriously inaccurate: sometimes they are so accommodating that you can get any reading you like by leaning in the right direction.

A BMI of 25–30 means you are 'overweight'. When doctors say someone is 'obese', it's not a vague term of abuse: it's simply defined as having a BMI over 30. A BMI over 40 would make you 'very obese'. Figure 10 shows you the acceptable weight range for your height.

Those who have built up very big muscles by weight training may be in the 'overweight' range although they are not fat. On the other hand, many people in the normal weight zone could do with more muscle and less fat.

A weighty problem

A growing proportion of the UK population is obese (BMI over 30). In 1980 about 8% of the adults were obese and by 2003 the proportion had almost trebled to 23%. And it's still rising! This is alarming – especially if you manufacture lifts. Obesity is the extreme end of the spectrum; many more people are overweight. Mortality shoots up as

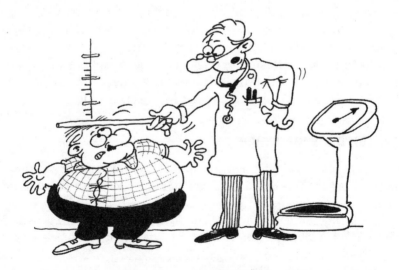

'Your weight is fine; it's your height that's the problem.'

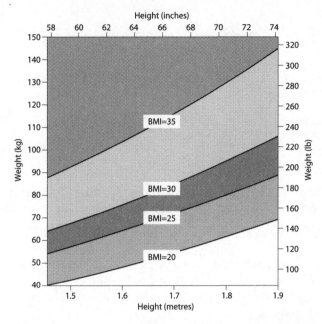

Figure 10 What you should weigh. The BMI weight/height diagram.
Use the chart or do this calculation to find out your BMI:
divide your weight in kilograms by the square of your height in metres.

Your BMI score:

below 20: underweight; **20–25**: ideal; **25–30**: overweight;
30+: seriously overweight – you need to see your doctor

the BMI rises above 30; the risk of heart disease is increased fivefold, and of diabetes twentyfold. Many other medical problems – such as high blood pressure, stroke, gallstones, respiratory disease, arthritis and hernias – occur more commonly in people who are overweight or obese. It could be twenty years before an obese person runs into medical problems and, for this reason, the effects of obesity have sometimes been underestimated in the past.

If you have raised blood pressure or cholesterol, losing excess weight is vital. In some cases this will solve the problem and avoid the need for drugs.

Why are we getting fatter?

Here's a simple fact: if you take in more energy (calories) than you use up, the spare energy will be stored. The body's main energy store is fat.

◆ Eating more fat and refined carbohydrate while being less active
  has resulted in more people getting fat

◆ In general, fat people don't have slow metabolism but disordered
  metabolism

◆ Occasionally, weight gain results from lack of thyroid hormone

◆ Increased waist circumference means fat inside the abdomen and is
  strongly linked to risk

◆ The metabolic syndrome comprises: increased waist circumference,
  unbalanced blood fats, raised blood pressure and insulin resistance

---

So if you don't use up all the calories you eat, you must get heavier. And if you burn more calories than you take in, you get lighter. This is inescapable. Energy cannot be created or destroyed. That's the first law of thermodynamics.

So what's changed? Why have Western societies got fatter during this century? There have been two notable changes. First, we get more of our calories from fat these days, often combined with refined carbohydrate. Secondly, we are using fewer calories; we're much less active. Technology sees to that. We travel door-to-door by car and floor-to-floor by escalator. We are even spared the effort of opening doors. Adjusting the TV by remote control still means lifting a finger; perhaps future sets will respond to our thoughts.

The metabolic myth

Many overweight people complain that they have a slow metabolism: 'If I so much as look at a lettuce leaf, I put on a pound.' The popular idea that fat people have low metabolic rates is completely false. The bigger the body, the more energy it uses just to stay alive. In other words, the bigger you are, the higher your resting metabolic rate. Not only that, but as soon as you start moving your body, you use up more energy than someone who has a smaller body to move.

Mind you, we are discovering more and more about the ways in which metabolism can be disordered in overweight people, particularly when there is excess abdominal fat. You will read more about that, and what you can do about it, in the coming pages.

And people who weigh the same won't necessarily have the same metabolic rates. One of the most important things to understand is that muscle uses more energy than fat. If you stay the same weight but increase your lean body mass (that is to say, you increase your muscle and reduce your fat) your metabolic rate will rise. So when you lose weight, you must make sure you lose fat – not muscle – or you'll find it impossible to keep the weight off.

If you have been fighting a losing battle with your weight, I hope this book will change all that. Just occasionally, it turns out that the metabolic rate has been slowed down by inadequate production of thyroid hormone. Your doctor will be happy to check whether you have this problem. If you have, it's simply corrected by taking a daily thyroid supplement.

Fats and figures

Are you an apple or a pear? Our figure is largely determined by the distribution of fat on our body. The typical female figure is 'pear-shaped' – excess fat being stored on the hips and thighs. An obese man typically stores most of his fat on the abdomen, making him 'apple-shaped'. Despite these stereotypes, women often develop excess abdominal fat, especially after the menopause.

Being apple-shaped is a much greater health hazard than being pear-shaped. 'Central obesity', the medical term for a fat belly, is strongly linked with coronary heart disease; it also increases the risk of premature death, high blood pressure, stroke, diabetes and gallstones.

One way of looking at the problem is to calculate the waist–hip ratio (that is, the waist measurement divided by the hip measurement). A ratio greater than 1 in a man, or 0.8 in a woman, would indicate an increased risk of coronary heart disease. For example, a man measuring 40 inches round the waist and 32 inches round the hips would have a ratio of 40/32 = 1.25, putting him at increased risk.

What a waist

Recently doctors have been using the simple waist measurement to pick out people at risk. It was Professor Michael Lean (so aptly named) who first suggested this. Writing in the *British Medical Journal* in 1995, Professor Lean and colleagues proposed that a simple, single waist measurement could identify people who needed to lose weight.

Why should waist circumference be so important? Here's the point. A fat tummy doesn't just mean fat under the skin. It means fat in and around abdominal organs like the liver. This visceral fat is strongly linked with insulin resistance, high blood pressure and abnormal blood fats (dyslipidaemia) – all part of the metabolic syndrome which affects perhaps a third of our population.

In fact, a wealth of research now points to the metabolic syndrome as the key to our Western epidemics of diabetes and heart disease. Central obesity is indeed central to the metabolic malaise that impairs sensitivity to insulin, deranges blood fats and clogs up arteries.

You see, visceral fat, the fat that is hidden within and around abdominal organs, is not inert lard. It behaves as an active organ, releasing a host of chemical messengers that mess with your metabolism. That's why it's essential to get rid of your toxic waist. The individual fat cells are called adipocytes and the chemicals they release are called adipokines.

Among all these nasty adipokines, there is one good guy – a protein called adiponectin. You want your adiponectin levels to be as high as possible. But the more visceral fat you have, the lower your levels of adiponectin.

As adiponectin falls, and other adipokines rise, biochemical changes have a number of very unwelcome effects: tissues become less sensitive to insulin, causing a rise in blood glucose and insulin levels; background inflammation goes up; the concentration of protective HDL-cholesterol falls; arteries become more susceptible to blockage by thrombosis and atherosclerosis; blood pressure rises.

You might think that with all this biochemistry going on, a tape measure is a pretty crude and unscientific tool for measuring risk. Not so. You can measure the fat in the abdomen with a highly sophisticated CT scanner. The result is very closely related to the reading on a tape measure. Your waist circumference really is a good indication of the amount of visceral fat hidden inside your abdomen. And as we've seen, excess fat in your abdomen is not dead weight; it's a living liability.

It's understandable, then, that research over recent years has confirmed what Professor Lean proposed: the simple waist circumference is even more closely linked to the risk of diabetes, heart disease and stroke than BMI or total body fat (as a percentage). An analysis in *Circulation* in 2007 concluded that every 1 cm increase in waist circumference meant a 2% rise in risk.

So often, complicated and expensive tests are done while the insight offered by a simple tape measure is ignored. What a waste.

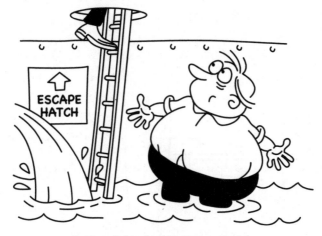

Excess abdominal fat increases risk.

How big should my belly be?

For a woman, a waist over 32 inches (81.3 cm) means some increased risk; over 35 inches (88.9 cm) risk becomes very significant. The equivalent values for a man are 37 inches (94 cm) and 40 inches (101.6 cm). And anyone who's taller lying down is in real trouble.

To measure your waist circumference (Figure 11), pass a tape measure around your bare tummy – just above the pelvic bone on each side, and parallel to the floor. Remove all the slack, without indenting the skin, breathe out, and take a measurement. It's worth repeating the process to make sure your readings are consistent.

People are often advised to place the tape measure just above the hip bone. I worry that they may misunderstand 'hip bone' and take a hip measurement – disastrous! Anatomically, the structure your tape measure should be just above is called the iliac crest of the pelvis.

The tape measure doesn't lie (unless you use one that stretches) but you can easily delude yourself by misplacing it or pulling it too tight. You know you've got a problem when the tape's too short. And if you think you don't need to measure your waist because you buy trousers with a 36-inch waist, think again! Most of us buy trousers at least 2 inches below our true waist measurement, and we've all seen bellies hanging over belts.

Even if your waist is at the top of the normal range, it's time to take action now, before things get worse.

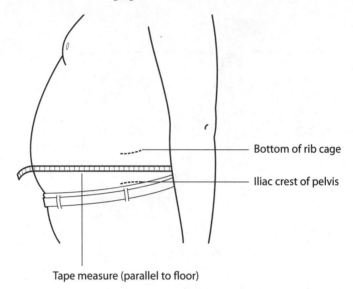

Bottom of rib cage

Iliac crest of pelvis

Tape measure (parallel to floor)

Figure 11 Measuring waist circumference.

ACTION POINTS

◆ Don't 'go on a diet'; change to a healthy way of life

◆ Set realistic goals; aim for a weight loss of 1–2 lb/week (0.5–1 kg)

◆ Don't weigh yourself more than once a week

◆ Eat as little saturated and trans fat as possible

◆ Choose low-GI carbohydrates and limit portions to keep down GL

◆ Eat more low-fat, protein-rich plant foods (e.g. tofu, beans)

◆ Don't go hungry. Eat regular meals

◆ Finish meals with fruit and carry a suitable snack (e.g. banana)

◆ As you get older, get smaller plates

◆ Cut down alcohol. It contains 7 cal/g

Dieting can damage your health

So, you've decided to take yourself in hand and lose that flab. What should you do? Go on a diet, right? Wrong! Think about it. Haven't you been here before? How many times have you been on a diet, lost weight and put it back on again? Yo-yo dieting is bad for you.

Whenever you 'go on a diet' that involves an unnatural pattern of eating – whether it's having meal replacement bars or eating nothing but yoghurt and grapefruit – you will lose weight initially as long as your calorie intake is less than your energy expenditure, but you cannot continue this unnatural behaviour for very long. Your diet comes to an end. Inevitably, the weight returns. And it's worse than that: if your diet has reduced your metabolic rate, the pounds will pile on even faster. All you have lost is your self-esteem.

Crazy diets are big business. Millions are drawn in by the promise of rapid weight loss, only to have their hopes dashed when the scales go back to their old ways.

Any diet involving a sudden reduction of calorie intake is likely to produce a substantial weight loss, typically about five pounds, in the first week. But don't get too excited. That's not five pounds of fat. It's mainly the water that goes as the body draws on energy stored as glycogen (a carbohydrate). You won't continue to lose weight at that rate (and you certainly shouldn't try as it would be very bad for you).

Very low calorie diets (VLCDs), in which meals are replaced by a broth, milkshake or snack bar of essential nutrients, certainly produce weight loss in the short term. Unfortunately, as well as losing fat, you can lose good lean muscle tissue on these diets. That's a disaster. You want more muscle, not less. And don't forget that muscle burns more calories than fat does; when you start eating proper food again, it will be that much harder to control your weight. Very low calorie diets may have a place under close medical supervision in the management of very obese people – where weight loss is a matter of life and death.

The Atkins Diet, a 1970s craze condemned by the American Medical Association, has enjoyed a resurgence of publicity and popularity. If you cut out carbohydrates and replace them with fat and protein, you go into 'ketosis' – the body's starvation mode. You may experience nausea and fatigue (not to mention bad breath). Short-term weight loss is quite possible, but those who stay on a diet like this are inviting kidney problems, cancer and heart disease.

If you are really keen to try the Atkins Diet, I strongly recommend that you modify it. You could cut out bread and potatoes, but keep up your fruit and vegetables. By all means increase your consumption of protein from **lean** sources such as grilled chicken, turkey and fish. Make sure your poultry is skinless and if you want to have more red meat, it must be very lean. Many people following the Atkins Diet are consuming vast quantities of saturated fat, and the long-term effects of that could be catastrophic.

The cabbage soup diet may come with a warning that you shouldn't continue the diet for more than a week, but you don't really need to be told: ferocious flatulence will soon blast you back to reality. Restricting yourself to one or two foods is nutritional nonsense. Any weight loss is the result of calorie reduction, which could just as well be achieved on a balanced diet.

What about drugs?

If you are struggling to lose weight, the idea of taking a pill to shift the pounds may be appealing. There are plenty of useless gimmicks to spend your money on. Fortunately, if you follow the advice in this book, you can lose excess weight gradually and safely. Drugs, of course, can never be a substitute for making the right lifestyle changes to maintain your ideal weight. And you'd be wise to steer clear of diet clinics that dish out pills (including thyroid hormone) for cash. Obesity is a serious problem and sometimes, under medical supervision, drugs can help to tackle it.

The appetite suppressants dexfenfluramine, fenfluramine and phentermine have been linked with serious side effects such as damage to heart valves, so I'm sure your doctor won't give you any of them.

Xenical (orlistat) can be prescribed for obese people who first lose 2.5 kg (5½ lb) over four weeks by changing their diet and being more active. It works by interfering with fat digestion so that 30% of the fat you eat passes through the bowel without being absorbed.

It's important to eat a low-fat diet while taking Xenical or you'll be dashing to the toilet with fatty diarrhoea. Of course, if I prescribe the drug, I always explain the need to avoid high-fat foods like chips. Sometimes a very obese patient will say, 'No problem. I never eat foods like that anyway.' Two weeks later, the patient returns and complains, 'That drug's awful. It gives me terrible diarrhoea – every time I have chips.'

Alli is an 'over-the-counter' version of orlistat, containing half the dose of prescribed capsules.

Reductil (sibutramine) is an appetite suppressant that works by boosting the action of certain chemical messengers (serotonin and noradrenaline) in the brain. It can cause a rise in blood pressure and pulse rate; these should be carefully monitored and sometimes treatment has to be stopped. Reductil is not licensed to be used for longer than a year. Unfortunately, weight may return at the end of a course of treatment.

Acomplia (rimonabant) was launched in the UK in 2006 and is extremely interesting. Being the first drug to selectively block cannabinoid type 1 (CB_1) receptors, Acomplia's novel mode of action gets closer to the root of our Western epidemics – obesity, diabetes and heart disease – than other drugs used for weight reduction.

Working on the recently-discovered endocannabinoid system, Acomplia is, in effect, an anti-metabolic-syndrome drug. Appetite is reduced by blocking CB_1 receptors in the brain. In addition, Acomplia blocks CB_1 receptors in visceral fat, in the liver and in muscles; adiponectin levels go up, insulin resistance is reduced, and regulation of glucose and blood fats improves. Blocking CB_1 receptors in the gut also increases satiety.

In theory, then, taking Acomplia should not only help people to lose weight, but also to lose visceral fat and reverse some of the effects of the metabolic syndrome on blood fats and glucose.

This was put to the test in a series of clinical trials under the RIO (Rimonabant In Obesity) programme. Around 6700 overweight and obese patients, including some with diabetes, took part. On Acomplia 20 mg, they lost an average 6.5 kg (about one stone) over a year, and those that continued treatment for two years kept the weight off. Weight loss was accompanied by a reduction in waist circumference of about 6.5 cm. In all the trials, Acomplia improved the balance of blood lipids. For example, in RIO-Lipids, HDL-cholesterol increased by 19.1% and triglycerides reduced by 12.6% (see Chapter 19). In RIO-Diabetes, patients on Acomplia 20 mg achieved much better control of their diabetes.

You'd expect this degree of weight loss to improve blood cholesterol and glucose levels. But the improvement in cholesterol levels and diabetic control seen in the RIO trials is roughly double what you could expect from the weight loss alone. The additional benefit produced by treatment with Acomplia can be put down to improvement in adiponectin levels resulting in reversal of some of the biochemical features of the metabolic syndrome.

Unfortunately, like any drug, Acomplia isn't suitable for everyone. It's not recommended for people suffering a major depressive illness or taking antidepressants. If you become depressed while taking Acomplia, you should stop treatment and consult your doctor.

Whether you are prescribed a drug or not, there is a huge amount you can do for yourself. To lose weight steadily, increase your adiponectin levels and shrink your waist, you need to make the right changes.

How to take control of your weight

Nothing to lose?

The first question is whether you need to lose any weight. Figure 10 shows you if you are in the acceptable weight range for your height. If you are, you may still have excess fat, especially around the abdomen; your tape measure will tell you (Figure 11). In fact, it is more hazardous to have a BMI in the normal range but excess visceral fat than to have a higher BMI with a normal waist circumference.

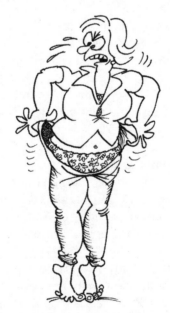

**'This diet's useless. I've been at it all day
and I still can't get into these jeans!'**

Your task is to reduce the flab and increase the muscle while staying in the desirable weight range – to tone up. If you follow the advice on diet and exercise in this book, you will do just that.

I use the word 'diet' extensively in this book. It's a good word, but it's a word that's been hijacked by the diet industry. I use it, of course, to refer to a normal pattern of eating and drinking, a way of life. This has nothing to do with the abnormal behaviour of 'going on a diet'. If you adopt the balanced diet explained in this book, you will control your weight **permanently** as well as reducing your risk of heart disease and cancer.

If your weight is **below** the normal range for your height, you certainly don't need to lose weight. Gaining weight may just be a matter of eating more food; but make sure you keep the balance right (see Chapter 13). You should see your doctor if you are very underweight. This is particularly important if you have lost weight recently. If you are afraid of putting on weight, even though the chart shows you are underweight, it may be that you are developing an eating disorder; the sooner you seek help, the better.

Setting goals

We all like quick results. We get instant tea and instant credit; why not instant weight loss? This desire for rapid results explains the commercial success of diet gimmicks. It also explains why diets fail.

If your goal is to lose half a stone before your holiday in two weeks, you can do it. If you imagine that the weight will stay off, you'll be disappointed. After a series of diets producing rapid weight reduction, and followed by rapid weight gain, you become despondent. You're setting the wrong goals.

But let's be realistic. If you're overweight, you don't really want to lose a few pounds for a few weeks, and then put them back on again. You want a permanent solution to the problem. So don't go on a diet.

Let's suppose for a moment that your weight has been around 12 stone for a long time but you should be 10 stone. This means that the way you are eating and drinking at the moment is feeding a 12-stone person. If you go on a diet until you reach 10 stone, and then go back to your normal habits, your weight will return to 12 stone. If you adopt the lifestyle of a 10-stone person, you can stay at 10 stone – for good.

Once you discover that a properly balanced low-fat diet can be exciting, varied and delicious, you won't want to go back to your old ways! If you follow the plan in this book, you will feel much better about yourself and enjoy a new vitality.

Setting realistic goals is essential. Figure 10 will show you how much weight you need to lose to get into the ideal range. But don't be in a hurry. If you lose one to two pounds (half to one kg) a week (or up to half a stone, or 3 kg, a month), you can reach your target weight and stay there. Sudden, severe weight loss is likely to reduce muscle as well as fat, making things harder in the long run.

Even if you remain overweight and fail to get down to the ideal range, losing 10% of your body weight is really worthwhile and brings measurable health benefits. In fact, if you lose that 10% of your weight gradually by following the plan in this book, you will lose 30% of your visceral fat in the process!

Don't weigh yourself more than once a week. It's pointless to pat yourself on the back or to get despondent because of day-to-day fluctuations that have more to do with fluid balance than anything else. In fact, monthly weighing makes more sense.

Reduce fat intake

This is the first step towards losing weight and slimming your waist.

Fat is the most concentrated source of calories that can pass your lips. Every gram of fat delivers nine calories (or strictly kilocalories) of energy. That's more than twice as much as carbohydrate (sugar and starch) or protein. Both carbohydrate and protein provide only four calories per gram.

Forget calorie counting. A calorie counter and calculator will do about as much for your appreciation of food as a ruler and stopwatch will do for your love life. There's more to food than calories.

If you eat a lot less fat, you are bound to be eating fewer calories; there's no need to count them. But nature abhors a vacuum and if you cut down on fat, you will automatically eat more of something else. If you replace the fat with either carbohydrate or protein, remember, gram for gram you will be consuming less than half the calories you were getting from fat. Traditional advice is simply to replace the fat with complex carbohydrate. But if you don't make the right choices, a reduced-fat diet could still leave you struggling to slim your waist.

Choose well – go low-GL

As we saw in Chapter 6, your choice of carbohydrate-rich foods makes all the difference when it comes to controlling your blood glucose and insulin levels. Just because a food such as bread or potato is made largely of complex carbohydrate (starch), it doesn't mean it will release its energy slowly. If you eat 50 g of carbohydrate in the form of a baguette (GI 95), the impact on your blood glucose will be similar to that of eating 50 g of pure glucose.

A food with a lower GI number releases its energy more slowly, but its effect on your blood glucose levels depends on how much of the food you eat. GL takes into account the amount of carbohydrate in a portion of the food (see page 77).

In general, refined carbohydrate foods (such as white flour, white bread and sugar) are unhelpful: not only has processing raised the GL, it has also stripped away nutrients like chromium, zinc and B vitamins which are essential for your metabolism, including blood glucose control.

If you cut out refined carbohydrates and make low-GL choices (such as beans, lentils and whole grains), you will avoid unhelpful surges in blood glucose; your metabolism will readjust and you will become more sensitive to insulin; visceral fat will be mobilised for fuel and your waist will start to shrink; noxious adipokines will diminish, adiponectin will increase, and the vicious cycle will be reversed.

Very low-carbohydrate diets miss the point. Although you can temporarily lose weight by cutting out carbohydrates, you could also lose weight by cutting off your leg; your body will function much better with good quality sources of carbohydrate.

In particular, diets so low in carbohydrate that they induce ketosis cannot be justified. A randomised trial published in the *American Journal of Clinical Nutrition* in 2006 compared a very low-carbohydrate diet (5% of energy from carbohydrate) which induced ketosis (see page 189) with a moderately low-carbohydrate diet (40% of energy from carbohydrate) on which there was no ketosis. The two diets were equally successful in reducing body weight, but the very low-carbohydrate diet had more unwanted effects on metabolism (e.g. raised LDL-cholesterol) and on mood.

In praise of protein

Protein, being made of amino acids, is rich in nitrogen. The recommended daily intake of protein is enough to replace the nitrogen you lose (in the urine, for example). But perhaps there's a case for eating more protein than this minimum requirement.

For a start, we have seen that the weight loss achieved on very low-carbohydrate diets can't be put down to ketosis; maybe it has something to do with the high protein content of such diets.

This was put to the test by David Weigle and his colleagues in a study published in the *American Journal of Clinical Nutrition* in 2005. Keeping the carbohydrate intake constant (50% of energy), they compared a diet that supplied 15% of the calories as protein (not unusual) with one in which 30% of the calories came from protein (a high protein content, typical of that in low-carbohydrate diets). Everybody in the study tried both diets. They did better on the high-protein diet: they lost more weight and body fat, and felt less hungry.

In fact, over the last few years, evidence from lots of studies has led to the conclusion that protein is particularly good at suppressing appetite. For years, some fad diets have claimed that eating more protein helps you to lose weight; only recently do we have strong scientific evidence to support this. (The findings of one or two small studies do not make strong evidence; it is only when a good number of different research groups find the same thing that we can be confident.)

Foods differ in their ability to induce 'satiety' – a feeling that you have eaten enough. One way researchers have investigated this is to give people meals that contain the same number of calories, but different proportions of protein, fat and carbohydrate (starch or sugar). In the hours that follow the meal, the people are asked to score their satiety on a chart, perhaps every 15 minutes, to see which meal is best at keeping hunger pangs at bay.

Another approach is to allow people to eat in the hours that follow the meal – and carefully measure the calories consumed.

Having sifted through lots of these investigations, I think it would be fair to say this: when it comes to suppressing appetite, protein is at least as good as complex carbohydrate (starch) and probably better; low-GI carbohydrate (e.g. wholegrain pasta) is better than high-GI carbohydrate (e.g. white bread and sugar); fat is poor.

One of the problems with comparing the effect of protein on satiety with that of starch, and pooling the findings of lots of studies, is that starch can take many different forms. When starch delivers a low GL, it will do more for satiety than high-GL starch. Also, the protein and fat content of a meal reduce the ability of the starch to raise blood glucose (i.e. they reduce its glycaemic effect).

Research comparing protein with carbohydrate and fat has revealed another very interesting difference. Whenever you eat food, your body has to expend energy to process it, and heat is produced as a by-product. This is called the thermic effect of the food, or thermogenesis. It turns out that the thermic effect of protein is higher than that of carbohydrate or fat. In other words, your body uses up more calories to process the protein you eat than it uses to process carbohydrate or fat.

The extra calories used up by thermogenesis after a high-protein meal are too few to make much contribution to the weight loss seen after a few weeks on a high-protein diet. Using a few extra calories a day for years, however, could make a significant contribution to weight maintenance.

It seems that most of the extra weight loss achieved by boosting the protein content of a diet can be put down to the positive effect of protein on satiety.

A possible additional benefit of increasing protein intake when you are losing weight is that it may help to prevent loss of muscle; you just want to lose fat, remember. A study published in *Obesity* in 2007 investigated the effects of calorie restriction in 46 overweight and obese women aged 28 to 80. As the women lost weight, a high-protein diet (30% of calories from protein) preserved lean body mass (muscles and organs) better than a 'normal' diet (18% of calories from protein). Also, although calories were restricted on both diets, the women felt less hungry on the high-protein regime.

The OmniHeart Study (page 269) showed that a diet in which 25% of calories came from protein had metabolic advantages over the carbohydrate-rich DASH diet. Replacing some carbohydrate with protein improved the impact on blood pressure, lipids and cardiovascular risk.

Check your balance

It may be that you have done well by following traditional advice to cut down fat and increase complex carbohydrate. Even if you have seen a reduction in your weight and total cholesterol, it's important to check the balance of blood lipids – to make sure you haven't pushed your HDL down and your triglycerides up. Following conventional wisdom can result in a high-GL diet that doesn't suit everyone – especially those struggling to reverse features of the metabolic syndrome.

If you have found it difficult to lose weight – or more particularly to slim your waist – on a low-fat, high-carbohydrate diet, you will probably be more successful if you shift the balance of nutrients. The pictorial representation of a balanced diet on page 138 is a good

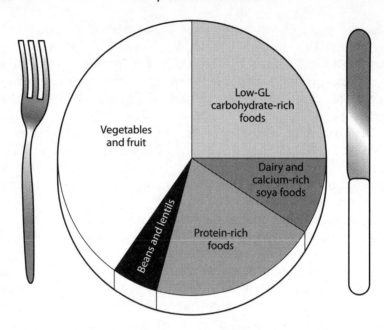

Figure 12 Shifting the balance.

starting point, but perhaps your plate should look more like Figure 12 This variation on the conventional balanced diet (Figure 9) is a big improvement for many people, especially those with the metabolic syndrome who are struggling to slim their waist.

Of course, vegetables and fruit contribute a little to your carbohydrate intake; dairy products and calcium-rich soya foods will boost your consumption of protein; beans and lentils are vegetables but also excellent sources of protein.

Figure 13 shows the macronutrient breakdown to aim for. Being selective with carbohydrates, while replacing some of them with protein – and keeping up your intake of mono-unsaturates – makes for better control of your blood glucose, appetite and energy levels. The alcohol is optional, of course; if you drink one or two units a day on six days of the week, it will contribute about 5% of your total calorie intake. You'll trim your tummy more rapidly if you drink less.

But how can you possibly adjust your diet – which consists of real food and drink, not dollops of macronutrients – to achieve the percentages shown in Figure 13? It certainly isn't a matter of common sense or intuition. Relax. It's all been worked out for you and it's handed to you on a plate in the Action Plan. Just follow the 28-day plan in Chapter 28; before long, getting the right proportions will be part of your new routine.

Achieving this balance of macronutrients will 'reset' your metabolism, readjust your lipids, raise your adiponectin levels and reverse the vicious cycle; you will start burning visceral fat and losing inches from your waist.

It is essential to choose low-fat sources of protein, especially when you are increasing your protein consumption. Use plenty of fish and shellfish, skinless chicken and turkey breast, tofu and other soya products, Quorn, very low-fat dairy products, beans, lentils and chickpeas. Eggs are useful too (see page 152). By all means have red meat sometimes, but make sure all visible fat is removed (or your fat intake will shoot over that 25% mark in no time).

The MUNCH plan (Chapter 28) provides 25% of energy as protein – but a high proportion of this protein comes from plants.

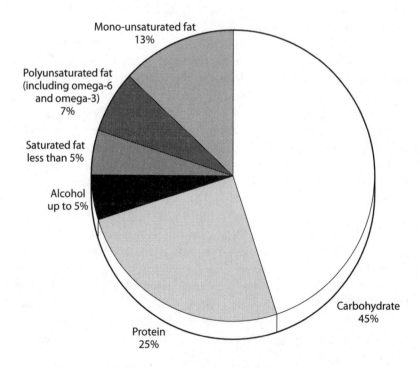

Figure 13 Balancing macronutrients to banish your toxic waist.
The pie chart shows the percentage of total energy intake supplied
by each macronutrient.

A word of caution

Short-term studies on higher-protein diets are very encouraging: they show helpful metabolic changes, loss of body fat, and accelerated reduction in waist circumference; such diets also appear to be safe for most people. We do not, however, have a lot of information about the long-term effects of a high protein intake.

There could be complications if your kidneys are abnormal to start with, according to a report from the Nurses' Health Study in 2003. The analysis showed no problem in women with normal kidney function. But in women with mild kidney disease, a high intake of protein (notably non-dairy animal protein) was linked with a faster rate of decline in kidney function.

Another concern about staying on a high-protein diet is that it may increase loss of calcium in the urine and raise the risk of kidney stones. Again, this seems to be associated with a high consumption of animal rather than plant protein. Drinking eight glasses of water a day, whether you're on a high-protein diet or not, helps to prevent stones forming in the urinary tract.

Years of losing extra calcium in the urine, and not getting enough in your diet to replace it, could result in a significant loss of calcium from your bones. To avoid osteoporosis (brittle bones), it is vital to maintain an adequate intake of calcium and vitamin D, for example by having three servings of low-fat dairy or calcium-rich soya products a day.

You should be particularly cautious about eating a high-protein diet if you have diabetes or kidney disease or a tendency to form kidney stones. Please seek advice from your doctor, who will already be monitoring your kidney function, before making any major changes to your diet.

Doctors now obtain a very useful indication of kidney function called 'estimated glomerular filtration rate' (eGFR) from a simple blood test. Since laboratories have been providing this information, we have been discovering many more people with mildly impaired kidney function. Most people with a moderately reduced eGFR (30–59) don't die of kidney failure; they eventually die, like most of us, from diseases of the heart and circulation. So, if you have a low eGFR, it is especially important to gain tight control of other risk factors, such as cholesterol and blood pressure, with drugs if necessary.

The thing is, you could have a low eGFR without knowing it and if you have, it should be monitored – especially if you plan to raise your protein intake. No doubt, your doctor would be happy to check your eGFR, cholesterol, triglycerides and glucose on one (fasting) blood sample, as well as measuring your blood pressure and waist circumference. I'm sure both you and your doctor will be delighted to document an improvement after three months on this plan.

Please remember that however successful you are, we do not yet have enough evidence to recommend obtaining 25–30% of your calories from protein indefinitely. If you follow this plan, no matter how long for, don't forget to include enough plant sources of protein (e.g. tofu, soya 'milk', Quorn, quinoa, beans, lentils, nuts and seeds) and drink plenty of water. Once you have reached your target, you could eat a little less protein and a little more low-GL carbohydrate.

◆ Fat contains 9 cal/g; sugar, starch and protein have only 4 cal/g

◆ You can be free from calorie counting

◆ Protein and starch suppress appetite better than fat does

◆ Low-GL carbohydrate keeps hunger at bay longer than refined carbohydrate

◆ Shifting the balance of protein, fat and carbohydrate can aid weight loss

◆ Be wary of high-protein diets if you have diabetes, kidney disease or a history of kidney stones

◆ Very high protein consumption for years may be unsafe

◆ Diets high in plant proteins are safer than those high in animal proteins

---

Akin to Atkins?

I hope you understand by now how very different this plan is from the Atkins Diet.

Some people lose weight in their first few months on the Atkins Diet. This is partly explained by the calorie reduction that goes with avoiding a food group. If you're on the Atkins Diet and you're offered a biscuit at your coffee break, you say, 'No thanks. Have you got any meat?' Your colleague doesn't have any meat at that point, so that's another lot of calories avoided.

Apart from that, in my opinion, their success can be put down to the high protein intake and low glycaemic load – which you can just as well achieve without depriving yourself of nutritious, low-GL carbohydrate foods or swamping your arteries with saturated fat.

It is far better for your health to keep saturated and trans fats to a minimum, while making sure you get enough of the essential omega-3 and omega-6 fatty acids, in addition to mono-unsaturated fat which helps to keep up your protective HDL-cholesterol (see Chapter 19).

Your metabolism also works more efficiently if you are not running short of micronutrients supplied by whole grains and needed by myriad enzymes, including those crucial to glucose and fat regulation. And why ditch the fibre that keeps your bowel out of trouble and lowers cholesterol?

It's hard to stay on a very low-carbohydrate diet for months on end. A more balanced diet – designed to regulate metabolism, weight and waist size – can become a way of life.

Plan ahead

Use the meal plans and tables in Chapter 28 to make a shopping list. Before starting your new way of eating, you need time to get rid of unhelpful foods, and stock your cupboards and fridge with foods that will help you banish your toxic waist for good.

Eaten plenty? Give it twenty

If you've finished your meal and still feel hungry, have a glass of water and do something else before you have another helping. It could be that your body needs a little more time to send all the signals to your brain that say you've had enough. Twenty minutes after that last mouthful, you may find the hunger's gone – and you'll be glad you didn't squeeze in another plateful!

Feast, don't fast

If you try going hungry, you won't last long. Foods rich in protein or unrefined carbohydrate (such as pulses and whole grains) will keep hunger pangs away more efficiently than high-fat foods.

Finish meals with fruit and always have helpful snacks to hand (e.g. fruit, celery or carrot sticks, a few almonds, rye bread and hummus). A banana in the handbag or briefcase could save you from that chocolate éclair (but if it's too ripe, it'll make a mess in your bag and deliver a high GL). In fact, healthy snacking during the day will help you control weight and cholesterol much better than going for long periods without food.

Don't skip breakfast and lunch. Have three meals and two or three snacks a day.

Size doesn't matter. Or does it?

As long as you eat the right foods, you can eat as much as you like, can't you? No. You can eat non-starchy vegetables freely; as long as they are not cooked or served with fat, you are unlikely to overdo it.

But eating a low-GL diet means selecting the right foods and eating the right quantity. There is a connection between the size of the person and the size of the portion.

Switch to the right foods, prepared in the right way, and you're more than half way there, but if you persistently eat too much of the right foods you will never reach your ideal weight. As we get older, and less active in most cases, we burn up fewer calories. If you keep on eating at 50 exactly the same as you were eating at 20, 'middle-age spread' is inevitable.

Certainly, one of the great things about getting the balance right, and eating far more vegetables but much less fat, is that you can enjoy a full plate of food and still control your weight. Even so, you may need to get smaller plates.

On your marks. Get set . . .

Sprinting is not always advisable, but exercise is essential. You cannot hope to control your weight permanently without including some form of exercise in your routine. If this is a completely novel concept for you, don't start running; it's best not to take the body by surprise.

Walking is ideal, if you have working legs. Start from your present level of activity and build up gradually. This may mean walking to the TV set to turn it on instead of using the remote control. Soon you could be doing half an hour's brisk walking a day and this will make a real difference. It's not so much that the pounds drop off with a little bit of exercise. They don't. But regular exercise increases your metabolic rate – not only while you're exercising but also when you're not – and reduces insulin resistance. In fact exercise is essential if you want to reverse the metabolic syndrome and avoid the decline to diabetes. It also helps to build up muscle tissue as you lose weight. And, as we've seen, muscle burns calories more efficiently than fat does.

Congratulations!

If you've discovered the benefits of healthy eating and you're including aerobic exercise in your daily routine, you might well congratulate yourself. But, as you raise that glass of celebratory champagne, it's worth remembering that alcohol has seven calories in every gram – calories you could well do without if weight is a problem.

Light drinking can have its benefits (see Chapter 11) but a **heavy** drinker may well become just that – and much of the extra weight is often carried in a 'beer gut'. Alcohol, it seems, increases the storage of fat on the abdomen where it is particularly linked to coronary risk.

Keeping it up

Or should that be down? Having lost some weight, it's all too easy to find it again. You are discovering that a really healthy diet is delicious, varied and satisfying. You are finding that exercise can be enjoyable. It can make you feel good about yourself. So this is not a weight-loss programme of so many weeks before returning to normal life. This **is** normal life – a much more satisfying life because you are in control. Here are a few extra tips to help you stay that way.

- Remember that when you weigh less you need less food, unless you increase your activity enough to compensate.

- Recognise the danger times and work out a strategy to deal with them. If you tend to overeat at the end of a stressful day (and then feel guilty or depressed), do a relaxation exercise when you get in or go for a short walk or pedal your exercise bike for 20 minutes. Don't worry about exercise making you hungry; it will often take the edge off your appetite if you exercise before eating.

- If you do overeat, or slip up and eat a high-fat meal, simply go back to your normal, low-fat way of eating straight away (i.e. at the next meal). You are not 'on a diet', so there's no need to overreact and give up as if you had 'broken the diet'.

- Sort out a dozen very low-fat, quick and easy recipes that you (and your family) enjoy. Always keep the ingredients in stock. Fall back on these old favourites whenever you're not sure what to cook.

- When cooking your favourite recipes, make extra portions and keep them in the freezer as a standby.

● Sit at the table to eat meals. Don't watch TV at the same time: tests show this can lead to overeating. Relax and enjoy your food. But stop eating before you feel absolutely full. Round off the meal with fruit. Treat yourself to varieties of fruit that you really enjoy.

SUMMARY OF THE SUCCESSFUL LONG-TERM WEIGHT CONTROL PLAN

◆ Set realistic goals

◆ Lose 1–2 lbs (0.5–1 kg) a week at most

◆ Reduce fat intake. Choose low-fat foods. With meat, remember: slim, trim and skim (Chapter 5). Grill, bake, boil, steam, poach or microwave, but don't fry

◆ Eat more low-fat, high-protein foods like fish, tofu, Quorn, quinoa and pulses

◆ Obtain friendly fats from nuts, seeds and oily fish

◆ Reduce intake of refined carbohydrates like sugar and white flour

◆ Choose unprocessed, low-GL foods, particularly pulses and whole grains such as rye and oats

◆ To keep down GL, reduce portion size of carbohydrate-dense foods like pasta; limit bread, rice and potatoes

◆ Eat more fruit and vegetables. At main meals, cover at least half the plate with vegetables, preferably of three different colours

◆ Don't go hungry. Have three meals and two or three snacks a day

◆ Always have healthy low-fat snacks, such as sticks of raw vegetable and hummus, to hand

◆ Include exercise in your daily routine

◆ Go easy on alcohol, and avoid sugary drinks, but drink plenty of water (six or more glasses a day)

◆ Keep going. Once your low-fat, low-GL lifestyle becomes a habit, you'll find you prefer it. And that'll be a big weight off your mind

Chapter 19

Control your cholesterol

'The lard starts forming on the guest even before he gets
out of his car, and by the time he rises flushed from the
table, he can be used to baste an ox.'

S J PERELMAN (1904–79) *Letter***, 1975**

In Chapter 4 we saw how countries with high average cholesterol levels have high rates of heart disease, and how your personal risk of having a heart attack is reduced by getting your cholesterol down. Remember that LDL-cholesterol is the 'bad' one while HDL-cholesterol is 'good'. We learnt that:

LOW-density lipoprotein (LDL) cholesterol should be LOW

HIGH-density lipoprotein (HDL) cholesterol should be HIGH

In this chapter we find out how to achieve it.

Checking your cholesterol

You could check your cholesterol level with a fingerprick test at your doctor's surgery, on the high street or even at home with a DIY test kit. The accuracy of these tests is variable and it would be unwise to base the whole direction of your life on a single reading of this kind. You can be more confident about accuracy if your doctor arranges for a blood sample to be taken from a vein and analysed in a hospital laboratory.

◆ Total cholesterol can be measured without fasting

◆ An overnight fast is needed to tell your triglyceride and HDL levels

---

◆ Recommended levels:

- Total cholesterol less than 5.0 mmol/l

- LDL-cholesterol less than 3.0 mmol/l

- HDL-cholesterol more than 0.9 mmol/l

Samples taken when you haven't fasted are suitable for measuring total cholesterol (but not for telling you how much of it is HDL-cholesterol or LDL-cholesterol). The total cholesterol is not significantly altered by a 12-hour fast and a non-fasting or 'random' level is useful as a screening test to pick out people at high risk.

Triglycerides are quite different. The level of these fats in the blood shoots up and down according to what you've been eating in the last few hours. So measurement of triglycerides is pointless unless you've been fasting for 12 hours. This is one of the easiest fasts you could do. You can finish a banquet at 9 p.m., have blood taken at 9 a.m. the following morning and tuck into breakfast immediately afterwards. You can drink water during the fast, but avoid other drinks.

Measurement of triglycerides and HDL-cholesterol on a fasting blood sample allows the LDL-cholesterol to be calculated (in mmol/l) with this formula:

$$\text{LDL-chol} = (\text{total chol} - \text{HDL-chol}) - \frac{\text{triglycerides}}{2.19}$$

This formula is not accurate if the triglyceride concentration is above 4.5 mmol/l.

So, if your doctor arranges a fasting lipid profile, it will usually tell you your blood levels of the following:

- Total cholesterol;

- HDL-cholesterol;

- LDL-cholesterol;

- Triglycerides.

There are times when measuring cholesterol levels can be misleading; for example, it is advisable to wait **three months** after pregnancy, surgery or serious illness, including a heart attack, before having a cholesterol test. (Levels measured just after a heart attack, within 24 hours, are usually considered reliable.) Similarly, you should not have your cholesterol checked within **three weeks** of having flu or a similar illness because the result may be artificially low (unless this is for an insurance medical in which case perhaps it is the ideal time to have the test).

ACTION POINTS

Before having a cholesterol check:

◆ Wait at least 3 weeks after flu

◆ Wait at least 3 months after surgery, major illness, or pregnancy

---

On the level

When your cholesterol result is available, no doubt your doctor or practice nurse will give you individual advice. Here are some guidelines on the level.

Total cholesterol less than 5.0 mmol/l

If you are in this group, you are the proud owner of a 'normal' cholesterol level. But wait. Before you order that Indian takeaway to celebrate, remember you are not immune to heart disease. For a start, your cholesterol level goes up and down a bit and you might have caught it at a low point. And heart disease does strike some people in this group; you need to consider the other risk factors discussed in this book. Some people imagine that it doesn't matter what they eat because they have had a normal cholesterol reading. They're wrong. This book explains how a good diet will protect you – or a bad diet will put you at risk – in a number of ways that are nothing to do with your cholesterol level.

Total cholesterol 5.1–6.4 mmol/l

This is too high. Mind you, if you're in this group, you're in good company: the average cholesterol level for the UK population is about 5.9 mmol/l (5.8 for men and 6.0 for women). And about two-thirds of the population have undesirable lipid profiles! But you don't want to be among them. You're reading this book because you want to escape the epidemic of heart disease. Of course, you may not have escaped; you may already have heart disease. In that case, even a mildly raised cholesterol level must be taken very seriously; there is a strong argument for taking a cholesterol-lowering drug (see page 326) as well as changing your diet and lifestyle.

If you are overweight, that's the first thing to put right (see Chapter 18). In many cases, making the changes that bring you gradually down to your ideal weight will sort the cholesterol out as well. Avoid all unnecessary fat, have lots of lentils, beans, soya (e.g. tofu) and whole grains, feast on fruit and vegetables, include fish at least twice a week and you will do well.

If you are on the skinny side, you should still keep saturated fat intake as low as possible but there's no need to be afraid of olive oil, rapeseed oil, hazelnuts, almonds, walnuts, avocados and oily fish. I wouldn't recommend a high-fat diet, though, as this may raise the risk of thrombosis.

Total cholesterol 6.5–7.8 mmol/l
This is significantly raised but if you come into this group you are not a freak: levels in this range are very common in the UK (but, then, so are heart attacks). It's definitely time to tackle all your risk factors and adopt a healthy lifestyle.

Total cholesterol above 7.8 mmol/l
Don't panic. Calmly and rationally check that your will is in order. No, I'm not serious – although this is always worth doing if you haven't done it. If your cholesterol level is in this range, it is certainly very high but it doesn't mean you will necessarily die young (as you will realise if you are already 85). Indeed, if you were to check cholesterol levels among the residents of an old folks' home, you would find a good few with levels around 8 mmol/l. Just how serious this is depends what other risk factors are present. If the high cholesterol is your only risk factor, you may well make it to the old people's home; but if you smoke and have high blood pressure as well, you probably won't (unless you make some changes).

Whatever the case, attaining your ideal weight and adopting the diet and lifestyle recommended in this book will significantly reduce your risk of heart disease. If you already have heart disease and a very raised cholesterol, then it's essential to get it down – right down (preferably below 5 mmol/l). Drug treatment will be needed, as well as a good diet.

If your cholesterol level turns out to be something like 10 or 11 mmol/l, then it's just as well you had it measured. You may well have the genetic disorder called familial hypercholesterolaemia (FH), which affects about 1 in 500 of the population. Untreated, most of these people will develop heart disease at a young age. Drug treatment to lower cholesterol is life-saving and other members of the family should have their lipids checked.

Before making any drastic decisions like taking a cholesterol-lowering drug for the rest of your life, you should have at least two measurements including a full fasting lipid profile. Your doctor will also want to use some of the blood to check liver, kidney and thyroid function to make sure your raised cholesterol is not the result of some other disease. It's helpful to spend three months trying to lower your cholesterol by changing your diet although people with familial hypercholesterolaemia, vascular disease or diabetes will need drug treatment as well.

There are multitudes who do not have a serious metabolic disorder and yet have cholesterols above 7 mmol/l. They will not solve the problem by making a few sensible changes like switching to sunflower spread. Most could achieve a spectacular reduction by following the advice in this book.

◆ Some people have inherited disorders that cause very high cholesterol levels and need drug treatment as well as diet

◆ People who already have heart disease should get their total cholesterol level below 5 mmol/l – with drugs if necessary

◆ A good diet is essential, whether drugs are used or not

◆ The importance of a high cholesterol depends on the other risk factors present

Getting the low down

You will remember that the aim of the game is:

To get the LOW-Density Lipoprotein (LDL) down LOW.

Because most of the blood cholesterol is LDL-cholesterol, it is generally the case that if your total cholesterol level is too high, so is your LDL-cholesterol; reducing the total cholesterol will bring down the LDL-cholesterol as well.

How low should you go? Aim for an LDL-cholesterol of 3.0 mmol/l or less; if you have other risk factors such as high blood pressure, this is all the more important. Those who already have heart disease should get it down to well below 3.0 mmol/l – with the help of a statin drug in most cases.

Some people, mostly women, have a raised total cholesterol reading even though their LDL-cholesterol level is satisfactory. This is because they have extra high HDL-cholesterol levels and in these cases it doesn't matter that the total is a little high.

Want to get the low down? Here's the plan.

Keep saturated fat intake as low as possible
Avoid: fatty meats and poultry skin; meat products (e.g. sausages, luncheon meat, beefburgers, pies, pâté, etc.); full-fat dairy products (use skimmed milk products instead); manufactured cakes, biscuits and puddings; dressings and sauces (unless very low-fat); fried foods; lard, suet, dripping, ghee, palm oil, coconut oil and 'vegetable oil'; crisps and similar savoury snacks; chocolate, fudge, toffee and butterscotch; coconut, etc.

Favour friendly fats
Use olive oil or rapeseed oil for dressings and cooking, including home-made cakes and biscuits. Avoid 'vegetable oil', e.g. buy sardines in olive oil. Include nuts like almonds, hazelnuts and walnuts, and seeds such as flax, sunflower, sesame and pumpkin seeds. If you use a fat spread, consider changing to one fortified with plant sterols or stanols (Flora pro.activ or Benecol). Keep the overall fat intake low unless you need to gain weight.

Eat fish at least twice a week
Include oily fish (e.g. salmon, sardines, pilchards, mackerel, herring)

but have any fish you fancy. Every time fish replaces fatty meat or meat products, it's helping to keep the LDL-cholesterol low (not to mention the effect of fish oil on triglycerides and thrombosis risk). If you don't fancy any fish, try recipes that disguise it.

FISHING FOR ALTERNATIVES

I have recommended that you eat fish – preferably, at least twice a week. If you hate fish, you are not impressed with my advice.

Of course, if you hate fish as a rule, you may find the odd exception to prove it. It could be tuna salad that's uniquely acceptable, or perhaps monkfish kebabs. (Never tried them? Then how do you know you don't like them?) If you're finicky about fins, you can have a well-disguised fillet. A fish cake or pie or casserole could throw you off the scent. Or it may be that nothing less than very strong curry is adequate to disguise its fishy origin for you.

If all these strategies disgust you – if you feel you could never enjoy any form of fish – what then? Of course, you will choose other foods from the high-protein group, such as beans, pulses, nuts, tofu, Quorn and, if you're not a vegetarian, lean meat. But what about those valuable fish oils that supply essential omega-3 fatty acids?

Unless you're a vegetarian, you might choose to take a supplement of fish oil (see page 104). Valuable plant sources of omega-3 (in the form of alpha-linolenic acid) include walnuts, pumpkin seeds, linseeds, flaxseed oil and rapeseed oil.

Eat at least five portions of fruit and vegetables a day

Five is the minimum; nine is fine. In fact, you can munch away freely on extremely low-GL vegetables (Table 29) – as long as you haven't added any fat – and very low-GL fruit such as berries. With other fruit and with root vegetables, be guided by GL (Table 10). Olives and avocados provide useful mono-unsaturated fat, but you need to keep to small portions unless you're underweight. Large amounts of soluble fibre will help to lower LDL-cholesterol but, more to the point, you'll be eating the fruit and vegetables in place of something containing saturated fat, which would raise it. And beans (including soya products), peas, lentils and chickpeas are high-protein foods that can be used in place of meat.

The secret combination

The importance of reducing saturated fat intake is clear. In addition, we have seen that certain foods can help to lower blood cholesterol levels. Soya protein, soluble fibre, plant sterols and almonds have all been shown in different studies to produce some reduction in cholesterol. What would be the result of combining all these in one diet? Would their cholesterol-lowering effects add up, or might some of them cancel each other out?

David Jenkins and his colleagues in Toronto decided to put this to the test. People entering this study were already eating a low-saturated fat diet. As well as being low in saturated fat, the test diet – or 'portfolio' diet as they dubbed it – included (for a 2000-calorie diet) 46 g/day of soya protein, 18 g/day of soluble fibre (from oat bran, barley and psyllium), and 2 g/day of plant sterols (in a fat spread). The diet was also rich in vegetables (including aubergine, okra and pulses) and provided 28 g (1 oz) of almonds a day.

The results were dramatic. The portfolio diet reduced LDL-cholesterol by 29%. This drop in cholesterol was similar to that achieved with one of the less powerful statins. The combination had 'unlocked' the body's natural ability to lower cholesterol.

Maintaining the high

If you have switched to a very low-fat diet with a high carbohydrate content, your HDL-cholesterol may have dropped a little. In addition, you may remember that mono-unsaturates are rather better than polyunsaturates at maintaining the level of HDL-cholesterol. Ideally, your HDL-cholesterol should be above 1 mmol/l.

You may also find that your triglyceride level has risen in response to a high-carbohydrate diet. The combination of low HDL-cholesterol and high triglycerides – known as dyslipidaemia – is a feature of the metabolic syndrome (page 313) and is commonly seen in diabetes.

In some parts of the world, people have low levels of HDL-cholesterol because most of their energy comes from carbohydrate; they have very low saturated fat intakes, low levels of

LDL-cholesterol, and low rates of heart disease. But a low HDL-cholesterol linked with excess visceral fat or other risk factors is very undesirable. Small changes in HDL-cholesterol have a big impact on risk.

If your HDL-cholesterol has dropped on a low-fat, high-carbohydrate diet, you may do better by shifting the balance of nutrients to include more mono-unsaturated fat and more protein (see page 196).

Here are some tips worth trying if your HDL-cholesterol is struggling to get above 1 mmol/l.

- Add some good sources of mono-unsaturated fatty acids to your diet, such as olive oil, rapeseed oil, olives, avocados, hazelnuts and almonds.

- Eat more lean protein. Include fish and skinless chicken breast, but also plenty of protein-rich plant foods such as pulses and tofu.

- Cut down any unnecessary sources of polyunsaturates, e.g. sunflower, safflower, soya or corn oils; sunflower spread or sunflower seeds.

- Eat a low-GL diet (see page 77). Cut down on high-GI foods such as baguettes, white bread and instant rice; eat more low-GI foods like beans and lentils. A **small** portion of spaghetti tossed in a little olive oil (delicious with garlic) would be a better choice than baked potato with sunflower spread.

- Check your waist circumference and, if necessary, follow the advice in Chapter 18 to reduce it.

- If you smoke, you must stop. Apart from all the other harmful effects, smoking depresses HDL-cholesterol.

- Take more exercise. Aerobic exercise raises HDL-cholesterol levels. Twenty minutes three times a week is better than nothing, but you may need a lot more than this to make a significant impact on your HDL concentration.

- A little alcohol (e.g. one or two units a day) can help to lift drooping HDL levels.

- If you are taking a non-selective beta-blocker (such as propranolol), it may be reducing your HDL-cholesterol and raising your triglycerides. This would be something to discuss with your doctor.

If your HDL-cholesterol is below 0.6 mmol/l, and especially if you have a family history of heart disease, you should have specific medical advice about this.

Where do triglycerides fit in?

We've seen that triglycerides are fats. They are to be found in our food and in our flab. If we want a meaningful measurement of the level in our blood, the sample must be taken after a 12-hour fast.

Fasting triglyceride levels above 1.5 mmol/l are considered abnormal, but the link between raised levels and coronary heart disease is not as clear-cut as it is with cholesterol. For one thing, high triglyceride levels are commonly found in people who have other problems that raise their risk of heart disease (such as obesity, diabetes and high blood pressure). There is no doubt that the combination of high triglycerides and low HDL-cholesterol, which is often seen in people with metabolic syndrome and diabetes, is undesirable. Some families have a hereditary metabolic disorder that results in high cholesterol and triglyceride levels (familial combined hyperlipidaemia) and a high incidence of heart disease.

Heavy drinking is a common cause of raised triglycerides and many people could rapidly bring their level down to normal by cutting alcohol consumption.

Triglyceride levels above 5.0 mmol/l are very high. As levels rise above 11 mmol/l the blood plasma looks like milk and there is a risk of pancreatitis – a life-threatening illness.

If your fasting triglyceride level is above 1.5 mmol/l:

- Get down to your ideal weight and waist circumference (see Chapter 18);
- Follow the tips to raise your HDL (page 215);
- Eat more oily fish. Fish oils help to reduce triglyceride levels;
- Eat a low-GL diet (see page 77);
- Cut alcohol consumption down to a maximum of one unit a day;
- Keep up a regular aerobic exercise programme;
- Have your blood glucose level measured to exclude diabetes;
- Get your blood pressure checked.

If your triglyceride level is above 5.0 mmol/l, you need specific medical advice.

◆ It's sensible to be settled on an improved diet for 3 months before rechecking your cholesterol

◆ Once you've established a normal lipid profile by changing your lifestyle, there's no need to keep checking your cholesterol level – as long as you keep checking your lifestyle (see Action Plan)

◆ If you are taking a drug to lower your cholesterol, your doctor may wish to do a blood test every 6–12 months

---

What about all the cholesterol in my food?

Frankly, there isn't much. In an average day of munching your way through all those grams of carbohydrate, protein and fat, you will eat less than half a gram of cholesterol. Let's suppose you are eating 400 mg of cholesterol a day and, without making any other changes, you cut that in half to 200 mg a day. That might reduce your blood cholesterol by about 0.2 mmol/l. Impressed?

Now perhaps you can see why all that talk of a 'low-cholesterol diet' is rather silly. And those eye-catching food labels saying 'Low in cholesterol' are playing on the fact that people don't understand this.

How much of the cholesterol that we eat ends up in the blood? This varies. If you were to eat a whole plate of triglycerides, they would all be digested and absorbed from the intestine into the bloodstream (if you didn't vomit before they had the chance). Cholesterol's different. The amount you absorb is largely determined by your genes. In a group of 94 normal men and women, Bosner and colleagues found that the proportion of cholesterol absorbed from the intestine ranged from 29% to 80% (average 56%). Also, soluble fibre and plant sterols in your intestine might reduce absorbtion.

Clearly, cholesterol in your food doesn't influence your blood cholesterol level as much as saturated fat does. Nevertheless, if you are eating a lot of cholesterol and absorbing a high proportion of it, the impact can be significant. A cholesterol-lowering diet should contain no more than 300 mg of cholesterol a day.

So why have I hardly mentioned ways of cutting down dietary cholesterol in this book? That's simple. Much of the cholesterol is found in foods rich in saturated fatty acids. By cutting down your saturated fat intake, you will automatically reduce your consumption of cholesterol.

Here are some foods with a particularly high content of cholesterol:

- All offal such as liver (including liver pâté);

- Fish roe (including taramasalata);

- Egg yolk;

- Egg mayonnaise;

- Some shellfish such as shrimps, prawns, crayfish, lobster, squid and cuttlefish.

I can't get my cholesterol down

You've made radical changes to your diet. The healthier lifestyle is beginning to be second nature and you're feeling better for it. Three months on, you wait eagerly for the result of your cholesterol test. What a terrible disappointment, then, when it turns out to be much the same as the last one. You pick yourself up and go away for another three months. When the next test is no better, despite every effort to get your cholesterol down, it gets you down instead.

I hope this is not your experience. I hope you are one of the majority of people who can make very satisfying reductions in cholesterol levels as long as they make big enough changes to diet and lifestyle.

If you are having difficulty, it is very helpful to keep a dietary diary for a week. Write down *everything* you eat and drink for seven days. I sometimes ask patients to do this and it often shows up areas that can be improved. Your doctor, practice nurse or dietitian would probably be happy to go through it with you.

There will always be some who have a genuine 'metabolic resistance' to cholesterol reduction. Oh yes, many who are placed in this category are deluding themselves and their physicians and, if they were actually to follow the recommendations in this book, their cholesterol levels would come tumbling down. Others, though, are battling with a genetically programmed overproduction of cholesterol, which cannot be fully controlled by changing the diet.

If you are one of these people, I have something very important to say to you: don't get despondent and decide that the healthy diet is a waste of effort. It isn't.

First, if you achieve even a small reduction in your cholesterol level, this is worthwhile. Remember that every 1% reduction in total cholesterol results in *at least* a 2% (probably 3%) reduction in risk of coronary heart disease.

Secondly, even if you were unable to bring about any reduction at all in your cholesterol level, the healthy diet and lifestyle would still be vital. Cutting down saturated fat and eating more fish will reduce the risk of thrombosis (which can cause a heart attack); the diet and lifestyle recommended in this book may help to control blood pressure (and raised blood pressure makes a high cholesterol more dangerous); antioxidants from fruit and vegetables can stop fatty plaques forming in arteries. These are just a few of the ways in which a healthy diet can protect you even if it doesn't bring down your cholesterol.

Your doctor may recommend drug treatment to lower your cholesterol if it stays high on a good diet – especially if you have other risk factors or have already developed heart disease. Some people imagine that the drug does all the work and a healthy diet is no longer needed. You know better.

◆ Cut down saturated fat and you needn't bother about the cholesterol content of most foods

◆ Avoid large quantities of offal, fish roe and egg yolk, which have a very high cholesterol content

◆ A healthy diet will help to protect your heart even if it has a disappointing effect on your cholesterol level

Chapter 20

Exercise

'I like long walks, especially when they are taken
by people who annoy me.'

FRED ALLEN

Why bother?

OK, so regular, vigorous exercise might add four years to my lifespan. What's the point when I'll have spent those four years doing vigorous exercise? So says the cynic.

Is there any scientific evidence that exercise can help us to avoid heart disease – and perhaps prevent the heart attack that could shorten a life, not just by four years, but by 40 years in some cases?

◆ Physically active people are much less likely to have a heart attack than inactive people

◆ Being athletic in your youth doesn't protect you in middle age

◆ Fitness has a short shelf life. You need to stay active

◆ Exercise raises HDL-cholesterol, reduces thrombosis risk, strengthens bones, muscles and the heart and reduces stress

◆ When you are unfit, strenuous exercise can be dangerous

◆ It is more dangerous not to exercise than to take regular exercise of the right intensity

Are you a sitting duck?

It was over half a century ago that Morris and his colleagues presented some early evidence. In 1953 they published a paper in *The Lancet* drawing attention to the fact that bus drivers, who spent all day sitting down, had more heart attacks than bus conductors who ran up and down stairs collecting fares. Similarly, when they investigated postal workers, they discovered that clerks had more heart attacks than postmen who delivered mail.

Twenty years later, Morris and his team were investigating the leisure time activities of male civil servants aged 40–64 (or, at least, the activities they would admit to). Men who reported taking part in vigorous physical activity on the initial survey (1968–70) suffered less than half the coronary heart disease of their less active colleagues over the next eight and a half years.

Dock workers in San Francisco were monitored for 22 years by Paffenbarger and Hale, during which time 11% died of coronary heart disease. The risk of dying from heart disease was 80% higher for those with the less energetic jobs compared with the men doing heavy work (which was defined as using up more than 8500 calories a week at work).

A very different social group, graduates from Harvard, were also studied by Dr Paffenbarger and his colleagues. Those who expended less than 2000 calories a week on leisure time activities had a 64% higher risk of a first heart attack than their more energetic contemporaries.

An interesting discovery was made about the graduates who had been keen athletes at college: they were just as likely to get heart attacks in middle age as their sedentary classmates. To protect against heart disease, regular exercise had to be continued through adulthood. The inactive student who took up regular exercise after leaving college had a lower risk than the college athlete who rested on his laurels (or anything else comfortable he could find to sit on).

This observation – that only continuing exercise protects against heart disease – was confirmed by Morris and his colleagues in a later report on the British civil servants. So, if you think you've done enough exercise to last a lifetime, think again!

Pooling the results of the many studies on this question that have now been published, it looks as though not exercising will more or less double your risk of dying from a heart attack.

The object of the exercise

What can we hope to achieve by exercising? Staying alive by avoiding a heart attack is a pretty good start. It is likely that exercise reduces coronary risk in a number of ways.

- *Reducing blood pressure* A number of research groups have shown that regular exercise can lower blood pressure.

- *Raising HDL-cholesterol* Many investigations have shown that aerobic exercise raises the level of protective HDL-cholesterol and lowers triglycerides. This results partly from increased activity of an enzyme called lipoprotein lipase in trained muscle. The changes are small and a lot of regular, vigorous exercise is needed to make a significant impact.

- *Preventing thrombosis* It is likely that regular exercise reduces the risk of blood clots forming in the circulation. This may result partly from changes in platelets and also from reduction in levels of the clotting factor, fibrinogen. The finding that exercise must be continued to protect against heart attacks would be explained by an effect on blood clotting.

- *Exercising the heart muscle* Like other muscles, the heart benefits from training. A fit person has a slower heart rate because the heart beats more efficiently. As a result, when extra demands are made during exertion, the heart can cope without straining.

The benefits of exercise don't end with the cardiovascular system. Here are some of the other objectives we can expect to meet with a regular exercise programme.

- *Weight control* Exercise is an essential ingredient in any weight-loss programme and helps you to stay at your ideal weight. It increases the metabolic rate, not just while you are exercising, but for some hours afterwards as well.

- *Increased lean body mass* If you exercise regularly while losing weight, things are even better than your scales would have you believe. You will be losing fat and gaining muscle; muscle is heavier than fat (but much better at burning calories).

- *Reduced diabetes risk* Type 2 diabetes – the sort that usually comes on after the age of 40 but is now occurring in some obese children – is caused by insulin resistance (page 186). Regular exercise (e.g. 150 minutes a week), combined with a good diet, helps to reverse features of the metabolic syndrome and prevent diabetes. If you already have diabetes, exercise will help to control it.

- *Giving up smoking* Several studies have indicated that a regular exercise programme helps smokers to quit.

- *Improved mobility* Keeping fit is good for all of us but maintaining the mobility of muscles and joints is especially helpful for older people.

- *Stronger bones* Exercise can help to protect bones against osteoporosis – the brittle bone disorder that causes fractures in so many post-menopausal women.

- *Reduced stress* Exercise is a good stress reliever.

- *Improved sleep* Vigorous physical activity can help to promote sound sleep (but you should avoid exercise just before bedtime or it may have the opposite effect).

- *Feeling good* Getting physically fit can increase your vitality and sense of wellbeing, and help you to work more efficiently.

Running the risk

You may remember Jim Fixx, the American jogging enthusiast who dropped dead while doing his daily run. So, what are the risks of running and other forms of vigorous exercise?

An investigation by Siscovick and colleagues in Seattle, Washington, was reported in the *New England Journal of Medicine* in 1984. The researchers interviewed the wives of 133 men (aged 25–75) who had suffered a cardiac arrest (which means that the heart suddenly stopped beating). They recorded what the men had been doing at the time of the cardiac arrest and their normal pattern of vigorous exercise. Exercise patterns in the community were established by interviewing the wives of a random sample of healthy men.

The conclusions were alarming. Men who were normally inactive were over 50 times more likely to die during vigorous exercise than at other times. The men who took regular exercise were also at increased risk while exercising but for them the risk of dying during exercise was only five times greater than at other times. Perhaps you think that exercise sounds pretty dangerous even for the man who takes it regularly, but the overall risk for the active men in the study was only 40% of that for the inactive ones.

The message is clear. Vigorous exercise is dangerous for middle-aged and older men who aren't used to it. No doubt the same goes for women. Of course, if you never take any vigorous exercise at all, your risk of dying during vigorous exercise is zero. Indeed, it is safer not to take any exercise than to surprise the body occasionally with a burst of vigorous activity. This is especially dangerous when there is added stress; it's just not worth running for that bus unless you are used to running.

The balance of risks is firmly in favour of taking regular exercise. In other words, your risk of heart disease and sudden death is substantially reduced by regular exercise – as long as you take sensible precautions.

What precautions should I take?

Take it gradually
This is particularly important if you are over 40. Walking is a good way to start if you have not been exercising. Gradually increase the distance and pace. If you want to progress to jogging, start with one-minute jogs, followed by a few minutes of walking. If you use an exercise bike, start on an easy setting and be content with a few minutes at first.

Take it easy
Your exercise session should make you puff and pant a *little*, but you should not get so breathless that you are unable to carry on a normal conversation.

Take notice of your body
If it hurts, don't do it. When your body gives warning signals, slow down or stop. Particularly if you have any chest pain, nausea, palpitations or dizziness, ease off. In fact, Jim Fixx was suffering from coronary heart disease and had been ignoring warning symptoms.

Take time to warm-up and cool-down

Starting your exercise slowly and gently allows muscles to become more flexible and less liable to injury. Cool-down by reducing your exercise intensity for some minutes before stopping. It's as simple as walking around after running, or pedalling slowly on your exercise bike. This gives your circulation time to readjust after sending extra blood to working muscles.

Take your pulse

Your heart rate can tell you whether you are exercising too hard for safety or not hard enough to get fit. You should aim to keep your heart rate in the target range for your age once you have warmed-up. The cool-down will allow your heart to settle gradually towards its normal rate.

You can feel your radial pulse on the thumb side of your wrist. Alternatively, the carotid pulse is easily felt by pushing the index and middle finger of one hand gently into the neck beside the larynx (voice box). If you count the number of beats in 10 seconds and multiply by six, it will tell you the number of beats per minute (Figure 14).

Your 'maximum heart rate' is calculated by subtracting your age from 220:

$$\text{Maximum heart rate} = 220 - \text{age.}$$

For example, if you are 40 years old, your maximum heart rate is 180 beats per minute. Your target heart rate for exercise is 70% of this (126) and the target range is 65–75% of the maximum heart rate (117–135).

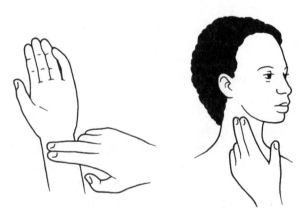

Figure 14 Taking your pulse at the wrist and the neck.

I am sure you will have no difficulty following this example to calculate your own target range but Table 20 gives you an indication.

Table 20 Target heart rate for exercise

Age (years)	Target range (beats/min) 65–75% max. rate
20	130–150
30	123–142
40	117–135
50	110–127
60	104–120
70+	97–112

If you are very unfit, you will get your heart rate into the target range just by walking. Having said that, remember that if you are just starting an exercise programme, there is no hurry to get up to the target range. It is more important to ease yourself in gently. Don't go above your range.

For those who like gadgets and have money to spare, an electronic heart rate monitor could be a good investment. This saves interrupting your exercise session to feel your pulse, and can be programmed to tell you whenever you go outside your target range.

Take plenty of fluids

Doctors are always telling people to drink plenty of fluids – to which you would be entitled to reply, 'What else would I drink?' Of course, to a physicist or chemist, a fluid is a liquid or a gas; but we are definitely talking about liquid here. In fact, water is hard to beat. You can lose an awful lot of fluid (including water vapour from your lungs) during half an hour of exercise. Drink plenty of water before, after and, if necessary, during exercise. This is even more important in hot weather.

Take your doctor's advice if you have a medical problem

Any exercise video or DVD will tell you to see your doctor before doing the exercises. That lets the video company off the hook if you do yourself in. Of course, doctors would be overwhelmed if everyone went for a check-up before doing any exercise. Everyone should take exercise of some sort and you're more likely to need medical attention if you don't.

If you have a medical problem – such as asthma, bronchitis, emphysema, high blood pressure, heart disease, back pain or arthritis – the right exercise will be positively helpful but it's wise to check whether your doctor has any specific advice for you.

Take the right equipment

I suppose this is obvious if you exercise by rock climbing, but even for walking you need a decent pair of shoes. It is particularly important to have good exercise shoes to cushion the impact for activities like jogging and step aerobics.

Take a couple of hours to digest your lunch

By all means take exercise shortly before meals; this can take the edge off your appetite and help you to avoid overeating. Don't take vigorous exercise straight after meals. Extra blood is diverted to the gut for digestion and your heart won't welcome the increased demands of exercise.

Take a break if you're unwell

Don't undertake energetic exercise if you have a fever or flu-like illness. Your heart will already be working harder as a result of the fever and some viruses affect the heart muscle.

If you have to take a break for more than a week, remember to ease yourself in gradually when you start exercising again.

Well, if that's about as much as you can take, why not take five?

Take heart

Although it is wise to take all these sensible precautions, we must return to the fact that the risks of not exercising are much greater than the risks of taking regular vigorous exercise. Occasionally, someone dies of a heart attack while jogging; but he might have died ten years earlier without exercise. And think of all the people who die while lying in bed: nobody seems concerned that that's dangerous (although it is if you do it for days on end).

Death during recreational exercise is very uncommon. It has been estimated to account for 4.46 deaths per 100 000 of the male population per year in Rhode Island. Most of these deaths are due to coronary heart disease and, of course, this book is all about preventing that.

How much exercise do I need?

This apparently simple question has generated much debate among researchers. Does the exercise have to reach a particular intensity before it does any good? Or can you make up for low intensity by doing it for longer? What's the minimum you can get away with?

I mentioned that heavy work, in Dr Paffenbarger's study of San Francisco dock workers, was defined as using more than 8500 calories a week at work. Well, you would need to walk or run over 85 miles (137 km) a week to burn up all those calories. Could you fit that into your leisure time? Don't worry. Other studies have shown much more realistic schedules to be beneficial.

Your aim should be to get fit and stay fit. By doing this, you will significantly reduce your risk of coronary heart disease.

Two scientists (Wenger and Bell) tested a range of different exercise programmes to see how good they were at getting people fit. The programmes differed according to the intensity, frequency and duration (in minutes) of the exercise sessions, and the length (in weeks) of the programme. Monitoring the heart rate (as described above) is a simple means of measuring intensity. They found that the benefit increased progressively as the frequency and duration of the exercise sessions and the length of the programme went up. Other researchers have confirmed this.

If you are finding it difficult to lose weight, despite improving your diet and walking briskly for 30 minutes a day, you may need to work the duration up to 60 minutes. Sometimes it is more convenient to divide your daily exercise into two sessions.

Very intensive exercise should not be a daily routine. You need a day to recover after a vigorous workout, so three times a week is ideal.

ACTION POINTS

◆ Take 20–30 minutes exercise a day (e.g. brisk walking)

◆ Always increase exercise time and intensity gradually

◆ Don't get too breathless to carry on a conversation

◆ Stop exercising if you get pain, nausea, dizziness or palpitations

◆ Stay within your target range

◆ Warm-up and cool-down

◆ Drink plenty of water

◆ Don't take vigorous exercise straight after a meal

◆ Avoid strenuous exercise while you're unwell

Does a half-hearted effort do any good?

Wenger and Bell found that the intensity of the exercise had to be at least 50% of the individual's maximum capacity to provide effective fitness training. As long as this minimum intensity is reached, it looks as though you can make up for a lower intensity of aerobic exercise by doing it for longer.

A sensible aim would be to spend half an hour a day, on six days of the week, on an activity that gets your heart rate into your target range. Apart from all the benefits of being fit, you would cut your risk of heart disease in half – and that's nothing to be half-hearted about!

What sort of exercise should I do?

You should do some form of **aerobic exercise** that you can keep up for at least 20 minutes without stopping. Aerobic exercise is any activity in which the large muscles in the arms and legs are moving rhythmically; the muscles use more oxygen so you have to breathe more frequently and deeply to get extra oxygen into the blood; the heart works harder to increase the delivery of oxygenated blood to the muscles.

'Anaerobic' exercise refers to 'static' or 'isometric' muscular effort: instead of moving rhythmically, the muscles strain against resistance.

Examples are weightlifting and tug-of-war. This sort of exercise can increase muscle strength but is no help to you in the prevention of coronary heart disease. It should never be done instead of aerobic exercise but is an optional extra for fit people. Those who already have coronary heart disease should avoid anaerobic exercise.

Exercise your choice

There is a wide range of aerobic activities for you to choose from. Here are some examples.

- Walking

- Running/jogging/running on the spot

- Climbing stairs

- 'Aerobics' and 'step aerobics'

- Cycling/using a stationary exercise bike

- Swimming

- Rowing

- Dancing

- Tennis/squash/soccer/rugby football/basketball, etc.

- Skating

- Skiing

To be effective, your aerobic exercise needs to be done several times a week and kept up. It clearly helps if you enjoy it but it also needs to fit into your daily routine. There aren't many people in a position to go skiing that often.

Swimming is excellent if you can do it; drowning is not helpful. It's never too late to learn. A supervised swimming pool is, of course, safer than rivers, lakes or the sea. Because of the support provided by the water, swimming is particularly useful for people with problems such as back pain, arthritis or obesity. It's a great family activity too. Mind you, unless you have your own swimming pool, you need to be well organised to go often enough to make this your main form of exercise.

Dancing could be anything from a slow waltz to an all-night party.

Ballroom dancing can provide useful exercise, especially for older people; unless you are very unfit, you will need something more vigorous than a waltz to stretch your cardiovascular system. I used to like disco dancing but would rarely be seen at a club these days. I will confess, strictly in confidence, that I enjoy dancing to disco music in the privacy of my own home – often using a step to increase the intensity.

Music certainly makes any repetitive movement more fun. Avoiding monotony in your exercise routine is more than half the battle. For some people an aerobics class is the answer. Others, like me, prefer to strut their stuff away from the public gaze. There's no shortage of workout videos; my wife seems to have most of them. To be fair, she uses them. I've no objection to watching American fitness guru Kathy Smith in her leotard, but I prefer a less structured workout. Do what suits you.

Sex? Yes, even sexual intercourse is exercise. But remember: you're aiming for at least 20 minutes of rhythmic activity. In fact, the average union of a married couple is considered equivalent to no more than climbing two flights of stairs. That won't satisfy the heart.

Squash is not a game for the unfit. Once the competitive spirit takes over, you don't realise how hard you're pushing yourself. An investigation into 60 sudden deaths connected with squash playing, reported in the *British Heart Journal* in 1986, showed that coronary heart disease was the certified cause of death in 51 cases. You may have been a superb squash player in your youth but fitness has a short shelf life; by the time your racquet has collected dust gradual retraining is due.

Fit in 30 minutes a day?

So, having chosen my aerobic exercise, I could get fit in 30 minutes a day; but how can I fit in 30 minutes a day? Days are too short.

This can be a real problem. Usually, though, once you've decided that exercise is important to you, you can work out ways of fitting it into your schedule.

In the first edition I explained how I would get home from work in the evening, put the kettle on, and pedal the exercise bike for 20 minutes or so while watching TV. Well, since then we've invested in a high-quality treadmill and I've changed my routine. I get up earlier and do over 30 minutes' brisk walking on the treadmill (watching early morning TV) before having my shower. I find it easier to keep going energetically for half an hour on the treadmill than on the exercise bike. This routine works better for me because I can keep to it seven days a week (and still get up later at weekends).

Sometimes I use the exercise bike as well, doing intermittent upper body exercises while pedalling. (Yes, I can ride my exercise bike 'no hands'.) I'm under no illusion: this routine won't turn me into an athlete; but, so far, it's been enough to keep me alive.

Do you remember the study by Wenger and Bell that showed increasing benefit as the frequency and duration of exercise were stepped up? Aim for half an hour a day; if you can do more, so much the better – 20 minutes three times a week is the bare minimum.

Now it may suit you better to do your exercise in the evening. Or perhaps you have exercise facilities at work and you can go in your lunch hour. If you stay in hotels a lot, there may be a gym or swimming pool but you can always dance, skip or run on the spot in the privacy of your room. The important thing is to find a formula that suits you. If you choose something that is extremely inconvenient or unpleasant, there is very little chance that you will keep it up. That's pointless.

If you stick to your routine, your brain will assist by producing morphine-like hormones (endorphins), which can help to get you hooked on exercise. There are a few people for whom exercise has become the sole purpose of their existence, resulting in social dysfunction. I'm not advocating that!

In addition to my treadmill routine, I try to snatch a few minutes of activity here and there throughout the day. After all, our bodies are designed to move but modern technology – which provides us with cars, escalators, washing machines and remote controls – spares us (or denies us) activity at every turn. There are lots of ways that you can put some movement back into your life. Here are some of them.

- Use stairs instead of lifts and escalators. If you must use an escalator, walk as well.

- If it's not far, forget the car.

- When you do use the car, park and stride: park well away from your destination (which is often easier) and walk the rest.

- When you use public transport, ride and stride: get off a stop earlier, or forget the taxi from the station.

- Go to work on your legs, not on an egg. (Sorry if I've baffled younger readers.) Walk to work if you can.

- Buy a large dog and train it to throw sticks for you.

- If you have children, prise them away from the TV or computer and play energetic games with them. Children, too, are suffering the consequences of inactivity these days.

I won't suggest that you do all your washing by hand or generate your electricity with a treadmill; but you can use your ingenuity to put technology in its place. It is an irony that technology contrives to spare us our every move with no end of labour-saving schemes, yet bids to save us from decaying through disuse with high-tech exercise machines.

One high-tech device you may find useful is a pedometer. It's worth buying a reliable model; you don't want one of those dodgy ones that credit you with 400 steps for driving the kids to school. If possible, before you part with your money, check it counts 30 steps correctly (choosing a short circular route so you don't get arrested for shoplifting).

The recommended 10 000 steps a day is roughly five miles. If, like many people, your daily routine doesn't take you above 6000 steps, adding a 30-minute brisk walk could get you up to the target.

Exercise is easy: you can walk it

Unlike me, you may be able to get all the vigorous activity you need without any exercise machines. (As well as the bike and treadmill, we have a huge 'multi-gym' at home; you wouldn't believe the exercise I get dismantling it and humping it around every time we move house.)

Brisk walking is hard to beat. Although many of us have forgotten this, it can actually be used as a means of transport. Make sure you have good, comfortable shoes. Aim for a speed of four miles per hour (6.4 km/h) if you are able-bodied. Start at a very gentle pace if you are unfit and gradually increase the Frequency, Intensity and Time of your walks until you are **FIT**.

How can you tell how fit you are? Well, for a start, if you haven't been physically active in your job or your leisure time, you can confidently say you are unfit without doing any sort of exercise test. On the other hand, if you are a keen athlete doing regular training, you will be fit and no doubt have a slow resting heart rate to confirm it. A 'normal' resting heart rate is around 72 beats per minute; very fit people may have a rate below 50 beats per minute. (If you have a resting

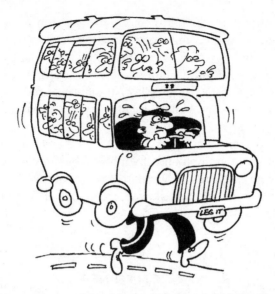

You can use your ingenuity to put technology in its place.

pulse of 40 beats per minute but get tired walking from the kitchen to the lounge, your slow pulse is unlikely to mean you are fit; it's more likely you have 'heart block' and might benefit from a pacemaker. See your doctor!)

There are various standardised exercise tests designed to measure your fitness level. For example, the Canadian Home Fitness Test involves stepping up and down two 10 cm (4 in) steps at a speed that depends on your age. Either a metronome or a prerecorded audiotape giving one beat per step is used to set the pace. The pulse is taken after three minutes and very unfit people have to stop then; others continue for a further three minutes and the fitness rating depends on the pulse at that stage.

Most readers attempting this would probably have to make do with steps of the wrong height and, without an age-appropriate prerecorded tape, it would be impossible to get the speed right. These factors would completely invalidate it as a standardised fitness test and I think it would be positively unhelpful to provide you with a score table.

What you can do, though, is to document your improvement as you train. Using any steps that you have at home (such as the bottom two stairs or a proper aerobics step) and stepping up and down at a fixed rate (such as the beat of a particular piece of music) you can take your pulse after three and six minutes. As always, stop if you have any warning symptoms, become too breathless to converse, or find your pulse above your target range after three minutes. As long as you keep the conditions exactly the same on each occasion, you can make a valid comparison of your fitness level at different times. As you train, your resting pulse – and your pulse after a standard amount of exercise – will slow down.

Yes, getting fit and staying fit can be a walkover. Learn complicated exercises and sports physiology if you wish, but all you need to *learn by heart* is your *target range*. No matter what your walk of life, if you can include 30 minutes of brisk walking in your daily routine, you'll soon be there.

ACTION POINTS

◆ Choose an enjoyable aerobic exercise that fits into your daily routine

◆ Use stairs, not lifts and escalators

◆ Use legs more and wheels less

Chapter 21

Smoking

'A custom loathsome to the eye, hateful to the nose,
harmful to the brain, dangerous to the lungs, and in the
black, stinking fume thereof, nearest resembling the
horrible Stygian smoke of the pit that is bottomless.'

JAMES I (James VI of Scotland) (1566–1625)
A Counterblast to Tobacco, 1604

Like the 'wisest fool in Christendom', as James I was dubbed, most people realise that smoking is bad for you. Few understand how bad.

◆ Everybody knows smoking is bad for you; few understand how bad

◆ Smokers have more heart disease, artery damage, strokes, cancer, bronchitis, emphysema, osteoporosis and wrinkles

◆ Smoking in pregnancy harms the baby

◆ Smoking doesn't just increase risk; it is always harmful

◆ Pipe smoking is a bit less dangerous than cigarette smoking – but only if you've never been a cigarette smoker

---

Smoke alarmism?

If you are a smoker, you may feel persecuted. Non-smokers, like me, constantly bemoaning the social evils of the weed make it ever harder to have a relaxing cigarette in public without sensing the icy glare of someone's disapproval. We fill people's heads with the notion that even passive smoking is more dangerous than bungee jumping. In pursuit of our moral crusade, you tell yourself, we dramatise the dangers of this time-honoured pleasure.

After all, it was back in the sixteenth century that Sir Walter Raleigh came across those fine flowering plants from the genus Nicotiana. What was anyone supposed to do with a find like that? Isn't it only sensible to take a bunch of the dried leaves, roll it in a piece of paper, stick it in your mouth, and set fire to it – then inhale the smoke?

The truth is that, with over 4000 different chemicals now identified in that smoke, it would be a hard job to exaggerate the ill effects of smoking. They are so far-reaching. Here are a few facts.

- About 114 000 deaths in the UK each year are related to smoking.

- Approximately half of these deaths are caused by damaged arteries.

- Smokers are much more likely to die of a heart attack than non-smokers. The more you smoke, the bigger the risk. INTERHEART showed a clear stepwise increase in risk as the number of cigarettes smoked went up. Smoking up to five cigarettes daily increased the risk of a heart attack by 40%; 40 a day increased it by a massive 900%.

- Risk factors multiply: raised blood pressure or high cholesterol are much bigger hazards in a smoker.

- Smokers are more likely to have a stroke.

- The death rate from aortic aneurysm (weakness in the wall of the body's main artery, which can result in fatal haemorrhage) is ten times higher in men smoking more than 25 cigarettes a day than in non-smokers.

- Blockage to arteries in the legs leading to pain, and even gangrene and amputation, is not an uncommon problem but it rarely arises in those who have never been smokers.

- Women over 35 taking the oral contraceptive pill have a very low risk of suffering a heart attack or stroke – unless they smoke!

- Like heart disease, cancer (of which there are many types) is a major killer. Lung cancer is one of the commonest forms and is caused by smoking; it's very rare in non-smokers.

- Apart from lung cancer, smoking is to blame for many other cancers as well. Cancers of the lips, mouth, throat, larynx (voice box), oesophagus (gullet), bladder, kidney and pancreas are all more common in smokers.

- Chronic bronchitis and emphysema – serious lung diseases that can lead to sufferers fighting for breath – are caused by smoking in the great majority of cases.

- Smoking in pregnancy is extremely harmful; it results in a smaller baby with a reduced chance of survival.

- Osteoporosis, in which the bones become brittle, is made worse by smoking. A study published in the *British Medical Journal* in 1997 concluded that women who continued to smoke after the menopause were more likely to break their hips; by the age of 80, the risk was 71% higher in smokers.

- Digestive problems in smokers range from reduced ability to smell and taste food through to difficulty healing duodenal ulcers.

- Wrinkles are an outward sign of the accelerated ageing processes throughout a smoker's body. In fact, 'smokers face' has been described in the *British Medical Journal*; it features increased wrinkling and wasting of the skin together with grey discoloration.

Are you putting up a smoke screen?

Did you hear about the smoker who read a very persuasive article about the dangers of smoking? It affected him so deeply that he gave up – reading, I mean. Sometimes smokers say they enjoy smoking and don't want to stop. After all, this sounds better than admitting that you can't stop. Unfortunately, when you hide behind a smoke screen, you end up fooling yourself.

There are lots of other arguments that smokers put forward in the hope of convincing others, and themselves, that it's reasonable to continue smoking.

Any smoker will draw comfort from the sprightly 85-year-old who smokes 20 a day and still outwalks his old dog on the way to the pub. No wonder this exceptional example is imprinted on the memory and invoked whenever the hazards of smoking are raised. It's far more comfortable, of course, to forget all those who died in their fifties or spend the last miserable year of life attached to an oxygen cylinder. I would like to make two additional observations: (a) this fortunate pensioner would have been fitter still without cigarettes – perhaps running a marathon, and (b) the dog has very little incentive to get to the pub.

Understandably, many smokers are concerned that they will put on weight if they stop smoking. A small weight gain may occur initially (both because of a change in metabolism and because some people eat more). Weight gain is certainly not inevitable, even though you may find food tastier and more enjoyable as a non-smoker; following the advice in this book will allow you to control your weight – permanently. But to suggest that you might as well keep smoking rather than put on weight is complete nonsense. You'd have to gain about ten stone before it started to match the risk of smoking 20 a day!

Then there's the argument that says: 'I might be knocked over by a car tomorrow, so why worry about the dangers of smoking?' Of course, it's true that any of us could be killed on the roads but, as a smoker, it's overwhelmingly more likely that your death will be caused by smoking; you may even combine the two spectacularly and have a heart attack while driving.

This idea that smoking is a risk but it's a gamble you're prepared to take is another piece of self-deception. Smoking is often depicted as a game of Russian roulette: if you're unlucky you get lung cancer, but, if fate smiles on you, you get off scot-free. Rubbish. The smoker always incurs a penalty; damaged health is a certainty.

We cannot predict which smokers will die before the age of 60 from a heart attack or a stroke or cancer. But you don't need a crystal ball to see that any smoker's body would function better if it weren't being poisoned.

It's an unfortunate fact that many people do give up smoking – after they've had a heart attack. Many others don't get the chance to think again at that stage. Bismarck wisely said, and I'm paraphrasing the German here, 'A fool learns from his mistakes; I learn from other people's mistakes.'

The age of innocence

I have every sympathy with older folk who took up smoking at a time when the dangers weren't appreciated. Although James I had made an accurate assessment almost 350 years earlier, it wasn't until about 1950 that science made the connection between smoking and lung cancer. Since then, so much more has been learnt about the deadly path that smokers are on. What a tragedy that young people still flock like lemmings to join them!

'I never smoked a cigarette until I was nine,' protested W C Fields, apparently.

Children, of course, will always experiment. I cannot have been more than nine myself when I acquired a plastic pipe from a Jamboree Bag and thought what fun it would be to smoke tea leaves in it. I only tried it the once. Young people often find their first cigarette unpleasant, but peer group pressure ensures they persist until they've mastered the weed – or rather, it's mastered them.

Meanwhile, the cigarette makers hide behind platitudes about the individual's right to choose. They shield themselves with spin-doctors (medically qualified in some cases) employed to conceal or confuse the conclusions of research. This smouldering fuse is running out: surely manufacturers are soon to be smoked out to face an army of the aggrieved, all making claims for compensation.

To the young, though, middle age and ill health seem remote. If you tell a teenaged girl that smoking will kill her, she'll probably laugh a lungful of smoke in your face; but if her boyfriend tells her he'd rather kiss an ashtray, that'll get her worried.

Don't the young and impressionable deserve protection from the greedy – from those who glamorise this ghastly deathtrap? Why would legislators hesitate?

'This vice brings in one hundred million francs in taxes every year. I will certainly forbid it at once – as soon as you can name a virtue that brings in as much revenue.'

NAPOLEON III (1808–73), French emperor

Just a pipe dream?

Smoking doesn't just shorten your life – it shortens your cigarettes. Even so, giving up may seem too hard. Perhaps you've thought about changing to a pipe to reduce your risks. It is true that pipe and cigar smokers who have never smoked cigarettes have a lower risk of heart

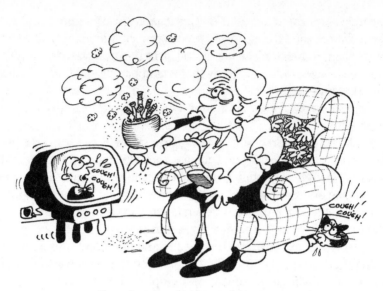

Changing to a pipe is not the answer.

disease than cigarette smokers. That's because those who've always smoked cigars or a pipe usually don't inhale the smoke; not surprisingly, they still have high rates of mouth cancer.

Perhaps you've already made the change from cigarettes to a pipe and now congratulate yourself on doing what you could to help your heart. Unfortunately, pipe smokers who've switched from cigarettes continue to inhale. And a scientific paper on the risks of 'secondary pipe smoking' would give you no comfort at all. Put that in your pipe and smoke it.

The big smoke

Whatever you choose to put in your pipe, it will be hard-pressed to beat the range of toxins released by burning tobacco. Of course, I don't really recommend changing to a different fuel; at least the tobacco smoker has the benefit of intensive research into the diseases he is inducing.

The 4000 or so different chemicals in tobacco smoke include well-known poisons such as arsenic, cyanide and benzene. **Free radicals** speed up ageing processes (such as thinning and wrinkling of the skin) as well as damaging the lining of arteries and triggering production of cancer cells. Quite a number of **carcinogens** (cancer-producing substances) have been identified in tobacco smoke, not to mention the many chemicals with unknown effects.

Some ingredients of the smoke act as **irritants** in the lung, provoking increased mucus production and paralysing the lungs' self-cleaning mechanism. Other chemicals are absorbed into the bloodstream and carried all round the body. Two of these – **nicotine** and **carbon monoxide** – are known to be particularly important.

Nicotine reaches the brain within a few seconds of inhaling tobacco smoke and is largely to blame for a smoker's dependence on cigarettes. This is why nicotine replacement therapy can help you to stop smoking. Nicotine has some effects on the circulation, constricting blood vessels and raising the heart rate. Sometimes people worry about the dangers of nicotine therapy – in pregnancy, for example. But it's far safer to take nicotine by itself than in combination with over 4000 other chemicals in cigarette smoke; and much better than failing to quit.

Carbon monoxide, of course, is the silent killer that strikes when the flue on a domestic gas appliance malfunctions; people just wake up dead. It is now removed from car exhaust fumes, which are no longer used for suicide (except in soap operas). No doubt it plays a key role in the deaths of millions of smokers. Oxygen is carried round our bodies by the red pigment in blood called haemoglobin. Carbon monoxide can combine with haemoglobin more easily than oxygen can (to form carboxyhaemoglobin). As a result, the blood is able to carry less oxygen to organs such as the heart and brain.

The combined effects of nicotine and carbon monoxide increase the heart's requirement for oxygen while reducing the supply. In addition, the clogging of arteries with fatty deposits is accelerated and (because of effects on platelets and fibrinogen) the blood clots more easily. It would be difficult to design a drug that paved the way for a heart attack more efficiently.

Do unto others . . .

Roy Castle, the much-loved entertainer, died of lung cancer. He was not a smoker. During his years in show business, he'd been subjected to an awful lot of smoke from other people (especially in smoky clubs).

'Passive smoking', or involuntary smoking, is dangerous. A Japanese study published in the *British Medical Journal* in 1981 showed that the non-smoking wives of heavy smokers had an increased risk of lung cancer. Since then, many research teams have confirmed the higher rate of lung cancer in non-smokers living with smokers. An analysis of 37 published studies was reported in the *British Medical Journal* in October 1997. The conclusion was that living with a smoker increases a non-smoker's risk of lung cancer by 26%. In addition, cancer-producing substances from tobacco can be found in the blood and urine of these involuntary smokers.

Coronary heart disease, too, is commoner in passive smokers. It is true that there is more nicotine and carbon monoxide in the 'side-stream' smoke (which comes off the end of the cigarette) than in the 'mainstream' smoke (which is drawn through the cigarette by the smoker). Even so, the extent of the risk to non-smokers has been an unwelcome surprise.

The evidence from 19 published studies of heart disease risk in life-long non-smokers who live with a smoker was analysed in the *British Medical Journal* in 1997. The risk of coronary heart disease in these involuntary smokers was 30% higher than the risk in non-smokers who did not live with a smoker.

It turns out that studies of this sort have underestimated the dangers of passive smoking. Non-smokers who don't live with a smoker are frequently exposed to cigarette smoke outside the home. In an investigation published in the *British Medical Journal* in 2004, researchers used a sensitive blood test (serum continine level) to give an accurate measure of exposure to cigarette smoke. They found that passive smoking raised the risk of coronary heart disease by 50 to 60%. Research published in *Circulation* in 2007 demonstrated that passive smokers had raised blood levels of homocysteine and fibrinogen – two substances linked with an increased risk of heart disease. One estimate blames passive smoking for 62 000 heart disease deaths a year in the USA.

Despite the inevitable bleating of the tobacco industry, the dangers of environmental tobacco smoke are established beyond doubt. Employers have a clear duty to provide a safe working environment for their employees. July 2007 saw the introduction of the smoking ban in England (following bans in Scotland, Wales and Northern Ireland), making it illegal to smoke in nearly all enclosed public spaces and workplaces. Dangers aside, most non-smokers find it very unpleasant, or even disgusting, to breathe in second-hand tobacco smoke.

Smoking parents put their children at risk. Smokers' children are more likely to suffer sudden infant death syndrome ('cot death'), respiratory infections, asthma attacks and middle ear problems. Children with a smoking parent are also more likely to become smokers themselves.

◆ The 4000 chemicals in cigarette smoke include nicotine, carbon monoxide, free radicals and substances that cause cancer

◆ Living with a smoker increases a non-smoker's risk of lung cancer by 26%, and of heart disease by 30%

◆ It has been estimated that passive smoking causes 62 000 deaths from heart disease every year in the USA

◆ Smokers' children suffer more asthma attacks, respiratory infections, ear problems and cot deaths; they are more likely to become smokers

Is it too late to stop?

No. It's never too late to give up smoking. Perhaps you think the damage has already been done and, yes, if you've been smoking for years, a lot of damage has been done. But a lot can be undone. In a study on British doctors, the increased heart disease risk from smoking was cut in half in the first two or three years after stopping; after 10 years the risk had returned to that of a non-smoker! Some benefit is immediate. For a start, you'll be supplying the blood with oxygen instead of carbon monoxide. And the increased risk of blood clots is soon reversed.

If you have already developed chronic bronchitis or emphysema, you can't undo the lung damage; but it is essential to stop smoking immediately or you will go downhill fast.

Smokers who already have coronary heart disease have everything to gain by giving up (cigarettes, I mean, not the will to live). If you have already had a heart attack, you are much less likely to have another one if you stop smoking.

Kicking the habit

If you are a smoker, and in your right mind, you want to kick the habit before you kick the bucket. Most smokers would like to stop. But it's not that easy, is it? Millions have done it, though, and there's no reason why you shouldn't join them.

Here is a plan that can help you do just that. This approach has already helped thousands to become successful ex-smokers.

Ready . . .

So, you're ready to stop smoking. Congratulations. Realising that smoking is bad for you and deciding that you'd like to stop just won't do. You must decide that you are *going to stop* and that you are ready to do it now.

Steady . . .

Hold it right there. Don't throw away your cigarettes just yet. I know. Once you've made the decision to stop, you want to get on with it right away, before you change your mind. If you prepare yourself properly before you stop, you are much more likely to succeed.

Fix the date when you will become a non-smoker – one or two weeks ahead. It could be an ordinary working day or at a weekend. Don't choose a day when you will be under extra pressure.

Tell people about your decision, especially friends who don't smoke; they can be a great support. The more people you tell, the more committed you will feel. If a friend or colleague wants to give up with you, so much the better. A smoking partner will make life much more difficult for you and it really is ideal to give up together. Joining – or even setting up – a self-help group and working through this programme with others is often more successful than going it alone.

Make a list of all the benefits you will enjoy as a non-smoker. Put it on your dressing table or by your dentures or wherever else you can read through it every day. This should be your own personal list but it might include any of these:

- I will age less quickly – inside and out;

- I will be putting oxygen into my blood, instead of carbon monoxide;

- I will feel generally more healthy;

- I will be better at sport;

- I will reduce my risk of heart disease, cancer, stroke, bronchitis and emphysema;

- I won't have bad breath, yellow fingers, smelly hair and smelly clothes;

- I will have less trouble with catarrh, coughs and chest infections;

- I will be able to smell and taste my food better;

- I will have more money to spend on other things;

- I will no longer be a nuisance and a health hazard to others;

- I will not damage my unborn child;

- I will not provoke asthma attacks, catarrh and ear infections in my children;

- I will no longer be encouraging my children to smoke;

- I will be more attractive;

- I will feel more in control.

Keep a 'smoking diary' – a record of every cigarette you smoke – for one week before you stop. This can be either a little notebook or simply a piece of paper but it must be kept with your cigarettes.

It is helpful to make out a chart for each day (Figure 15). Whenever you reach for a cigarette, simply note the time, what you are doing, who you are with, and how much you feel you need that cigarette. Complete this before you smoke the cigarette.

It will soon become clear if you smoke every time you have a coffee, or go to the pub, or meet your lover. Work out how you will avoid each of these situations when you stop smoking. Rating the importance of every cigarette shows you where you will need to be extra careful.

Try to analyse why you have smoked each cigarette. Is lighting up a pure habit – something you do automatically? Or is there a real craving, which starts soon after the last cigarette? Perhaps tension is a trigger and you use cigarettes as a way of trying to calm yourself down.

During this week or two of preparation, you can start cutting out the cigarettes that are easy to avoid. I'm not recommending cutting

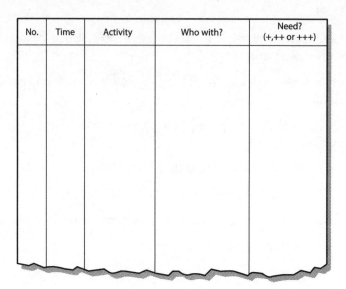

No.	Time	Activity	Who with?	Need? (+,++ or +++)

Figure 15 A smoking diary. Keep a record of every cigarette for a week
before you stop.

down as a way of giving up; it usually fails. After all, you are going to become a non-smoker on the chosen date. In the meantime, when you are offered cigarettes, you can practise refusing and explaining what you are doing. Anyone who teases you or tries to force cigarettes on you is someone to avoid. You may find it helpful to put an elastic band round your cigarette packet, possibly retaining your smoking diary, so you have to think twice before taking a cigarette.

·You can collect your cigarette ends in a glass jar (but make sure the marmalade is finished). Each evening hold the jar, have a good smell, meditate on the disgusting contents, and rejoice that you will soon be rid of all this.

Stop!
When your chosen day arrives, your waking thought will no doubt be 'What's that strange bleeping noise?' Once you've realised that it's the alarm clock, and it really is time to get up, your next thought should be 'I'm a non-smoker now!' Yes, this is your first day as a non-smoker. Of course, that's not strictly true: you were actually born a non-smoker. (If God had intended anything else, why would he surround us with water in the womb?) Today you will return to your natural state.

Bleary eyes permitting, read through the list of benefits you will now enjoy as a non-smoker. Have a good stretch and tell yourself that you don't need to smoke, and you don't want to.

Perhaps the postman will bring you some cards from supportive friends, congratulating you on becoming a non-smoker or, at least, from yourself, if you were thoughtful enough to post some the day before.

You must now live as a non-smoker. Rid your house or flat of cigarettes, lighters and ashtrays. Ask other people not to smoke in your home.

If you get a strong craving for a cigarette, don't worry. That intense feeling won't last very long. Go and get a glass of water or a raw carrot, or mow the lawn, or take the tortoise for a walk. Take a long, deep breath and think of all the lovely oxygen you're getting into your lungs; breathe out slowly and dwell on the deadly carbon monoxide you're getting rid of. Repeat the deep breathing until the craving has passed.

You are expecting some withdrawal symptoms; you know that your body has got used to a regular supply of nicotine. Cravings, irritability, headaches and sleep disturbance are all common but settle as the body readjusts itself over a couple of weeks. Some people don't notice any withdrawal symptoms.

What about nicotine patches? Nicotine replacement therapy, with skin patches, chewing gum, nasal spray, or inhalator, can be very helpful – especially for heavy smokers with strong cravings. You can now obtain these preparations on an NHS prescription. All that nicotine patches can do is to smooth out the physical withdrawal from nicotine. Plenty of people who are determined to stop smoking sail through the nicotine withdrawal without patches. On the other hand, those who think the patches will be a simple solution often fail. Don't expect them to patch up worn-out will-power. They won't.

Zyban (bupropion) won't give up smoking for you either, but it is helpful for some smokers who are determined to stop. It works on chemical pathways in the brain that are involved in nicotine dependence. Zyban isn't suitable for people with epilepsy, eating disorders or certain psychiatric conditions. The tablets are normally taken for two months and smoking is continued until the 'quit date' – usually the eighth day. Champix (varenicline) is an alternative drug that also acts on receptors in the brain to relieve nicotine craving and withdrawal.

It's essential that drug treatment is combined with some form of emotional support. Ask your doctor or pharmacist about local NHS services for smokers. Apart from nicotine dependence, you are dealing with a habit – a behaviour that has been automatic for some years. The habit can still haunt you long after you've got through the physical withdrawal from nicotine. This is where your smoking diary comes in. Avoid activities and situations that were strongly linked with smoking.

Here are some guidelines that are particularly important in the first two weeks after you stop smoking.

- *Avoid alcohol* You probably think this is a really rum suggestion. Your spirits need lifting more than ever, now that you're coping with nicotine withdrawal, and I suggest going without alcohol as well! The long and the short of it is that most smokers light up when they drink alcohol. Also, alcohol anaesthetises the will-power.

- *Avoid coffee and tea* This might seem to add insult to injury, but check your smoking diary. How often do you drink tea or coffee without smoking? If you have reached for your cigarettes every time you've had a coffee, day after day, year after year, you'll be making it very hard for yourself if you keep drinking coffee while adjusting to life as a non-smoker.

- *Drink plenty!* There are lots of suitable drinks – such as water, fruit juice, diluted fruit juice, squash and herbal tea. You must keep well hydrated.

- *Change your ways* Use your smoking diary to avoid being trapped by routines that were strongly linked with smoking. If you would normally light up at the end of your evening meal, get up; wash up, if necessary, but don't sit there missing your cigarette.

- *Weigh your change* Or, at least, collect the money you would have spent on cigarettes – perhaps in a glass jar. You'll soon have enough to treat yourself to a celebratory meal out – and now you can enjoy it without being tormented by cigarette smoke!

- *Change your weight* Yes, if you need to lose weight, there is no reason why you shouldn't do so after giving up smoking by making sensible changes in your diet (see Chapter 18). Above all, there is no need to succumb to the weight gain that everybody fears. Have plenty of healthy snacks to hand (such as raw carrots, celery sticks, sugarsnap peas, apples) and avoid comforting yourself with sweets and biscuits. Whenever you're not sure what to do with your hands, get a glass of water.

● *Wait, you'll change!* At this stage, you may think 'I can't go on like this, craving after cigarettes for months on end'. But it's not like that. If you can get through one day as a non-smoker, you can get through every day. Just take one day at a time. Like Old Nick himself, nicotine holds many in bondage; but you are breaking free, and you'll soon change from being an addict to being in control.

You've given up now. Don't give up now

It was Mark Twain who pointed out that it was easy to give up smoking – and that he had done it hundreds of times.

Now you've come this far, the last thing you want is to throw it all away. There's far too much at stake. You are a non-smoker now. Here are a few filtered tips to help you stay that way.

◆ The sooner you stop smoking, the better. But it's never too late to stop

◆ In the British Doctors Study, the increased risk of heart disease in smokers had disappeared 10 years after stopping

◆ If you already have bronchitis, emphysema or heart disease, stopping is even more urgent

◆ Benefits of giving up include: ageing less quickly; feeling better; reducing the risk of cancer, heart disease, stroke and chest problems; being more attractive; tasting food better; having less catarrh; saving money

◆ If you follow this programme, you could join millions of successful ex-smokers

- **A**void smoky social situations. Alcohol makes things worse by lowering your resistance. A party is a recipe for disaster. And beware the temptress, sending smoke signals across the room.

- **B**rush up daily on your list of the benefits that are building up now you've become a non-smoker. Brush your teeth thoroughly each morning – if you have any (teeth, I mean, not mornings) – and bethink how beautifully fresh your breath is becoming.

- **C**ontracts can help to strengthen resolve when cravings or irritating symptoms such as coughing come along. Consider a contract with yourself or a colleague, confirming your commitment to remain a non-smoker, come what may. Coughing can be a nuisance when you stop smoking but don't be tempted to treat it with a cigarette! Cilia are the microscopic hairlike growths that normally keep the lungs clean but have been crippled for years by smoke. Clearance of conglomerated muck commences as the cleaning system gets to work again; coughing is a sign of recovery.

- **D**istance yourself from smokers, now you are a non-smoker. Don't despise smokers, but do consider developing a discussion group for those who decide to drop the habit. Don't duck the issue, but decline cigarettes decidedly by declaring 'I don't smoke' and don't dither with 'Er, well, I'm trying to give them up'.

- **E**xercise regularly (but not excessively). Exacting experiments have exposed the fact that those who exercise are extra likely to remain ex-smokers.

- **F**ailure frequently follows from falling for 'just one fag' – perhaps as a reward for giving up so successfully. Five cigarettes later, all your good intentions have gone up in smoke!

Chapter 22

Blood pressure

Millions of people in the UK have high blood pressure, and many of them don't realise it. Blood pressure is a major risk factor: the higher your blood pressure, the greater your risk of stroke, heart attack, heart failure and kidney disease.

How can I tell if my blood pressure's high?

Some people assume their blood pressure is OK because they feel fine. Others think their blood pressure must be high because they have headaches or feel hot or get flushed. The inconvenient truth about blood pressure is that it simply doesn't declare itself like that.

Going red in the face might indicate all sorts of things but is often, quite wrongly, taken to be a sign of high blood pressure.

> **'I always take blushing either for a sign of guilt, or of ill breeding.'**
>
> **WILLIAM CONGREVE (1670–1729)**
> ***The Way of the World*, 1700, Act 1, Sc. 9**

You can have a very high blood pressure with no symptoms. You can have a normal blood pressure and feel terrible. The only way to find out your blood pressure is to measure it; everyone should have this done.

Perhaps it would be more convenient if we could monitor our blood pressure by the way we were feeling, but measurement of blood pressure these days is not nearly as inconvenient as it used to be. The first recorded measurement of blood pressure was carried out by an English clergyman called Stephen Hales in 1733. He connected a main artery from a horse to a vertical glass tube, using the windpipe of a goose. Blood rose to a height of eight feet three inches. I've seen some pretty antiquated surgeries in my time, but I'd be very surprised if your doctor has ever suggested doing this to you. Measuring blood pressure still involved cutting an artery right up until 1896 when Scipione Riva-Rocci introduced the arm cuff.

Nowadays, of course, checking your blood pressure couldn't be more straightforward. It's simpler than checking your cholesterol level – or even your bank balance in many cases. It's quick and cheap – and could save you, and the Health Service, a lot of trouble and expense in the future. It's painless: all you feel is a brief squeeze on the upper arm. And, at a time when the Health Service is feeling the squeeze, that seems a small price to pay.

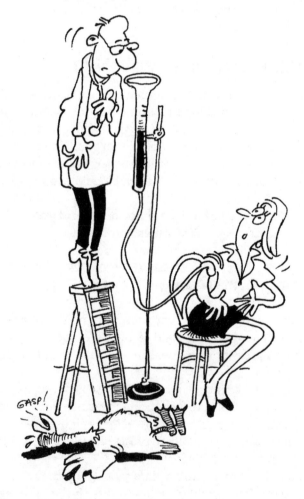

GASP!

I'd be very surprised if your doctor has suggested doing this to you.

◆ Blood has to be under pressure in order to circulate

◆ High blood pressure increases the risk of strokes and heart attacks
   – the higher the pressure, the higher the risk

◆ You might feel fine with a high blood pressure or terrible with a
   normal blood pressure

◆ All adults should have their blood pressure checked

Measurement of blood pressure

Your blood pressure results from the pump at the heart of your circulation forcing blood through a network of narrowing arteries. Your heart is a muscular pump that squeezes blood through one-way valves with every beat. It's a thankless task. Anyone who had a heart would feel at least a wave of sympathy on reflecting that it beats about 100 000 times a day, but if it so much as rests for just a few seconds, all hell breaks loose. Imagine trying to work the muscles in your legs this way. It takes a dedicated muscle to keep going like that – for life – and the heart muscle is specially adapted to the task.

This kind of pump could not maintain a completely steady pressure. Blood pressure rises to a peak level as the heart contracts, and falls to a minimum as the heart relaxes to refill with blood. Of course, the heart's one-way valves prevent any backward flow. You can feel for yourself the surge of pressure with every heartbeat; it is felt as the pulse in one of

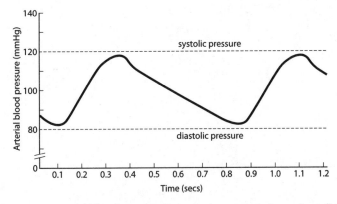

Figure 16 Arterial blood pressure. Pressure rises to a maximum (systolic)
and falls to a minimum (diastolic).

your arteries. So your blood pressure rises and falls as a wave – constantly varying between peak and trough (Figure 16). The **squeezing** phase of the heart's cycle is called **systole**; the **downbeat** phase in which the heart relaxes and **draws** in more blood is called **diastole**.

What does all this have to do with measuring blood pressure? Everything. You can now understand why two numbers have to be noted, and why the peak pressure is called the *systolic* and the minimum pressure the *diastolic*. The instrument used to measure these pressures is called a *sphygmomanometer* – at least, by those who can say it (Figure 17).

Figure 17 shows a traditional instrument that uses a column of mercury to indicate pressure. The cuff, which is wrapped around your upper arm, contains a tubular balloon that can be inflated, applying pressure to the brachial artery in your arm; this pressure is shown in 'millimetres of mercury' (mmHg).

The doctor or nurse taking your blood pressure will blow up the cuff enough to squeeze the walls of the brachial artery together so that no blood flows past that point. Don't worry. The cuff is then slowly deflated – long before your arm turns black – while any noises in the artery are detected with a stethoscope. The moment the cuff pressure falls below the systolic pressure in the artery, blood will push audibly past the cuff, and the operator will note the level of the mercury column at that moment – the systolic pressure in mmHg.

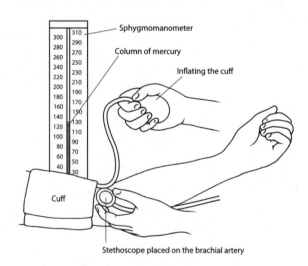

Figure 17 A traditional mercury sphygmomanometer.

As the cuff pressure is gradually reduced further, the tapping sound of blood forcing its way through the squashed artery will continue to be heard through the stethoscope. After all, as long as the cuff pressure is greater than the minimum artery pressure (the diastolic), the artery walls will be squeezed together between heartbeats – only to be forced apart again as the pressure rises in systole. The moment the cuff pressure falls below even the diastolic pressure, the artery will remain open all the time; the tapping sound of blood forcing the artery open disappears. At this point, the height of the mercury column is noted – and that gives the diastolic pressure in mmHg.

The systolic pressure reading (the high number) is written on top and the diastolic pressure reading (the low number) underneath. So, if your systolic pressure were 120 mmHg and your diastolic 80 mmHg, your blood pressure would be written down like this:

$$\text{Blood Pressure (BP)} = \frac{120\,\text{mmHg}}{80}$$

Your doctor or nurse would say that your blood pressure was '120 over 80'.

Safety in numbers?

Can a couple of numbers really be so important to our health and safety? The evidence is clear: the lower those numbers, the smaller the risk of a stroke or heart attack. As the average blood pressure falls, risk keeps on falling with it – right down to the point where you fall over. Obviously, you don't want your blood pressure that low. In other words, the lower your blood pressure, the better – as long as it's not so low that you suffer symptoms like falling over or feeling faint or dizzy.

And both numbers are important. Persistent elevation of either the diastolic or the systolic pressure increases the risk – even if the other number is normal.

Your blood pressure is constantly regulated by a complex system involving enzymes, hormones and nerves. Occasionally, high blood pressure is caused by some underlying disorder (such as a disease of the kidneys or adrenal glands). But in the great majority of cases no cause can be found; this is called 'essential hypertension'.

Genes play their part and a tendency to high blood pressure can run in families. Whatever your genetic background, your lifestyle can make all the difference. Eating too much salt, drinking excess alcohol, and being overweight or inactive can all push up your blood pressure.

If you have high blood pressure, you may also have other features of the metabolic syndrome. The numbers on that tape measure are crucial too, remember. Reverse the metabolic vicious cycle and get your waist measurement right down; your blood pressure will probably go down with it (see Chapter 18).

◆ The maximum pressure is called systolic and the minimum is called diastolic

◆ Both systolic and diastolic pressures are important

◆ Most cases of hypertension are 'essential' – no cause is found

◆ Sometimes high blood pressure runs in families

◆ Hormones and the nervous system are constantly regulating blood pressure

◆ Blood pressure is raised by eating too much salt, drinking excess alcohol, being overweight and not exercising

---

What if my number's up?

At last you get round to seeing your doctor to have your blood pressure checked, only to be told 'It's a bit up, I'm afraid'. If your reading's up, don't let it get you down. And don't give up. It's not over yet!

For a start, Table 21 will help you figure out your numbers.

Could it be a wrong number?

Phoney numbers are all too possible if careful attention is not paid to maintenance and correct use of the sphygmomanometer. The mercury column has been used to measure blood pressure for over a hundred years and I've seen a few instruments that looked as if they were there at the beginning. It's impossible to obtain accurate readings if the manometer is not properly calibrated or if the top of the mercury column is hidden behind oxidised mercury on the inside of the glass.

Electronic instruments that bleep and flash may seem more state-

Table 21 Blood pressure measurement

	Systolic pressure (mmHg)	Diastolic pressure (mmHg)
Ideal	under 120	under 80
Normal	120–129	80–84
Borderline	130–140	85–90
Raised	over 140	over 90
High	over 160	over 100
Very high!	200+	110+

of-the-art but that doesn't automatically make them more accurate. If you are thinking of buying one of these devices to check your own blood pressure, choose one that has been validated according to standards set by the British Hypertension Society (BHS) or the Association for the Advancement of Medical Instrumentation (AAMI). You can find information about validated instruments on the BHS website (www.bhsoc.org).

Automatic electronic blood pressure recorders are extremely easy to use and they eliminate the 'observer error' that occurs with mercury manometers. No doubt electronic devices will soon replace mercury instruments altogether, not least because mercury is considered an environmental hazard.

Even the most accurate of blood pressure readings is merely a snapshot – a record of one moment in a constantly changing scene. Your blood pressure varies throughout the day and probably falls to its lowest level while you're asleep. Anything from being in a hurry to having a very full bladder will push it up temporarily. It's the 'resting blood pressure' that counts; try to arrive in plenty of time for an appointment at the surgery so you can sit calmly for a few minutes before your blood pressure is taken. Of course, if you sit there fuming because the doctor's running late, this won't help at all.

You can see how misleading a single measurement of blood

pressure could be. A series of readings, taken on different occasions, allows decisions to be based on the average or mean blood pressure.

The mean machine

Think how useful it would be if there were a machine that would tell us the mean blood pressure over a 24-hour period of normal activity.

There is. The computerised ambulatory blood pressure monitoring machine is worn, usually for a period of 24 hours, while getting on with normal life. It automatically records the blood pressure at programmed intervals – usually every 30 minutes. Not only does this provide the mean systolic and diastolic pressures, it also allows analysis of the pattern of blood pressure variation during the 24 hours. For example, it seems that people who do not show the normal drop in blood pressure overnight ('non-dippers') are at increased risk.

These 24-hour blood pressure monitors are particularly useful for identifying those with so-called 'white coat hypertension'. These people have normal blood pressures most of the time. But as soon as someone comes along to measure the pressure, it shoots up. For most of these people, the blood pressure will go up whether the doctor is actually wearing a white coat or not, although it is said to occur a little less often when nurses take the reading (but I'm sure it all depends on what gets you going). It's completely normal to be a little apprehensive about seeing a doctor or having your blood pressure checked and this certainly doesn't mean that your blood pressure will necessarily be high. Even so, it may be that up to 20% of those with high readings actually have 'white coat hypertension'.

Those clever 24-hour machines cost around £1500 each so don't be surprised if your doctor isn't using one on everybody.

Cost is not the only good reason for restricting the use of these machines at the moment. Another problem is that most of the research that has enabled us to decide what levels of blood pressure are risky enough to require treatment has relied upon the conventional method of measuring blood pressure. We cannot assume, for example, that someone who always has high blood pressure readings at a clinic is necessarily at very low risk simply because a 24-hour record looks fine. When 24-hour recording has been used in more long-term studies, we will be clearer about its value in assessing risk. In all probability, as more data are gathered, this high-tech investigation will become routine.

Are you due for an age rise?

When you get to a certain age, lots of things start dropping. Blood pressure isn't one of them. I recall being told at medical school that the normal systolic blood pressure was given by 100 plus the person's age (120 mmHg at age 20; 160 mmHg at age 60). This rise in blood pressure with advancing age is so common in our society that we have come to regard it as normal.

Rural communities that have not adopted a westernised lifestyle escape this age-related rise in blood pressure. Their low-salt diets can take much of the credit.

◆ A blood pressure of 120/80 mmHg or less is ideal; 160/95 mmHg is high

◆ Blood pressure tends to rise with age but not in communities with extremely low salt intakes

◆ Readings on at least 3 separate occasions are needed to indicate the average blood pressure

◆ A 24-hour blood pressure monitor can help to identify 'white coat hypertension' (in which readings are only high in the surgery or clinic)

What does high pressure do to you?

We have seen that people with high blood pressure are more likely to suffer a stroke or heart attack. Why?

The wall of an artery is made up of three layers: a tough, fibrous, outer sleeve; a muscular, elastic middle layer; and a smooth inner lining. This smooth, low-friction lining is delicate; it can easily be damaged by the wear and tear of blood flow under pressure. Minor scuffs are soon put right by the body's maintenance service. But constantly raised blood pressure is more punishing and cholesterol builds up on damaged areas of the artery lining. When this process affects the coronary arteries, angina and heart attacks may follow. Narrowing of arteries in the brain can lead to a stroke; a haemorrhagic stroke, in which a damaged artery bleeds, is more likely when the pressure is high.

There are other ways, too, in which constantly high blood pressure can damage organs. After years of working extra hard, the heart's main pumping chamber (the left ventricle) can become enlarged and, eventually, heart failure may occur. Eye damage can result in impaired vision or blindness. Long-term effects on the kidneys may lead to kidney failure.

Can treatment really help?

We know that strokes and heart attacks are more common among those with high blood pressure. But this doesn't necessarily mean that lowering blood pressure will reverse the risk. The prevalence of train spotting may be higher among men wearing anoraks; but we cannot be sure that keeping them dressed in suits will reduce their train spotting. Raised blood pressure could be an anorak – an outward sign of a deeper problem within. Suppose it reflected a hidden metabolic disturbance, like insulin resistance, which was the real cause of strokes and heart attacks. Treatment of blood pressure could then be very disappointing.

Fortunately, we now have strong evidence from clinical trials that lowering blood pressure with any of the commonly used drugs reduces the risk of a stroke or heart attack.

Of course, it's not a case of most people having 'normal blood pressure' while a few are afflicted with 'high blood pressure'; it's a continuous spectrum. So how do we decide when someone has the medical condition of 'hypertension'? The late Professor Geoffrey Rose came up with a practical approach, defining hypertension as 'the level of blood pressure above which treatment does more good than harm'.

To treat, or not to treat?

That is the question being asked by doctors in every surgery up and down the land. The patient has returned for a fourth blood pressure check and, yet again, the reading is high. Should drug treatment be started?

If you have a mean blood pressure of around 200/110 mmHg, your doctor will, quite rightly, want to get it down quickly. You are likely to need drug treatment and it should not be unduly delayed.

On the other hand, if your blood pressure is more moderately raised, you may be able to avoid the need for drug therapy by making the right lifestyle changes (see below).

When there is no urgency about the situation, your doctor is likely to let you try to reduce your blood pressure without drugs for at least three months. If some progress has been made in that time, it's well worth trying for longer.

If your systolic pressure remains above 160 mmHg, or your diastolic above 100 mmHg, your doctor will probably recommend drug treatment. When raised blood pressure has already caused heart, kidney or eye problems, treatment would be started at lower levels of blood pressure (systolic 140 mmHg; diastolic 90 mmHg). If your blood pressure is staying between 140/90 mmHg and 160/100 mmHg, but you have no problems with your kidneys, eyes, heart or circulation, and no diabetes, your risk of having a heart attack or stroke is now used to decide whether or not to prescribe blood pressure treatment. Current guidelines recommend drug treatment if your risk of suffering from cardiovascular disease in the next ten years is at least 20% (see Chapter 25).

What difference does diabetes make?

If you have diabetes, it is even more important to avoid high blood pressure; your doctor will be trying to keep your reading below 140/80 mmHg. Diabetes is bad for the arteries, and one of the main aims of managing diabetes is to reduce the risk of heart disease. There is now strong evidence that people with diabetes do better if blood pressure is well controlled.

Managing high blood pressure

Management of blood pressure is not, in fact, just a numbers game – even though it was sometimes seen that way in the past. High blood pressure is a very important risk factor but it's not the only one. The aim is to treat the whole person – not the numbers on a digital device. Doctors realised a long time ago that high blood pressure is not a disease of the left arm. All risk factors need to be addressed.

Whether you need drug treatment or not, you must also change your lifestyle. Not only does this make your drug treatment more effective, and perhaps limit the dose you need, it also works in other ways to protect your heart and circulation.

Once you have started drug treatment of high blood pressure, you will normally need to continue for good. It's not a cure. You don't take a drug for a couple of months and settle your blood pressure forever. Occasionally, though, if significant lifestyle changes are made after treatment has been started, the drug can be stopped without your blood pressure returning to its previous high level. Of course, you must not stop your medication on your own because that is highly dangerous. Discuss it with your doctor who will want to keep an eye on your blood pressure, especially if any change in treatment is advised.

◆ Constantly high blood pressure is bad for arteries, and can damage your heart, brain, kidneys and eyes

◆ Lowering raised blood pressure reduces strokes dramatically and heart attacks significantly

◆ If you have diabetes, it is even more important to control high blood pressure

◆ Very high blood pressure should be controlled quickly and drugs will be needed

◆ Mildly raised blood pressure may respond to lifestyle changes without drugs

Drugs used to treat high blood pressure

Doctors today have a wide variety of drugs (see Table 22) that bring down blood pressure.

In fact, the first four letters of the alphabet could provide a useful mnemonic if you wanted to remember all the important classes of drugs used to treat high blood pressure:

ACE inhibitors
Angiotensin receptor blockers
Alpha-blockers

Beta-blockers

Calcium channel blockers

Diuretics

> ◆ Lifestyle changes reduce the risks, whether drugs are used or not
>
> ◆ Drugs have side effects, but it is usually possible to find a treatment that controls blood pressure without side effects

Table 22 Classes of drugs

Class of drugs	Examples
ACE inhibitors (angiotensin converting enzyme inhibitors)	captopril, cilazapril, enalapril, fosinopril, imidapril, lisinopril, moexipril, perindopril, quinapril, ramipril, trandolapril
Angiotensin receptor blockers	candesartan, eprosartan, irbesartan, losartan, olmesartan, telmisartan, valsartan
Alpha-blockers	doxazosin, indoramin, prazosin, terazosin
Beta-blockers	acebutolol, atenolol, bisoprolol, celiprolol, metoprolol, nadolol, oxprenolol, pindolol, propranolol, timolol
Calcium channel blockers	amlodipine, diltiazem, felodipine, isradipine, lacidipine, lercanidipine, nisoldipine, nicardipine, nifedipine, verapamil
Diuretics	Bendroflumethiazide, chlortalidone, hydrochlorothiazide, indapamide, metolazone, xipamide

Diuretics

Thiazide diuretics lower blood pressure by encouraging the kidneys to excrete more sodium and water, and by relaxing the muscle layer in artery walls.

Beta-blockers (beta-adrenoreceptor blockers)

The eminent Nobel Prize winner, Sir James Black, has made several landmark contributions to medicine. After all, he was my professor of pharmacology when I was an undergraduate at University College

London. Not only that, but he developed the brilliant idea of beta-blockers while he was working at Imperial Chemical Industries. Propranolol was the first one that could be taken by mouth and it is still in widespread use today. Since its birth in the sixties, there has been a beta-blocker baby boom. (I am referring to the many new beta-blockers, and not suggesting that these drugs boost fertility!)

These drugs block some of the body's responses to adrenaline and similar chemical messengers; they slow the heart rate but also lower blood pressure by reducing the output of renin.

Calcium channel blockers

This is not a reference to chalk cliffs collapsing into the Channel Tunnel. It's the name given to a group of drugs that block the passage of calcium through channels in cell membranes. The effect of this is to relax the muscle in artery walls, making the arteries wider and reducing resistance to blood flow.

ACE inhibitors

Don't get this term confused with the ACE *vitamins*: any drug that inhibited the action of those vital antioxidants would be little help to us in our battle against coronary heart disease. No, the full name of this family of drugs is *angiotensin converting enzyme inhibitors*. They hinder the activity of the renin-angiotensin system. As a result, artery walls become more relaxed and the kidneys allow more sodium into the urine.

Angiotensin receptor blockers

Like ACE inhibitors, the angiotensin receptor blockers work on the renin-angiotensin system but they block the angiotensin receptor instead of interfering with the production of angiotensin II. These drugs provide a useful alternative to ACE inhibitors (especially for people who develop a persistent dry cough on an ACE inhibitor).

Alpha-blockers (alpha-adrenoreceptor blockers)

These drugs make blood vessels dilate (get wider) by relaxing muscle tissue in their walls.

Side effects

All these drugs cause side effects in some people. Beta-blockers can trigger wheezing and must be avoided by people with asthma.

Diuretics sometimes provoke gout and, like certain beta-blockers, can have unwanted effects on the lipid profile. Calcium channel blockers may cause ankle swelling. Some people get a dry cough when using ACE inhibitors. Sometimes drugs used to treat blood pressure make it more difficult for a man to get an erection. Why suffer in silence? In fact, if you think your treatment is causing any side effects, please tell your doctor; it may well be possible to change to something that suits you better.

How does a doctor choose a drug?

Confronted with a patient with high blood pressure, and such a wide choice of drugs, how can a doctor make a rational choice? Let me immediately assure you that this is not merely a question of which pharmaceutical representative has just taken your doctor out to lunch. These days, most GPs are very well informed about the therapeutic options.

Diuretics and beta-blockers are the traditional first choices and, it must be said, most of the evidence that treating raised blood pressure is beneficial came from research using these drugs.

When NICE issued guidelines on treatment of hypertension in 2006, news reports led to a lot of confusion. Some patients thought beta-blockers had been declared dangerous or even banned. Beta-blockers are still very helpful for some people with high blood pressure, and NICE said nothing to contradict that.

Important evidence, which NICE took into account, came from the Anglo-Scandinavian Cardiac Outcomes Trial (ASCOT) which compared traditional treatment for hypertension with newer drugs. We know that reduction of blood pressure with a beta-blocker and diuretic prevents a lot of strokes and heart attacks; ASCOT showed that treatment with a calcium channel blocker and ACE inhibitor (amlodipine and perindopril) does the job more efficiently, producing a bigger reduction in cardiovascular complications and total mortality.

It's not that beta-blockers cause strokes, as some people thought after reading newspaper articles: beta-blockers are not as good at preventing strokes as some other drugs used for hypertension. Another very important finding is that people taking a beta-blocker, particularly in combination with a diuretic, are more likely to develop diabetes than those treated with a calcium channel blocker or ACE inhibitor.

So now, a beta-blocker wouldn't normally be the first drug we would choose to lower blood pressure, unless there's another good reason to use a beta-blocker (such as angina or a previous heart attack, a rapid heart rate, or migraine).

It's a matter of tailoring the therapy to fit the patient. For someone under 55, an ACE inhibitor would often be first choice. But black people tend to have low renin levels and respond less well to an ACE inhibitor (unless it's combined with another drug); a calcium channel blocker or diuretic may work better. The doctor is likely to start with a diuretic or calcium channel blocker for someone over 55, especially when there is isolated systolic hypertension.

Whichever drug is chosen first, it is often necessary to add others. If the combination of ACE inhibitor, calcium channel blocker and diuretic fails to control blood pressure, adding a beta-blocker will often be a good move. Alpha-blockers, as well as lowering blood pressure, relax the muscles at the outlet of the bladder. This can be very helpful for men with prostate symptoms, and disastrous for people with incontinence.

Good control of blood pressure without side effects can normally be achieved.

Should I take aspirin?

Aspirin reduces the risk of forming a blood clot in the circulation (thrombosis) and that's why a low dose (75 mg a day) is recommended for those who already have heart disease or have had a stroke caused by a blood clot in the brain. Also, some research suggests that aspirin can reduce the chances of developing certain cancers.

A lot of people have heard these claims and take an aspirin with their cornflakes just to be on the safe side. The trouble is that taking an aspirin every day increases the risk of bleeding – particularly from the stomach. If you have already suffered a thrombosis in an artery, the small risk from taking aspirin is overshadowed by the benefit. But if you've never had a problem with your circulation, the risk from taking the aspirin might be bigger than the risk you're trying to reduce. Wearing a steel bucket over your head could reduce your risk of being killed by a freak missile, but that's no use if you get run over because you can't see where you're going.

What if your only problem is high blood pressure – which does raise that risk of having a stroke or heart attack? You may have been confused by media coverage of one study showing that people with high blood pressure were protected by aspirin, followed by reports highlighting the risk of brain haemorrhage when people take aspirin if they have high blood pressure.

Well, aspirin is hazardous if the blood pressure is poorly controlled. The thing to do is to weigh up the risks and tip the balance in your favour. Above all, get high blood pressure (and other risk factors) under control. If you have high blood pressure, it's a good idea to take aspirin (75 mg daily) if *all* of these are true:

- you are at least 50 years old;

- your blood pressure is now well controlled (below 150/90 mmHg);

- you have diabetes OR there are already signs of blood pressure affecting your heart, kidneys or eyes OR your risk of a heart attack or stroke is at least 20% in ten years (see Chapter 25);

- aspirin doesn't upset you.

It's possible that the beneficial effects of aspirin on the circulation are cancelled by taking the anti-inflammatory drug ibuprofen at the same time. Researchers at Mount Sinai School of Medicine investigated the outcomes of using various drug combinations in high cardiovascular risk patients who also had osteoarthritis. In a randomised trial published in *Annals of the Rheumatic Diseases* in 2007, they found that patients who took ibuprofen as well as aspirin were nine times more likely to suffer a heart attack. In any case, combining anti-inflammatory drugs with aspirin increases the risk of stomach irritation and should be done only under medical supervision.

A lifestyle to lower the pressure

Making the right changes to your lifestyle may avoid the need to take blood pressure-lowering drugs altogether. If your blood pressure is normal now, the healthy lifestyle will help to keep it that way. When drug treatment is necessary, lifestyle remains crucial: getting it right helps the drugs to work better and protects your heart in other ways. If your doctor has prescribed a drug for your blood pressure, you must never stop it without medical advice.

Here is the **SAFE** way to lower your blood pressure. There are now many good studies to show that each of these changes can reduce blood pressure.

Salt

Cut down gradually and your palate will adjust to not adding salt in the kitchen or at the table. Season well with herbs, spices, pepper, garlic, mustard powder, vinegar, lemon, etc. Watch out for high-sodium seasonings like soy sauce. Remember that most of the salt consumed by the nation comes in processed foods. Read those labels and use fresh ingredients when possible (see Chapter 7).

Every day, eat at least four portions of fruit and four portions of vegetables (including plenty of pulses) to boost potassium and magnesium intake. Have two or three servings a day of very low-fat dairy products (see Chapter 5) to keep up your calcium.

Alcohol

Excess alcohol raises blood pressure; cutting down reduces it. The maximum allowance on any one day is 4 units for a man and 3 for a woman. But 1 or 2 units (e.g. 1 glass of wine) on most days would be better (see Chapter 11).

Fat

Losing that fat can lower your pressure. In fact one analysis predicts that a weight loss of 12 kg (less than 2 stone) will produce a fall in blood pressure of 21/13 mmHg – a very significant reduction. Of course, in any individual, the actual change in blood pressure will be influenced by other factors (such as salt and alcohol intake) which are changing at the same time (see Chapters 7 and 11).

To reduce body fat, the first move is to eat less fat (see Chapter 18). For the sake of your arteries, avoid saturated fat wherever you can.

Exercise

Move your body and master your pressure. Studies have now confirmed that when physical activity is increased, the resting blood pressure is reduced. Remember to increase very gradually from your present level of activity (see Chapter 20).

The DASH diet

This may sound like fast food for the gulp-and-go gourmet, but the DASH (Dietary Approaches to Stop Hypertension) trial was an

American research project that investigated the effects of different diets on blood pressure. Published in 1997, the study showed that a diet including 8–10 servings a day of fruit and vegetables (much richer in potassium, magnesium and fibre than the typical American diet) could lower blood pressure significantly. And when the calcium content of this diet was boosted by the addition of two or three servings a day of low-fat dairy products, the reduction in blood pressure was almost doubled. A follow-up study published in 2001, the DASH Sodium Trial, confirmed that the DASH diet lowered blood pressure most efficiently when combined with a low salt intake.

Following the general principles of the DASH diet, researchers went on to test three diets that contained different proportions of carbohydrate, protein and unsaturated fat. In the OmniHeart Study (Optimal Macronutrient Intake Trial for Heart Health), the higher-carbohydrate diet derived 58% of its calories from carbohydrate and was similar to the original DASH diet. This was compared with two diets in which 10% of the calories from carbohydrate were replaced with calories from either protein or mono-unsaturated fat.

All three diets produced improvements in blood pressure and lipids, representing a worthwhile reduction in heart risk. But the diets higher in protein and in mono-unsaturated fat achieved even better results than the carbohydrate-rich diet.

To improve your blood pressure now and in the future, follow this **SAFE** plan for salt, alcohol, fat and exercise. Don't forget to include at least eight servings of fruit and vegetables, and three servings of very low-fat dairy products, every day for maximum benefit.

Of course, it's important to support the **SAFE** plan to lower your pressure with the other recommendations in this book to protect your heart. In particular:

- Eat oily fish at least twice a week (but watch out for the added salt content of tinned fish). There is evidence that high doses of fish oil can reduce blood pressure and, in one study, giving fish oil was more effective when combined with salt restriction;

- Don't smoke! Your blood pressure goes up when you smoke a cigarette and, of course, the long-term effects of habitual smoking are disastrous.

And, if the pace of life is a problem, the next chapter, which deals with stress, should help to ease the pressure too.

ACTION POINTS

◆ Have your blood pressure checked (unless you have had a normal
reading in the last year)

◆ Follow this SAFE plan for salt, alcohol, fat and exercise:

  ● Eat at least eight servings of fruit and vegetables (including
  plenty of pulses) every day

  ● Have three servings of very low-fat dairy products a day

  ● If you have been prescribed a drug for high blood pressure,
  take it regularly and never stop it without medical supervision

Chapter 23

Stress

'Stress . . . The overpowering pressure
of some adverse force or influence.'

The Shorter Oxford English Dictionary

Is stress a cause of heart disease?

What is stress and how do we know whether one man's stress is bigger than another's? How do we measure it?

Is the busy business executive more stressed than the dustman – or is the executive thriving on challenges while the dustman is frustrated by lack of control over his life? Clearly, if you can't measure stress, or identify those with a lot of it, you can't tell whether the more stressed get more heart disease.

An early attempt to resolve this was made by Friedman and Rosenman in the 1950s when they developed their famous theory of personality types. The classification was simpler than ABC – just A and B, in fact. The type A person is hard-working, competitive, aggressive, impatient, never satisfied and always in a rush. He's the guy who finishes all your sentences for you because you take too long to find the right word. And he always turns the toilet roll to face the 'right' way. On the other hand, the type B personality is non-competitive, easy-going and relaxed.

Of course, this classification is a little too simple to accommodate the full range of humanity: most of us will display both type A and type B behaviour at different times. Even so, you can probably think of people who fit firmly into one category or the other.

A study of 3524 men aged 39–59 classified them according to personality type and studied the history of their heart disease over eight years. This was reported by Rosenman and colleagues in 1975 as the Western Collaborative Group Study. The researchers made an adjustment for the main risk factors (such as smoking) and concluded that those with a type A personality had double the risk of heart disease.

Later research found a much weaker link between type A personality and heart disease. Out of twelve studies reviewed by Kornitzer in 1992, seven showed no connection between type A personality and coronary heart disease.

A follow-up on the men in the Western Collaborative Group Study, after 22 years, in 1988, is astonishing. As a risk factor, type A personality appeared to have done a U-turn. The men who had developed heart disease in the first eight and a half years of the investigation had a lower death rate – one-third lower – if they had been labelled type A rather than type B at the outset!

What could have changed since the 1970s? In some studies, different methods of identifying type A behaviour may be relevant but this would not apply to the Western Collaborative Group Study. It could well be that the no-nonsense, high-achieving type A people have taken messages about healthy living to heart and been more successful at making lifestyle changes.

◆ Aggressive type A behaviour is bad for your heart but you can change this behaviour and reduce your risk

◆ Achieving goals, including lifestyle changes, can help your heart

◆ Psychosocial stress – such as lack of job control – increases heart risk

---

It probably is bad for your heart (not to mention your social life) to be aggressive, hostile and impatient, but some positive type A characteristics, such as devotion to work, do not appear to raise the risk of heart disease. A certain level of stress is quite normal and healthy, if balanced with relaxation; it can help you to achieve satisfying goals. So don't worry yourself sick about a little bit of stress.

Lifestyle changes can more than compensate for the risk attached to the 'wrong' personality. And, while you cannot transform yourself to become a different personality, you can certainly change the more destructive elements of type A behaviour.

Psychosocial stress

This is nothing to do with a gathering of Alfred Hitchcock fans. It's the term used to refer to stress that results from a person's *psychological* response to difficult *social* circumstances.

Among the women followed for 20 years in the Framingham Study, heart disease was linked with low educational level, low pay, and lack of holidays (even after physical risk factors had been allowed for).

The Scottish Heart Health Study found higher coronary rates in areas of high unemployment.

Having a job can be stressful too. The Whitehall II study reported in the *British Medical Journal* in 1997 involved 10308 male and female civil servants aged 35 to 55.

The researchers concluded that those with little control over their jobs were significantly more likely to develop heart disease. The findings applied equally to men and women. This helps to confirm the conclusions of other investigators. In fact, in a 1994 review, 17 out of 25 studies found a significant link between job control and cardiovascular risk. A study published in the *Journal of Epidemiology and Community Health* in 2007 showed that those experiencing unfair treatment at work had a higher risk of heart disease.

It seems that giving employees more variety in their duties, and a bigger say in decisions about work, could be to the benefit of public health.

◆ Stress releases adrenaline, speeds up the heart and primes the body for 'fight or flight'

◆ Some stress is normal; too much is damaging to health

◆ Stress reduction can help to lower blood pressure

How does the body respond to stress?

Faced with a hungry wolf at the entrance of his family cave, primitive man immediately produced a surge of adrenaline. His heart rate increased and he started breathing faster. This, together with diversion of blood from the skin and gut to the muscles, ensured all muscles were well supplied with oxygen – ready to fight a ravenous predator. No doubt, sudden confrontation by a fierce caveman produced the same stress response in the wolf, boosting its performance for a speedy getaway. Both wolf and caveman released extra fats and sugar into the blood to fuel fast-working muscles.

If he happened upon stampeding elephants, on the other hand, our courageous caveman did not confront them; he used his stress response to effect an escape. Even so, if it came to the crunch, his body had prepared by increasing the clotting power of the blood to min-imise bleeding.

You can see why this stress response is called the 'fight-or-flight' reaction and how useful it is for avoiding disasters. Even in modern life we are occasionally faced with a challenge requiring an immedi-ate physical response; it could be anything from a mugger to a volcanic eruption. But your body may have the same fight-or-flight reaction when you serve a cantankerous customer in a department store. In this case, fighting or running away, or even moderate bleed-ing, won't be very helpful.

And when you are sitting in a traffic jam – adrenaline and cortisol coursing through your arteries, fat and glucose mobilised, muscles primed for action – what is your body to make of it when, half an hour later, the only sign of physical activity is your turning of a few pages of the road atlas in the vain search for a short cut?

Frequent arousal of the stress response, especially without appro-priate exercise, will take its toll on health and, in the long term, raise the risk of heart disease. Of course, the risk will escalate if stress pro-vokes heavy smoking, overeating or excess alcohol consumption. Chronic stress – that is, stress which continues over a long period – can lead to anxiety, depression and a very wide range of physical symptoms (such as palpitations, chest pain, headaches, muscle pains and bowel upsets).

Can stress reduction lower the risk of heart disease?

Raised blood pressure is, of course, one of the main risk factors for coronary heart disease. We know that acute stress pushes up the blood pressure temporarily; it is not so clear whether chronic stress is an important cause of permanently raised blood pressure (hypertension). Several studies have used relaxation techniques, breathing exercises or biofeedback while monitoring blood pressure. Typically, up to ten people would attend sessions for ten weeks, each session lasting an hour or so. A review in the *Drug and Therapeutics Bulletin* in 1989 concluded that these methods could lower blood pressure and that, in some cases, the benefit could be sustained for years.

A study by Friedman and colleagues on people who had survived a heart attack was published in the *American Heart Journal* in 1986. The people who were given special counselling sessions to modify their type A behaviour (in addition to routine care) were less likely to have a further heart attack.

Stress busting

There's no need to be a victim of stress. You're the boss. Don't be fooled into smoking, eating all the wrong things, drinking too much alcohol, or overdosing on caffeine in response to stress. That's letting it get the better of you.

The positive 'arousal' that gives you the energy to achieve your best is good. Negative, energy-sapping anxiety is not. Here is a plan to turn the turmoil of stress into **REST**.

To conquer stress you need:

RELAXATION	Respiration. Breathing is essential
	Relaxation of muscle and mind
	Replay. Got it taped?
	Recreation
	Retiring – to bed, I mean
EXERCISE	
STRATEGIES for STRESS REDUCTION	Stress diary
	Solving problems
	Social skills training
	Sex
	Stroking a pet
	Saving time
TALK	Talking it through
	Taking advice
	Talking therapy

Relaxation

Rest and relaxation are essential. If you don't recharge your batteries, they go flat. This may happen insidiously until you suddenly discover that there's no juice left – just like the car that won't start one winter's morning.

Winston Churchill regularly made time for a rest – even when he had the Second World War to run. The **rest** is history.

'Just relax,' says the doctor, as he approaches you with a long shiny metal thing. It's rather difficult to relax to order, isn't it? Sometimes, the harder you try to relax, the more wound up you become – especially when relaxation is a matter of urgency, so you can fit in a few hours' sleep before making an early start the next day.

Relaxation is a technique that can be learnt. With practice, you get better at switching to relax mode whenever it's called for.

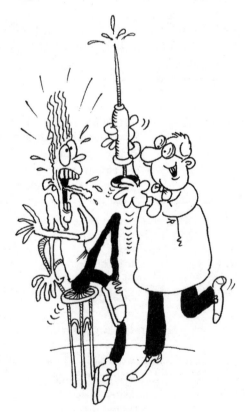

'Just relax!'

Respiration. Breathing is essential

Of course, those of us without respiratory diseases take breathing for granted. You just do it (about 17 000 times a day). You don't need to be told. But the way you breathe directly affects the way you feel – and vice versa. At times of stress, you take rapid, shallow breaths; you sigh and gasp. Regular, leisurely, 'abdominal' breathing helps you to unwind and feel relaxed.

Try placing your right hand on your abdomen – below the rib cage – and your left hand on your chest. Breathe out with a leisurely sigh, allowing all tension to flow away from you, and see the hand on your tummy move inwards. Breathe in through your nose and see how your tummy moves out while the hand on your chest stays still. Your diaphragm is doing its job. Keep breathing through your nose now, gently and calmly. Don't force extra-deep breaths. Let your tummy rise and fall with your body's natural rhythm. Feel the calm come over you as tension drains away.

Now you've got the idea of abdominal breathing, you can do it with your hands in any relaxed position – by your sides or on your lap. A few minutes of breathing like this is a good start to any relaxation exercise but you can also do it on the train, or at the dentist, or waiting for a job interview.

Relaxation of muscle and mind

'Damn braces: Bless relaxes.'

WILLIAM BLAKE (1757–1827)
The Marriage of Heaven and Hell, 1790–3,
Proverbs of Hell

Stress tenses muscles and primes them for action; releasing muscle tension tells the brain that all is well and allows your mind to become relaxed.

For a successful relaxation session you need a comfortable, warm room where you will be undisturbed for at least 20 minutes. You can do it sitting down but it is usually helpful to lie on the bed or floor, with your head supported by a pillow or cushion. If it's at all chilly, you should cover yourself with a blanket.

A relaxation session

Lying on your back, feet apart, arms relaxed at your sides, close your eyes and begin your abdominal breathing. Feel the tension leave you as you breathe out. Imagine the warmth of the sun caressing you as your body becomes heavy and limp. Your breathing becomes naturally slow and peaceful.

Now clench your right fist and tense the muscles of your right arm. This is what tension feels like; concentrate on it for a few moments. Release the tension, let your fingers go loose and feel how warm, limp and heavy the arm is becoming. Repeat this for your left arm.

Tighten the muscles in your right leg, lifting the knee a little. (Don't overdo it if you get cramp easily!) Concentrate only on your right leg. Feel the discomfort of tight muscles. As you breathe out, let the tension go. Feel the leg become heavy and warm as every part of it relaxes. Repeat this with your left leg.

Say 'relax' as you breathe out, and think of the tension ebbing away with each breath.

Lift your shoulders up – right up to your ears. Hold them there. Feel the tension in your chest, your neck and your head. Then, as you breathe out, let more and more of the tension go. Let the full weight of your head and neck sink into the pillow. Relax.

Tense your neck and throat muscles by pushing your head down into the pillow. Hold it for a few moments, then gently let the tension go, bit by bit, until it's all gone.

Pull your shoulders back a little, towards the floor. Notice the tension in the muscles of your back. Let the tension go again, sinking into the floor as you breathe out. Feel warm and heavy.

Pull your tummy in – right in – tensing the muscles of your abdomen. Note how your breathing is pushed up into your chest. Feel the tightness. Then, as you breathe out, let the tightness go. Relax. Let your breathing become calm and natural once again.

Tighten all the muscles in your face. Screw up your eyes, frown and clench your teeth. Feel the tension all over your face, in your jaw and in your head. How uncomfortable this is. How unnatural. Gradually, let all the tension go. Feel the warmth of sunshine on your face as your brow becomes quite smooth again. Let your mouth fall slightly open as every muscle is released.

Let your whole body feel heavy, warm and limp – sinking into the floor. Feel completely relaxed as you breathe gently and calmly, your tummy rising and falling. Now that you are relaxed, let your thoughts take you to a beautiful walled garden. As you enter the garden, smell the sweet aroma of the flowers. Feel the gentle, warm breeze on your face. Hear the birds singing and the brook babbling. Bask in the sunshine. There's nothing to trouble you here. You can come here whenever you want, once you've become relaxed.

When you are ready to leave, let your thoughts take you out of the walled garden. Slowly open your eyes and become aware of your surroundings. Have a really good stretch. Roll onto your side for a little while before getting up.

Replay. Got it taped?

'He who laughs, lasts.'

MARY PETTIBONE POOLE,
A Glass Eye at the Keyhole

Once you've learnt a relaxation exercise of this sort, you don't need any special equipment to practise it. To begin with, though, it's best to use a relaxation tape (or CD) and these are widely available. You could even record the above text if you like listening to your own voice (sad). A calm, soothing voice is much more helpful than a squeaky, tense one. A good professional tape or disk would be a sound investment.

Doing relaxation exercises once or twice a day gives you the best results. You soon become more aware of the tension that creeps into muscles at times of stress – and you know how to release it, with or without a tape.

Talking of audiotapes, it's worth mentioning that anxiety is often provoked by playing back a sequence of negative thoughts – over and over again. Do you sometimes catch yourself thinking 'I'll never cope; it's going to be awful . . . '? You need to stop the 'tape', take the cassette out of your head, and replace it with one full of positive thoughts: 'Of course I'll cope; I'll enjoy it; I've met bigger challenges than babysitting a hamster.' I realise that your worries may not be trivial at all. You may be worried sick about coping with disability or bereavement or about how you will support your family after redundancy. Just the same, the constant playing of negative thoughts feeds anxiety that can well up and hit you in surprising ways. Change the tape.

Recreation

Whether your hobby is gardening, playing Monopoly or rearing stick insects, the diversion is very refreshing and helps to trickle charge your batteries. Listening to music can be very relaxing and if you play an instrument, so much the better. (But, if you're a beginner, a sound-proof room could save some stress in other members of the family.) Where there's life there should be laughter, and a really good giggle is a great boost.

Retiring – to bed, I mean

> **'I love sleep because it is both pleasant
> and safe to use.'**
> ──────────
> **FRAN LEBOWITZ, *Metropolitan Life*, 1978**

Sleep is the ultimate rest (excluding death). If you can sleep like a log it's a great blessing. Sometimes, when stressed, the most we can manage is a few splinters. If you haven't yet twigged the root cause of your insomnia, these tips may help.

- Sleep requires a noise-free environment. If your neighbour uses a chain-saw all night, trying to sleep like a log is bound to go against the grain. Talk to your neighbour (when he hasn't got his chain-saw). If this fails, talk to your local Environmental Health Officer.

- It's difficult to sleep if you're uncomfortable. If you are around six foot six, and trying to sleep in a six-foot bed, is it any wonder you feel a bit hung over in the morning? Is your room too hot or cold? If it's pain that keeps you awake, a painkiller would be more appropriate than a sleeping tablet. (Just a small appendix to that point: I'm assuming here that you know the cause of the pain. But if it's appendicitis, appendicectomy would be more appropriate still.)

- Too much caffeine won't help, so watch the cola, coffee and tea – especially evening coffee. In fact, drinking coffee after 12 noon can interfere with your night's sleep.

- You may drop off easily after a few alcoholic drinks – only to wake early, unable to get back to sleep.

- Regular physical exercise can help you sleep better, but taking it late in the evening can keep you awake.

- An afternoon cat nap of a few minutes can be refreshing. But, just as eating between meals can cause trouble, so daytime sleeps can spoil your 'nappetite' at night. Try to limit them to 20 minutes maximum.

- Going to bed at wildly different times every night doesn't give your body clock a chance to settle down. Try to establish a routine.

- Don't necessarily expect eight hours' sleep a night. Didn't Mrs Thatcher thrive on four? Some people need more than others but we all need less as we get older.

- If an active mind is keeping you awake, do your relaxation exercise (unless the active mind is not your own, in which case ask your partner to stop talking). End up in your beautiful walled garden, or on the beach listening to the breaking waves. It beats counting sheep.

Exercise

Regular physical exercise is a vital part of your stress-busting pro-gramme. You can never really rest unless you've been active, any more than you can wake up unless you've been asleep.

An exercise session gives you an important break and perhaps a change of scenery but, as an antidote to stress, it goes much further than that. Aerobic activity, such as brisk walking for half an hour a day, deals with those stress hormones and burns off the extra fuel released for fight or flight. It also stimulates release of the body's natural tran-quillising proteins – endorphins – which help to bring about a feeling of wellbeing. Whatever you do, build up gradually from your present level of activity (see Chapter 20).

Strategies for stress reduction

There are various steps you can take to reduce the stress in your life.

Stress diary
You may find it helpful to keep a diary for a few days to identify your

main sources of stress. Is your relationship with a particular person causing trouble? Or are there certain events or tasks that you find especially stressful? Of course, on really stressful days, which could provide a lot of information for your diary, you'll be far too stressed to bother with a diary on top of everything else.

Solving problems

Once you've identified the problems, you can set about finding some solutions. A wise friend might see an answer that hasn't occurred to you.

If your wife is always in the bathroom just when you need to shave, getting up 15 minutes earlier could save a lot of frustration.

Or it may be that your husband snores – loudly. In some cases, simple measures such as taking less alcohol, or using a nasal appliance from the pharmacy (for the snorer), or ear-plugs (for the partner), or separate rooms (for the snorer, at least, even if everyone else has to share) will be satisfactory. If not, it's well worth seeking medical help before you end up in separate houses (or get serious complaints from the neighbours).

> **'Laugh and the world laughs with you,**
> **snore and you sleep alone.'**
>
> ———————————
>
> **ANTHONY BURGESS,**
> *Inside Mr Enderby*, 1968

Perhaps your journey to work winds you up, setting you off on the wrong foot. Leaving the house half an hour earlier could make all the difference. You might even be able to change your hours to avoid peak travel times. Consider using a different route, or changing to public transport, or car sharing or, if at all possible, walking to work.

If you get very edgy at work, your stress diary may help you put your finger on the main causes of tension. It could be one person who irks you. Sometimes a frank discussion will sort things out. On the other hand, working practices could be at fault; you may need the help of your union to deal with that.

The feeling that you have no control over the way you work can be very stressful. Remember that studies have consistently shown a link between lack of job control and coronary heart disease. It's not in anyone's interests to have a demoralised workforce with a poor sickness record. The scientific evidence suggests that workers should be given some say in decisions about their work. You are not powerless. A healthy and contented team is a productive team, and everyone wants that.

With any problem, apply the **ABC** of problem solving:

AVOID	*Can I avoid the problem?*	(Avoid rush-hour travel)
BEND	*Can I bend my ways?*	(Wear ear-plugs/get in the bathroom earlier)
CHANGE	*Can I change the problem?*	(Change work practices with the help of the union)

You won't find a perfect solution to every problem but a strategy to handle it better will reduce stress. Don't try to solve everything yourself: the support of friends, self-help groups or professionals can make all the difference.

Social skills training

Have you ever bought a set of encyclopaedias you couldn't afford because the salesman was so persuasive? Allowing yourself to be pushed into unwise decisions can cause a lot of stress. Assertiveness training helps people reduce stress by taking more control of their lives.

Being assertive does not mean being aggressive. Indeed, you will be far more effective if you are calm and polite but unshakeable.

This is one aspect of social skills training. Some people have serious problems when it comes to communicating and dealing with others; they need the special help of a clinical psychologist to learn these skills, but we all have room for improvement.

Do you accept another piece of Auntie Mabel's suet pudding against your better judgement? Many of us become overburdened with commitments because we don't like to say 'No'. Assertiveness training is founded on learning to value yourself. Role-play is used to practise self-assertion – for example, when complaining about a bad meal at a restaurant.

Sex

Satisfying sex soothes stress. Could sex actually save your life? Of course, if it weren't for sex, you wouldn't have a life to start with but does sexual activity prolong life? The Christmas 1997 edition of the *British Medical Journal* carried a paper by Davey Smith and colleagues suggesting that it does. In their study on middle-aged men, the researchers found the death rate to be 50% lower in men declaring frequent sex (twice a week or more) than in those reporting infrequent sex (less than monthly). Both total mortality and mortality from coronary heart disease were lower among those reporting more frequent sex.

Before I'm held responsible for a national earth tremor, or the inevitable baby boom to follow, I must point out that there are many unanswered questions about this study. It would be quite wrong to assume that frequent sex was the *cause* of the lower death rate. For a start, we would expect older men to have sex less frequently than younger men; they are also more likely to die. Again, being depressed, or extremely stressed, will increase your risk of dying: it will also put you right off sex. Further research is needed here.

In the meantime, let me recommend quality sex, in the safe setting of a committed relationship, as a good stress reliever. On the other hand, an extramarital affair increases stress: research has shown that it places a much greater strain on the cardiovascular system; it could provoke coronary death in those at risk.

Stroking a pet
Well, perhaps not the stick insects, but the companionship and physical contact of an animal friend is an effective stress reliever. Research has shown that single people who have had a heart attack tend to live longer if they have a pet. (A hamster is cheaper than a wife and doesn't answer back.)

Saving time
If only you could – save time, I mean. You know, the way you do with money. 'I don't feel like spending this time at the moment,' you could say. 'I'll put it in the time bank for now and spend it when I feel more motivated.'

You could have a time box on the mantelpiece for the odd spare minute; it would soon mount up. And when something had to be done urgently, you'd have all the time you needed put by. As long as you saved time sensibly, and didn't waste time, you could always take time out for leisure activities – just when it suited you.

Sadly, you can't. If you are in full-time employment and have a family to look after, there are never enough hours in the day. If you are unemployed, there may be too many. Both extremes are stressful. The answer is good time management. Here are some simple guidelines.

- Write down a plan for the day, ideally on the previous evening. (I know: you'd write it on a piece of paper.)

- Even if you are unemployed, a structured day is helpful; setting and achieving goals is satisfying.

- If you have too much to do, sort out the priorities. Not achieving goals is stressful.

  1 Some tasks may be important but not at all urgent. Work out the deadlines and plan to do the urgent jobs first.

  2 On reflection, some tasks are unimportant and can be scrapped altogether.

  3 Non-urgent tasks can be extremely important, even though you can't fix a date for the deadline. Making a will is an example; the deadline is very real. Include these tasks in your overall plan or they will always be squeezed out by the urgent things.

  4 Are there jobs on your list that would be better done by someone else? Delegate where appropriate. Hand back the jobs you should never have taken on.

- Make sure you allow enough time to complete each task on your plan for the day. Include time for travel, for the unexpected phone call and for appointments running late.

- Remember that all the routine jobs, such as dealing with your mail, take time and must be allowed for in your plan.

- Set aside time for relaxation and for physical exercise.

- Sometimes you can make better use of time by doing two things at once. While using your exercise bike, you can read a book. I used to play piggy-in-the-middle with my children as I pedalled – but I had to put the book down for that. (They're far too grown up for that now, so I have no-one to play with; in any case, I wouldn't try it on the treadmill.)

- Include time for social activities: playing with your children or grandchildren; sharing with your partner; or, if you live alone, having a drink with a friend or making a social phone call.

- Live a day at a time but have one eye on the longer term so those vital things that aren't urgent don't get left out.

Talk

'The telephone is a good way to talk to people without having to offer them a drink.'

FRAN LEBOWITZ,
Interview magazine, 1978

Talking it through

Have you ever thought that there's no point in talking about a problem because talking doesn't change anything? It isn't true, is it? It can be surprisingly helpful to talk things through with a friend. Even if your friend can't offer a solution, just talking about it helps to sort things out in your own mind.

And so many relationships break down because people allow feelings to fester instead of talking openly, honestly and kindly to each other. The most important words in the language are not, in fact, 'fatty acid' or 'antioxidant' but 'I'm sorry' and 'I forgive you'. Like all words, their power lies in the sincerity of the speaker.

Taking advice

Whatever the problem you are trying to cope with, there is bound to be a voluntary organisation or self-help group that can give you advice. There are always people who have worked through the same problem; they can be a great support.

Don't forget your local Citizens Advice Bureau. And if you are one of the many thousands of people sinking in debt, debt counselling can help you to surface again. Couples who can't resolve their differences should make a date with Relate, the relationship counselling service.

Talking therapy

Talking things over with friends and colleagues, and taking advice from those in the know, is likely to help. Some problems, however, need more formal talking therapy and perhaps the expertise of a psychiatrist, a psychologist or a psychotherapist. Your doctor will point you in the right direction.

If you follow this plan, you can **REST** assured that stress will be kept in its proper place.

ACTION POINTS

◆ Learn and practise relaxation. This chapter shows you how

◆ Replace negative thoughts with positive ones

◆ Develop an interesting hobby

◆ Get regular sleep; avoid excess caffeine and alcohol

◆ Exercise daily

◆ Identify your main sources of stress and apply the ABC of problem solving

◆ Plan your day (see 'Saving time')

◆ Talk and listen to the important people in your life

Chapter 24

The truth about women

'A woman who strives to be like a man lacks ambition.'

Graffito, New York, 1982

◆ Heart disease kills over 4 times more women than breast cancer in the UK

◆ Over 50 000 women die of heart disease each year

◆ Before the menopause, the low rates of heart disease in women are linked with the 'pear' pattern of fat storage, higher HDL and lower triglyceride levels

◆ Low iron stores in women before the menopause may reduce free radical attack on artery walls

---

Inspired by the suffragettes in the early twentieth century, women have protested their right to equality with men ever since. Their demands do not extend to an equal share of heart disease, any more than men have sought a fairer spread of breast cancer. After all, heart disease is a male affliction, is it not? Many women reading this book are concerned about a husband, partner, brother, son or father rather than themselves. And as P J O'Rourke observed, '. . . there is one thing women can never take away from men. We die sooner.'

For all that, the truth is that every year in the UK many more women die of coronary heart disease than of breast cancer – over four times as many. Heart disease kills over 50 000 women a year in the UK. No other single disease takes so many female lives. And yet, many people, including some health professionals, see it as a male disease.

True it is that when you hear of a tragic early death – a friend or neighbour struck down by a heart attack before the age of 50 – it is far more likely to be a man. Occasionally, you do hear the shocking news that a very young woman has died of a heart attack; it usually turns out that she was a heavy smoker. On average, heart disease strikes women a decade later than men.

Mind you, the seed of heart disease is sown in childhood, or even before (see Chapter 16), so it's never too early to adopt a healthy lifestyle.

Perhaps you're thinking: 'Well, I've got to die of something; it might as well be a heart attack. I'd prefer that to a slow death from cancer.' I agree that, given the available options, a quick heart attack seems quite desirable – especially if you could arrange to slip away in your sleep. But we can't make these arrangements and, rather than a quick death, heart disease could bring 20 years of disability. Don't invite it.

Why do women lag behind?

Men often complain that women drive too slowly. They certainly die more slowly – in the sense that, on average, they get round to it later in life than men, and not in the sense that they take longer to do it when the time comes. You could postulate a direct connection between their patterns of driving and dying. I mean, apart from the obvious point about driving more safely, you could focus on the fact that the main reason why women live longer is that they get heart disease later. Could it be that women lag behind both in driving and dying simply because type A behaviour is more prevalent in men behind the wheel, increasing their coronary risk?

It's an attractive theory but it doesn't fully explain all the facts. What about the main risk factors for heart disease? Perhaps lifestyle differences can explain why heart disease hits women a few years later than men. Prepare for a shock. As a sweeping generalisation, compared with men, women:

- Eat more saturated fat (as a percentage of calories);
- Eat less fibre;
- Are less active.

With the passing years, compared with men, women are more likely to:

- Become obese;

- Develop diabetes;

- Have raised cholesterol levels;

- Have high blood pressure.

Once we could at least have pointed to the lower rates of smoking among women. Not now. As the proportion of UK adults smoking cigarettes has dropped, women have clung to their percentage and have just about achieved equality with men – as if bidding for an equal share of smoking-related diseases. And more teenaged girls than boys now smoke.

With all these features pushing up the risk in women, is it not surprising that, on average, they get their heart disease a decade after men? What factors can we find to help explain why women lag behind? Here are some more generalisations about women that will count in their favour:

- HDL-cholesterol levels are higher;

- Triglyceride levels are lower;

- They are more pear-shaped.

We all have some body fat and women have more than men. As well as being an energy store it provides us with thermal insulation like the lagging on a hot-water cylinder. Although most women are very sensitive about the amount of 'lagging' round their bottom and thighs, it's much safer to carry it there; fat round the tummy (central obesity) brings a much higher coronary risk. Now perhaps you understand why women lag behind.

The lipid link

What lies at the bottom of the link between lower body fat and a lower risk of heart disease? Why do those who carry fat higher up have a higher risk? Studies attempting to get to the bottom of this mystery have found that carrying your fat lower down goes together with lower triglyceride levels and higher levels of HDL-cholesterol. This is the typical female pattern. Having a fat tummy – the classic male shape – is linked with the reverse lipid profile (high triglycerides and low HDL-cholesterol), which is much more hazardous for the heart.

An increased waist circumference is an indication of excess visceral fat (see page 186) which is not just lagging but biochemically active blubber, producing a range of unhealthy metabolic changes.

The metabolic syndrome comprises central obesity, high triglycerides, low HDL-cholesterol, raised blood pressure and insulin resistance (in which the body has to produce higher levels of insulin to get a response). Women with the metabolic syndrome, which can lead on to diabetes, have become more apple-shaped, with a high waist-hip ratio, and an increased risk of heart disease.

Don't forget your change

It may be all too easy to walk away from a shop without your change but, for many women, hot flushes and sweats are the frequent reminders that make the change of life unforgettable. This time in a woman's life, during which the ovaries are winding down and a variety of symptoms can result from falling oestrogen levels, is known as the climacteric or perimenopause. The menopause is the point in time when the periods actually stop – or the last menstrual period – but climacteric symptoms can go on for a long time before and after that.

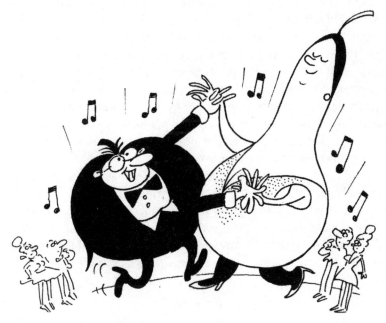

'They say opposites attract.'

Even those fortunate women who sail through the climacteric without any symptoms should not forget that the change is profound.

As oestrogen levels fall, various metabolic changes follow:

- LDL-cholesterol rises at the menopause;

- HDL-cholesterol falls, starting a few years before the last period;

- Changes in fibrinogen and Factor VII make the blood clot more easily.

These changes will all increase the risk of heart disease. However, the idea that the number of deaths due to heart disease *suddenly* increases at the menopause is not correct. There continues to be a steady rise in risk with increasing age.

The Iron Lady?

To leave the role of Prime Minister meant a huge change for Mrs Thatcher, but she had this comfort: her period in office was history – safe in the archives for ever. At the change of life, you have some consolation: your period is now history; you no longer experience the monthly bleed that sapped your strength; your risk of anaemia recedes and your store of iron builds up. But this inner store of strength could make a surprising contribution to your fortunes. It could result in more free radicals (see Chapter 9). Perhaps the slump in oestrogen secretion is the crucial change that pushes up your risk of heart disease. Even so, the danger from free radicals should not be overlooked. Attacking from within, like political rebels reacting to that iron hand, they damage arteries – those vital channels of support – starting a process that could prove fatal.

We all need iron. When you are young, you may lose so much with your periods that you need a supplement to help you to avoid anaemia. After the menopause you can normally obtain all the iron you need from your food, and you'd do well to give iron supplements a miss unless specifically advised by your doctor to take one. Iron shortage can crop up in old age as a result of a poor diet.

◆ Countries with high rates of heart disease in men have high rates in women too; the same risk factors affect both sexes

◆ Angina is as common in women as in men

◆ Women with heart disease are less likely than men to be correctly diagnosed

Heart disease in women

Heart disease is killing an alarming number of women in the UK. In fact, we're right near the top of an international league table – nothing to be proud of in this case.

When we compare the death rates for heart disease in men and women in different countries, several points stand out.

- The death rates are much lower in some countries than in others. For example, the problem in Japan is a tiny fraction of that in Scotland.

- In all countries, the death rates for women are lower than for men.

- Countries with high rates of heart disease in men have high rates in women too; the international rank order for men and women is similar.

- Women in the UK have higher death rates than the men in Japan, France and Spain.

Women are different from men. In particular, they get off to a good start with the protection that oestrogen gives them against heart disease. Comparing rates of heart disease in different countries tells us something very important: high rates in men go together with high rates in women; the rate in women always reflects the rate in men (Figure 18). Clearly, the same risk factors affect both men and women. The very low cholesterol levels in Japan make heart disease uncommon in both sexes. In Scotland, high levels of the risk factors result in high death rates in women as well as men.

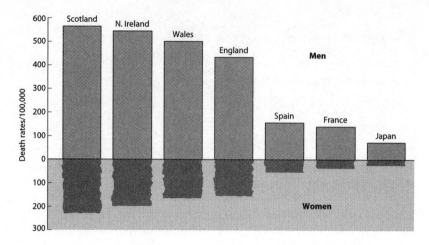

Figure 18 Death rates for heart disease. This chart is like a row of buildings on the water's edge – from the skyscraper full of heart disease victims in Scotland down to the single-storey building in Japan. In every country, the rate of deaths from heart disease in women is a reflection of the rate in men.

This is a vital observation. Even though so much of the research into heart disease has been done on men, we can be certain that women have everything to gain from the advice in this book.

Women who develop coronary heart disease are most likely to get angina. In fact, angina is as common in women as it is in men. Heart attacks occur more frequently in men. Mind you, women often have 'silent' heart attacks: the heart muscle becomes scarred without the normal symptoms of a heart attack.

Women with coronary heart disease actually have a rather worse prognosis than men with the disease. This is partly because the women will, on average, be older and more of them will have complications such as diabetes. It may also have something to do with the widespread myth that heart disease is a male problem. Research has shown that women with heart disease are less likely than men to be diagnosed and treated – even when the symptoms are the same.

Hormone Replacement Therapy

Oestrogen and progesterone – nature's double act

In nature, the opposing actions of these two female hormones produced by the ovaries are finely balanced to regulate the reproductive cycle. After the menopause when the ovaries stop working, reproduction is not an issue (but it might be if a woman ignores the advice to use some form of contraception for a year after the menopause as freak ovulation can occur). At this stage in life, it is the oestrogen that may be sorely missed.

Hormone replacement therapy (HRT) aims to replace the missing oestrogen. If oestrogen is given on its own to a woman who still has her womb, the lining of the womb (endometrium) grows thicker and the risk of cancer (endometrial carcinoma) is increased. This was a problem with early versions of HRT but modern preparations reduce the risk by including a progestogen. (A progestogen is a synthetic version of the natural hormone, progesterone.) If you have had a hysterectomy, you can use oestrogen by itself.

Why replace what nature has taken away?

The most effective treatment for women with symptoms of oestrogen deficiency – such as hot flushes, sweats and vaginal dryness – is oestrogen. Natural oestrogens (e.g. oestradiol) are used for HRT, rather than the more powerful synthetic oestrogen (ethinyloestradiol) used in the oral contraceptive pill.

In addition to relieving unpleasant perimenopausal symptoms, it was thought that HRT could help to protect against heart disease, osteoporosis, colon cancer and dementia.

Pause, O men

The menopause may be the preserve of women (although some contest that). But with the promise that HRT could protect against heart disease, is it any wonder that someone thought men too should have the benefit of oestrogen therapy? In 1973, the Coronary Drug Project Research Group set up an extraordinary clinical trial to compare four different cholesterol-lowering treatments in men, including two very high-dose oestrogen treatments. The trial was hampered by the number of men who dropped out when they developed breasts. The impotence wasn't very popular either.

Sadly, more recent studies give women pause too. Controlled trials have cast doubt on the protective power of HRT, while confirming that it can raise the risk of breast cancer and deep vein thrombosis (DVT).

Is HRT good for the heart?

Over the years, a number of large-scale observational studies have concluded that women who take oestrogen after the menopause are less likely to suffer from heart disease than those who don't. Overall, it looked as though women taking HRT enjoyed a 50% reduction in the risk of heart disease.

The Nurses' Health Study monitored many thousands of female nurses in the 1970s. The risk of heart disease in those who were taking oestrogen at the time of the survey was only 30% of the risk in those who had never taken it. Women who had used oestrogen therapy in the past had a 70% risk compared with those who had never done so.

The natural conclusion was that HRT protected the heart. But the problem with these observational studies is that the women who were prescribed HRT might have been healthier in the first place. For a start, health conscious women were more likely to request oestrogen replacement. And a doctor who suspected that HRT could increase risks (like the Pill) would be less likely to prescribe it for a woman with obvious risk factors (such as high blood pressure or obesity).

The only way to eliminate bias of this sort is to conduct huge randomised controlled trials. (These are known as 'prospective' as opposed to 'observational' studies.) The first results from such investigations caused a few shock waves.

The Women's Health Initiative (WHI) study in America published some findings in 2002. This was a properly controlled trial to investigate the effects of HRT in 16 608 women (aged 50–79) with no history of heart disease. Instead of confirming that the women on HRT were protected from heart attacks, it reported a few extra heart attacks and strokes among those taking oestrogen together with progestogen. (There were about seven extra heart attacks in every 10 000 women taking HRT for one year.)

The WHI Study published further results in 2004 – this time on 10 739 women (aged 50–79) who had previously undergone hysterectomy. These women had taken either oestrogen (without progestogen) or placebo (dummy tablets). The trial was stopped early, after less than seven years, because it looked as though oestrogen was slightly increasing the risk of having a stroke without offering protection against heart disease.

Another prospective study, dubbed HERS and published in 1998, examined the effects of HRT on women who already had heart disease. HERS stands for Heart and Estrogen progestin Replacement Study ('Estrogen' being the American spelling). In this investigation, the women who were taking HRT had just as many heart attacks as the women who weren't. A closer look reveals that the risk actually went up in the first year of taking HRT and reduced after that. Perhaps starting HRT was linked with an increase in blood clots before a slow protection against the build-up of fatty deposits could show up.

◆ Oestrogen replacement therapy relieves symptoms of the change

◆ Unless a woman has had a hysterectomy, HRT includes progestogen to protect the womb against cancer

◆ Oestrogen therapy raises HDL- and lowers LDL-cholesterol

◆ Oestrogen therapy is not suitable for men

Why should HRT protect against heart disease?

The original idea that oestrogen could protect women from heart disease came from the observation that heart disease is rare before the menopause. But, as we have seen, the risk of heart disease doesn't abruptly shoot up at the menopause; it rises steadily with age.

Mind you, a long-term study of the population of Framingham found that heart disease was more common in postmenopausal women than in premenopausal women of a similar age.

In addition, laboratory work suggests that replacing natural oestrogen after the menopause ought to protect against heart disease. Oestrogen therapy in women raises HDL-cholesterol and lowers LDL-cholesterol. Laboratory experiments have also shown that oestrogen can relax artery walls and improve blood flow.

It may be that weak natural oestrogens in soya protein, which seem to be good for the prostate glands of Japanese men, are also helping Japanese women to avoid hot flushes and osteoporosis. What part, I wonder, do these food oestrogens play in the heart protection that is linked with the Japanese diet?

Observational studies showing that women on oestrogen replacement therapy had much lower rates of heart disease seemed so promising. What a disappointment, then, that controlled trials – the acid test – failed to confirm the protective powers of oestrogen.

More bad news

Breast cancer, sadly, is all too common with up to 10% of women suffering the disease at some stage in their lives. Clearly, most women who get breast cancer while taking HRT would have got it anyway. It is now apparent that a few extra cases of breast cancer arise in women taking HRT for at least three years. For every 1000 women taking HRT for five years, there might be two extra cases of breast cancer, i.e. two cases that can be put down to HRT; after 15 years, you could expect 12 extra cases.

The Million Women Study published in the *The Lancet* in 2003 indicated that the risk of breast cancer with long-term use of HRT is significantly higher when oestrogen is combined with progestogen than when oestrogen is taken on its own.

In 2007, the Million Women Study collaborators published data confirming an increased risk of **ovarian cancer** among HRT users. In every 2500 women taking HRT for five years, there was an extra case of ovarian cancer.

There is an increased risk of **deep vein thrombosis** (DVT) while taking HRT, but for most women the risk remains low. The risk is higher in obese women and those who have had a DVT in the past. These factors should be taken into account when deciding whether to take HRT.

Colon cancer occurred less frequently among women taking HRT (oestrogen with progestogen) in the WHI Study, but when tumours were discovered, they were more advanced than those diagnosed in the placebo group.

Observational studies had suggested that HRT might offer protection against **dementia**. As a man, you might well opt to enter old age with two breasts and a sound mind, as opposed to a flat chest and no marbles. Unfortunately, controlled trials have failed to confirm that HRT can prevent or delay dementia.

It has been known for years that HRT can help to prevent **osteoporosis** (brittle bones) when taken for seven years or more. But even this has turned out to be disappointing. If you take HRT for, say, ten years, it will beef up your bones while you're taking it (at the expense of some increased risk of breast cancer, ovarian cancer and DVT). It used to be thought that, even after stopping HRT, you could take this extra bone strength with you into old age. Sadly, it now seems that the benefit to your bones wears off within a year of stopping oestrogen therapy. By the time you are really at risk of falling and breaking your hip, in your 70s and 80s, the extra bone strength has deserted you.

The good news is that we now have much better drugs for treating osteoporosis, or preventing it in people at high risk. So, after the age of 50, the case for using HRT to make your bones stronger is now much weaker.

Should I take HRT?

The average age for the menopause is 51. If you have an early menopause, at the age of 40, for example (which increases the risk of osteoporosis and heart disease), you should seriously consider taking HRT until you are 50. After all, you are just replacing what nature has withdrawn early; you needn't bother about the risks of older women taking HRT until you hit 50.

Oestrogen replacement is generally the most efficient treatment for troublesome menopausal symptoms. When it transforms the quality of your life, the benefits of taking HRT for a few years are likely to out-weigh the risks. If you opt for HRT, it's important to review the decision at least once a year with your doctor, as the balance of benefits and risks will change as time goes on.

On current evidence, we are unable to recommend HRT for the prevention of chronic diseases. Take heart. This book is full of other things you can do to reduce the risk of metabolic syndrome, diabetes, heart disease, stroke and cancer.

Chapter 25

Assessing your risk

Risk is a difficult concept. In this book, I talk about reducing your risk of having a heart attack – and about percentage reductions in risk. How do you assess the importance of a risk and decide whether it's worth changing your life for?

We all know that life is full of risks – such as the risk of being run over by a bus. Most of us will push this right out of our mind so we can get on with everyday life. Some will wear clean underwear, just in case. A few will avoid bus routes altogether.

It's easy to lose our sense of proportion, if we ever had one. A powerful TV programme can leave you anxious about being struck by a meteorite – so anxious, in fact, that you smoke your way to a heart attack. If people generally had a good grasp of risk analysis, the National Lottery would be a flop.

Relative risk

It may sound as though this section is on family history – or heart disease in your relations. Not so. **Relative risk** needs to be distinguished from **absolute risk**.

◆ A huge increase in *relative risk* (e.g. of being hit by a meteorite) may still leave you with a tiny *absolute risk*

◆ The risk of having a heart attack is high to start with when risk factors (such as high blood pressure and cholesterol) are present; doubling the risk by smoking is extremely dangerous

◆ Risk factors don't just add to the risk: they multiply it

◆ Having a high cholesterol level is far more serious if you have high blood pressure and smoke as well

---

Let's suppose you normally buy one entry for the National Lottery. One week you decide to splash out and buy two. By paying twice as much, you have doubled your chances of winning the jackpot. You have doubled the relative risk of winning – increased it by 100% – but the absolute risk remains so low it's not worth considering. The following week you go wild: you sell your classic collection of Barbie dolls and buy 100 entries. You've purchased a huge increase in your relative risk of winning top prize; it's now 100 times greater than it would have been with your normal outlay. But, contrary to popular delusion, your absolute risk of hitting the jackpot is still so low it isn't worth a second thought.

And if you were to double your girth – become twice as wide – I imagine that your risk of being hit by a small meteorite would more or less double (excluding complications like the fact that you would move more slowly, cover less ground, and be less likely to be in the 'right' place at the 'right' time). Despite this hefty rise in relative risk, however, you'd have a fat chance of hitting the headlines on that count. The absolute risk would be negligible.

By contrast, if your huge weight gain had also doubled your risk of coronary heart disease, a meteoric passage to the obituary column would be all too likely. Our background risk of heart disease is high in the UK. Anything that doubles the risk is significant.

Indeed, if you were now to take up smoking, further doubling this expanded risk, who knows? The next edition of your local paper could carry your obituary. This is how risk factors multiply. The bigger the risk to start with, the more dangerous it is to magnify it.

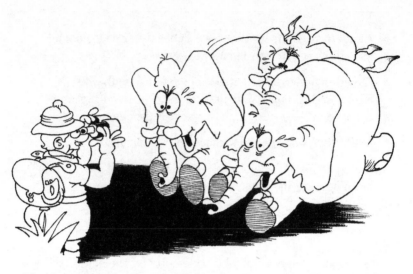

The bigger the risk to start with, the more dangerous it is to magnify it.

This is why some people get away with having one high risk factor – such as raised cholesterol. It is also why many others have heart attacks with 'normal' cholesterol levels – well below the national average of 5.9 mmol/l. An overweight, diabetic man of 40, whose mother developed angina at the age of 54, is off to a bad start. Perhaps his cholesterol level and blood pressure are only slightly raised. Now, if he smokes, he's not so much *adding* to his high risk as *multiplying* it. No wonder he is struck down with a heart attack before his 50th birthday when others, with higher cholesterol levels or blood pressures, go on to enjoy their retirement.

If you are at high risk, like this unfortunate man with diabetes, bringing in any unnecessary risk factors can be disastrous. By the same token, you have even more to gain than the low-risk person by making a few changes. Even a modest reduction in your relative risk can make a significant impact on absolute risk.

Like all family doctors, I have patients who are extremely anxious about their blood pressure. And yet they continue to smoke. A modest reduction in blood pressure, combined with giving up smoking, would cut risk more effectively than controlling blood pressure perfectly while ignoring everything else. As risk factors multiply, tackling them all is far more efficient than concentrating on one alone.

◆ If you have a family history of heart disease, it's all the more important to tackle the risk factors you can alter

◆ People with diabetes are more likely to get heart disease; controlling all the risk factors is extra important

◆ Some 'ageing processes' (such as the clogging of arteries and rise in blood pressure) can be prevented by the right lifestyle

---

Gene genie?

We cannot invoke some supernatural power to change our gene code or our gender. Does that mean that our fate is fixed – our destiny determined in our DNA?

Certainly, we can inherit a high risk of coronary heart disease. If one of your first degree relatives (a parent, brother, sister, son or daughter) developed the disease at a young age (below 50 for a male relative or 55 for a female relative) that gives you a risk factor that you cannot alter. Race, too, could raise your risk. Of the various ethnic groups within the UK population, Asians from the Indian subcontinent are at particularly high risk of heart disease. This seems to be linked with a genetic tendency to insulin resistance and diabetes.

If you're starting off with risk factors like this, which are beyond your control, you may be tempted to give up. What can you do about it anyway? In reality, if nature's dealt you a bad hand, there's everything to play for.

Perhaps you have relatives who developed diabetes in middle age – making them more prone to heart disease. You fear that you are set to suffer the same fate. A good diet and regular exercise could tip the balance in your favour; it might stop you getting diabetes. Even if you do get diabetes, the right lifestyle will limit its effects.

You know how risk factors multiply. You've seen that when the risk is high, changes in relative risk become more important. We have no gene genie (yet). And it doesn't take a genius to see that, when your genes are against you, you have all the more to gain by getting everything else on your side.

The risk factors

We've agreed that you can't do much about your age, sex or family history. You will remember these important risk factors, which are all affected by lifestyle:

- High blood cholesterol;

- High blood pressure;

- Smoking;

- Diabetes;

- Being overweight or obese;

- Lack of exercise.

Looking at the top three will tell you a lot. Supposing there are two men of the same age with no relevant family history. Finding out their cholesterol levels, blood pressures and smoking habits should tell you whether one of them is much more likely to have a heart attack in the next ten years than the other. It would also reveal the major changes needed to reduce that risk.

Simple methods of scoring coronary risk focus on these three top risk factors.

Of course, if one of the two men has diabetes, that will count against him. The metabolic effects of diabetes make heart disease more likely. Subtle changes in clotting factors and blood platelets make it easier for the blood to clot. Blood levels of triglycerides are often raised, while those of HDL-cholesterol are low. Central obesity and high blood pressure are common. Accelerated atherosclerosis may narrow arteries enough to cause angina or a heart attack.

Getting the diet right in diabetes is essential – not just to help control blood sugar but also to protect the arteries. The good news is that, if you have diabetes, you don't have to eat a *special* diet at all. The right diet is the same healthy, balanced diet that we should all be eating. Reducing saturated fat intake helps to prevent blood clots as well as controlling cholesterol. Eating a low-GL diet, with enough soluble fibre, lean protein and mono-unsaturated fat, improves the balance of lipids. Including enough fruit and vegetable provides antioxidants to prevent the oxidation of LDL that leads to atherosclerosis. An adequate intake of oily fish makes platelets less keen to clump together and lowers blood triglyceride levels. Reducing salt consumption helps to keep blood pressure down. I could go on. (No doubt you think I have already.)

In the same way, aerobic exercise, which is so important for all of us, is essential in the management of diabetes. It reduces body fat, keeps up HDL-cholesterol, improves control of blood pressure, and reduces the risk of heart disease.

With a healthy lifestyle, and sometimes a little help from drugs, all the risk factors in this list can be improved.

What about the ones you can't alter? Well, your sex and family history may stay much the same (the latter is more liable to change than the the former, if a relative has a heart attack, for example) but your age is guaranteed to change – for the worse, most readers will think. And, yes, the older you get, the more likely you are to have a heart attack.

Young at heart

The increased risk of coronary heart disease is not the only unwelcome effect of ageing, of course. We'd all like to stop the clock. We can't.

We can stop some of the changes that are just accepted as part of the ageing process. For a start, there's that rise in blood pressure which, you may remember, does not occur in communities that eat very little salt. Then there's the progressive narrowing and hardening of arteries – atherosclerosis – at the heart of Western vascular diseases. We see this insidious process as part and parcel of ageing, but it's quite possible to reach old age with arteries unscathed by atherosclerosis. Some people in the Third World do so. And antioxidants, which have a range of 'anti-ageing' actions, play a vital role in fighting off the ravages of time on arteries as well.

'You're as old as you feel,' they say. Many people feel just fine until the silent ageing of their heart becomes apparent. Exercising, not smoking, and eating as this book advises will do a lot to keep you young at heart.

ACTION POINT

◆ Have a Well-Person check to find out your risk factors.
   You will probably be able to arrange this at your doctor's surgery

Should I have my cholesterol checked?

By now you understand, I hope, how unhelpful it is when cholesterol gets all the attention. Sometimes people quote their 'cholesterol number' as if it were a complete statement of coronary risk. Knowing how risk factors interact with each other, you will want to avoid focusing all your attention on any one risk factor.

Even so, blood cholesterol level is a key risk factor. We've seen how the very low levels of cholesterol in Japan are responsible for low rates of heart disease. So, shouldn't everyone have a blood test?

Taking and processing blood samples from the whole population would use up an awful lot of time and money. Most experts agree that this would not be the best use of our limited resources. After all, we know that the average cholesterol level for the population is too high and that the great majority of people have a lot of room for improvement.

We have an epidemic of heart disease on our hands and you don't need to measure all those cholesterol levels to see that we desperately need the population to change its ways. If the nation were really to take the message of this book to heart, it would transform the health of our nation and relieve our National Health Service of crippling expenditure on obesity, diabetes and diseases of the heart and circulation (not to mention cancer).

Healthy living is vital for all of us, whatever our cholesterol may be.

If we don't measure any cholesterol levels, though, we won't identify those people who have special lipid problems requiring medical help. About two in every thousand people have familial hypercholesterolaemia and it takes drugs as well as lifestyle changes to save them from disaster.

You should certainly get your lipids measured if you have any of these problems:

- Angina or a previous heart attack;

- Blocked arteries in the legs causing pain on walking (claudication);

- Diabetes;

- High blood pressure;

- Fatty lumps under the skin and/or round tendons (xanthomas), fatty deposits in the eyelids (xanthelasmas), or an opaque ring round the cornea of the eye under the age of 50 (juvenile arcus), any of which *may* be a sign of an inherited cholesterol problem;

- Family history of high cholesterol levels;

- Family history of coronary heart disease (in a close male relative under 55 or close female relative under 65).

Having said all this, I believe one of the main benefits of measuring cholesterol is that it can provide motivation. There's nothing quite like a cholesterol reading of, say, 7.2 mmol/l for kick-starting that dietary overhaul that you've been meaning to get round to for the last few years. By the same token, it is not at all helpful if a 'normal' cholesterol result reassures you that you needn't bother about a good diet or healthy lifestyle. Remember that, like blood pressure measurement, because of biological and technical variations, two readings are better than one.

If you are already taking enough interest in the health of your heart to be reading this book, your doctor will doubtless be willing to arrange to check your cholesterol.

APT to underestimate?

There is agreement among experts that the benefit of lowering cholesterol has probably been underestimated. It is generally considered that a 1% reduction in cholesterol results in a 2% reduction in coronary risk – so that, if you reduced your cholesterol level by 10%, you would reduce your risk by 20%. In reality, a risk reduction of 3% for every 1% drop in cholesterol level is probably nearer the mark (that is, 30% reduction in risk for a 10% fall in cholesterol level).

And don't forget that if a change in diet produces a drop in cholesterol, that's only part of the story. The artery-clogging process of atherosclerosis will be affected, not only by the balance of lipids (LDL-cholesterol, HDL-cholesterol and triglycerides), but also by the supply of antioxidants and other micronutrients.

The build-up of cholesterol on artery walls is not a passive process like fat clogging up a drain pipe. Artery linings are constantly being damaged and repaired. The importance of inflammation in the growth of fatty plaques is becoming clearer. A blood test for high-sensitivity C-reactive protein (hsCRP) is a measure of inflammation. Raised CRP levels (perhaps reflecting inflammation in artery walls) are linked with higher rates of heart disease. No doubt, lots of factors in our diet (such as omega-3 fatty acids from fish oils) influence this inflammation.

Again, the significance of thrombosis is apt to be neglected: heart-attack risk is greatly reduced by cutting the risk of clots forming in the circulation. Your level of the blood-clotting protein, fibrinogen, seems to be an important coronary risk factor but it is difficult to measure so this is usually done only in research or in very specialised clinics. We know that diet has an important influence on blood clotting through effects on platelets, fibrinogen, factor VII and other clotting factors. The crucial importance of thrombosis is not just that a blood clot in a coronary artery is normally the final cause of a heart attack: thrombosis also plays a part in the gradual growth of cholesterol-laden plaques on artery walls. Of course, arteries that have been narrowed in this way are much more likely to be blocked by a clot.

This is how atherosclerosis and thrombosis work hand in hand to pave the way to a heart attack.

A good diet will protect your heart in many subtle ways that will not show up as a change in total cholesterol. It's possible to imagine two diets that offer quite different levels of protection against heart disease even though they are equally effective at lowering your cholesterol. There are three major ways in which a truly **APT** diet slashes your coronary risk.

Atherosclerosis   furring up of arteries is slowed down, stopped or reversed!

Pressure   blood pressure is reduced.

Thrombosis   blood clots are less likely to form in the circulation.

◆ The benefit of lowering cholesterol has been underestimated and a 10% cholesterol reduction could mean a 30% drop in risk

◆ An APT diet has major benefits for the circulation, reducing atherosclerosis, pressure and thrombosis – the three big players in the run-up to a heart attack

◆ Cholesterol is only part of the story and two diets might be equally effective at lowering cholesterol but have different effects on risk

The balanced, varied, delicious and exciting diet you've been reading about in this book does all these things. Table 23 shows some **apt** dietary changes, which help by holding back the three big players in the long run-up to a heart attack.

Table 23 APT changes in diet

Atherosclerosis	**P**ressure	**T**hrombosis
↓ Fat	↓ Fat (weight control)	↓ Fat
↓ Saturates	↓ Sodium	↓ Saturates
→ Mono-unsaturates	↑ Potassium	↑ Fish oils
→ Polyunsaturates	↑ Magnesium	↑ Garlic
↑ Starch	↑ Calcium	Moderate alcohol
↑ Soluble fibre	↓ Alcohol	
↑ Antioxidants	↑ Garlic	
↑ Garlic	↑ Fish oils	
Moderate alcohol		

A ready reckoner of risk

Figure 19 shows a chart that can be used to estimate the risk of developing cardiovascular disease (CVD) – i.e. having a heart attack or stroke or first attack of angina – within the next ten years. It is based on information gathered in the Framingham Study.

Health professionals use a chart like this (or the computer equivalent) to assess your risk of developing CVD in the future. This can help to decide whether drugs should be used to reduce the risk by lowering cholesterol or blood pressure. The chart is not designed for people who already have CVD or diabetes or those with an inherited high cholesterol level or very high blood pressure (persistently above 160/100 mmHg); where the risk is known to be that high, drug treatment will be offered anyway.

To use the chart, you need to find out your blood pressure and cholesterol level. You probably already know your age and sex (and whether you smoke)! Only the systolic blood pressure (the top figure) is used for the chart; an average of several readings is always better than one. The chart uses the ratio of total cholesterol to HDL-cholesterol (i.e. your total cholesterol divided by your HDL-cholesterol; but if you don't know your HDL-cholesterol level, you can assume it's 1.0 and simply use the total cholesterol number).

If you stopped smoking today, congratulations, but you should still read the chart as a smoker. The chart is based on a lifetime exposure to tobacco, not on whether you have a cigarette in your mouth at the time of the assessment. So, if you have stopped smoking within the last five years, it is better to read the chart as if you were a smoker.

Find the correct square for your sex, age and smoking habits (Figure 19). Now simply find where a horizontal line from your blood pressure on the left meets a vertical line from your cholesterol ratio at the bottom. The point where the two lines meet will fall within one of the three risk zones. Check the shading against the key to find out whether your 10-year risk is lower than 10%, between 10% and 20% or over 20%.

Your risk doesn't actually leap up once a decade, of course, any more than you suddenly become a year older on your birthday. The chart shows the risk you will acquire by the time you reach the top end of the age bracket (a bit like insurance companies always talking about your age at your *next* birthday). The risk indicated by the 60-years-and-over chart would be reached at the age of 69.

The main value of the charts is to decide whether drug treatment is needed in addition to lifestyle changes. It is based on observation of people who were not taking drugs to lower blood pressure or cholesterol. So it could be misleading if you read the chart using blood pressure and cholesterol values that have been reduced by drug treatment.

Where there is a significant family history of heart disease, the chart may underestimate risk. If a close female relative (mother, sister or daughter) suffered from coronary heart disease or a stroke before the age of 65, or a male relative (father, brother or son) before 55, you should multiply your risk score by 1.3.

The chart may underestimate risk in some ethnic groups. For South Asians, the risk is likely to be about 1.4 times the risk indicated by the chart.

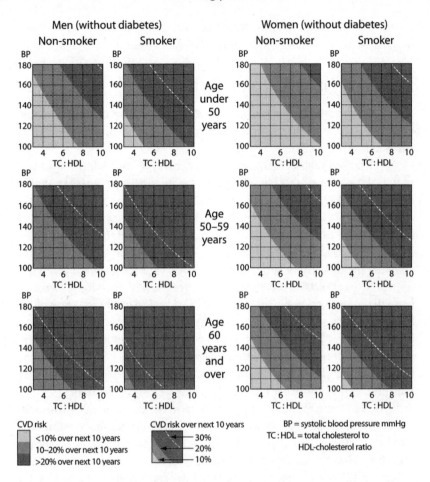

Men (without diabetes)   Women (without diabetes)

Non-smoker   Smoker   Non-smoker   Smoker

Age under 50 years

Age 50–59 years

Age 60 years and over

CVD risk
<10% over next 10 years
10–20% over next 10 years
>20% over next 10 years

CVD risk over next 10 years
30%
20%
10%

BP = systolic blood pressure mmHg
TC : HDL = total cholesterol to
HDL-cholesterol ratio

Figure 19 Reading your risks. Find the square that corresponds to your sex, age and smoking habits. Mark the point where a horizontal line from your blood pressure on the left meets a vertical line from your cholesterol ratio at the bottom. Use the key to read your approximate risk of having a heart attack or stroke in the next ten years. (This chart is not intended for those who are known to be at high risk because of existing cardiovascular disease or diabetes.)

Again, risk will be higher than suggested by the chart in women who had a very early menopause (see page 299.)

If you have a raised fasting blood glucose level, but have not as yet developed diabetes, your risk will be higher than the chart tells you. In diabetes, the fasting glucose level is 7 mmol/l or more; a fasting glucose below 6 mmol/l is normal. So a fasting glucose between 6 and

7 mmol/l is between normal and diabetes; this indicates insulin resistance and is often part of the metabolic syndrome.

Measuring your risk in centimetres

Your waist circumference is a very simple and useful guide to risk because it reflects the accumulation of metabolically mischievous visceral fat (page 187).

An enlarged waist circumference is central to the definition of the metabolic syndrome. Table 24 shows the new International Diabetes Federation (IDF) definition of the syndrome.

Alarmingly, perhaps, the IDF now considers a fasting glucose level of 5.6 mmol/l as high enough to qualify for the metabolic syndrome. In just the same way, the definition of diabetes has altered over the years to include lower glucose levels. This reflects research showing that the threshold for increased risk is very low. Before long, we'll all have diabetes! Seriously, though, any of us can so easily find ourselves on the slippery slide through the metabolic syndrome to diabetes and heart disease. Notice that a blood pressure of 130/85 mmHg, which most of us would pass as very reasonable, is high enough to count towards the metabolic syndrome; risk factors that seem to be mild or marginal can become significant when clustered with others.

If you have the metabolic syndrome, you're not alone; it's extremely common. This largely explains why we have epidemics of diabetes and heart disease. So, if you meet the IDF criteria, you want to get off the slide, don't you? It's time to take action. Slimming your waist (Chapter 18) is the first step; as you lose centimetres, you will gain sensitivity to insulin, and start to get your metabolism back on track.

The good news is that no matter how high your risk, you can reduce it.

A change of heart

A heart transplant is a drastic measure, for people with no other hope. Unless you have a rare kind of heart disease (such as a serious cardio-myopathy) there is a lot you can do to transform the outlook for your heart.

Michael was a 49-year-old bank employee. His wife had been trying to persuade him to have a check-up for some time but it was after a colleague died of a heart attack that Michael came to see me.

Table 24 The Metabolic Syndrome

International Diabetes Federation (IDF) definition

To meet the criteria for the metabolic syndrome, you must have:

◆ **Central obesity:** a waist circumference of 94 cm or more for a man; 80 cm or more for a woman*
   Plus any two of the following:

◆ **Raised triglyceride level:** 1.7 mmol/l or above (or specific treatment to reduce triglycerides)

◆ **Reduced HDL-cholesterol:** less than 1.03 mmol/l in men; less than 1.29 mmol/l in women (or specific treatment to raise HDL)

◆ **Raised blood pressure:** systolic BP 130 mmHg or above, or diastolic BP 85 mmHg or above (or treatment for previously diagnosed hypertension)

◆ **Raised fasting plasma glucose:** 5.6 mmol/l or above (or previously diagnosed Type 2 diabetes)

---

*These figures apply to Europid men and women. For other ethnic groups see Table 26.

He was not a pie-and-chips man. You wouldn't catch him at the greasy spoon. He was well aware that his diet wasn't perfect but he felt he'd made some healthy changes: cooked breakfasts were restricted to weekends; sunflower spread had replaced butter; he would often choose pasta dishes, especially in the staff canteen; chicken was frequently selected in preference to red meat; when convenient, reduced-fat products were included.

In fact, Michael was disappointed that, despite making these changes, his trousers were getting harder to do up. His wife had pointed out that love handles were one thing, but an overhanging balustrade was another.

His 20–30 cigarettes a day had been on the New Year hit list for as many years as he could remember. His busy schedule left no time for regular exercise. There was no history of heart disease in his close family but the sudden death of a colleague, just two years his senior, had really shaken him up.

After a few visits, we established that Michael's average blood pressure was 140/90 mmHg and his average total cholesterol level was 6.9 mmol/l, with an HDL-cholesterol of 0.9 mmol/l. So the ratio of total cholesterol to HDL-cholesterol was 7.7. He did not have diabetes. If you look at Figure 19 you can see that this would have given Michael a CVD risk of more than 20% over the following 10 years.

I asked Michael to complete a dietary diary for seven days. Spurred on particularly, it seemed, by his raised cholesterol level, he and his wife made some really big changes over the following four months. In Table 25 I have shown his entries for just one day on the original diet and, beside it, just one day on his changed diet.

With the help of the practice nurse, he gave up smoking. By leaving the car at home, and walking to and from the station, he included 40 minutes of brisk walking in his daily routine and bought an exercise bike to use at weekends.

Six months later, Michael told me he didn't feel at all deprived; he was enjoying his food more and feeling generally better. He had lost over one and a half stone in weight. His average blood pressure was now 120/80 and his total cholesterol was down to 5 with an HDL-cholesterol of 1. You will see that his CVD risk in ten years was now well below 20%.

Naturally, these simple charts based on the Framingham Study don't tell the whole story; they cannot necessarily reflect the benefits Michael derived from so many helpful dietary and lifestyle changes. And, of course, the longer he continues as a non-smoker, the more he stands to gain.

Now I must add a personal note here. No doubt, I am reducing my own coronary risk by enjoying a deliciously varied diet and an invigorating, healthy lifestyle. But I started with a fairly high risk. Perhaps I would have had a heart attack already if I hadn't made these changes. It's not unlikely that one day I shall have a heart attack. And the media mob will love that. They won't be able to contain their glee as they report, 'Dr Derrick Cutting – author of *Stop That Heart Attack!* – died of a heart attack today.' My wife will be left to face the mockery of the media on her own, so I'm addressing it now. If I've delayed that heart attack – stopped it from happening – for twenty, thirty or forty years, then that's a success, isn't it?

It just doesn't add up

Imagine a man who, like Michael, makes a series of lifestyle changes to reduce his coronary risk. Taking into account his age and the

Table 25 Extracts from Michael's dietary diary

	Tuesday (original diet)	**Thursday** (changed diet)
Breakfast	2 cups cafetière coffee (black) 1 slice toast, sunflower spread and marmalade Muesli (probably with coconut)	Shredded Wheat Bitesize with chopped dried apricots, raisins, sliced banana; skimmed milk Instant coffee, skimmed milk
Mid-morning	Coffee, 2 digestive biscuits Glass of water	Cup of tea, skimmed milk
Lunch	Fruit juice Lasagne, small portion chips Treacle tart, ice cream Coffee	2 glasses water Baked beans, 2 slices wholemeal toast (no spread) 1 bowl fruit salad 1 apple Cup of tea, skimmed milk
Afternoon	Cup of tea, whole milk Slice of swiss roll Banana	Glass of water Cup of tea, skimmed milk
Early evening	Bag of crisps (reduced fat)	2 slices wholemeal toast, low-sugar jam (no spread) 2 cups tea, skimmed milk
Dinner	Roast chicken quarter, roast potatoes, cauliflower cheese 3 glasses red wine Cheese (including reduced-fat cheddar), savoury biscuits, sunflower spread 2 cups cafetière coffee 3 chocolate mints	Salmon steak, broccoli, sweetcorn, peas, jacket potato with fat-free garlic and herb dressing (Kraft) 1 glass water 2 glasses red wine Summer pudding (fruit and bread) 1 cup filtered coffee Dates
Late evening	Hot chocolate (whole milk)	Home-made muesli (no coconut), skimmed milk

Table 26 Waist circumferences qualifying for the metabolic syndrome in various ethnic groups

Ethnic group		Waist circumference
Europeans (In the USA, higher values are used: 102 cm male; 88 cm female)	Male Female	94 cm 80 cm
South Asians	Male Female	90 cm 80 cm
Chinese	Male Female	90 cm 80 cm
Japanese	Male Female	85 cm 90 cm
Ethnic South and Central Americans		Use South Asian figures until more specific data available
Sub-Saharan Africans		Use European figures until more specific data available
Eastern Mediterranean and Middle East (Arab) populations		Use European figures until more specific data available

Adapted from the International Diabetes Federation (IDF) consensus.

It is the ethnic origin and not the country of residence that is relevant. Doctors in the USA use higher values for practical reasons (as such a large proportion of the population is above the lower threshold). If you happen to live in the USA, it is better to carry out your risk assessment using the figures for your ethnic group.

number of cigarettes he was smoking a day, we estimate that giving up smoking has reduced his risk by 50%. He then takes up an exercise programme that brings him another 50% reduction in coronary risk. Changes in his diet result in a 15% drop in cholesterol level, conferring a risk reduction of at least 30% (probably 45%). If we add these up, we're well over 100% already and there are other factors we haven't even considered yet. If he has removed more than 100% of his original risk, his new risk must be less than zero. It just doesn't add up.

Of course, there's a very basic flaw here. You don't just add up percentage risk reductions to find the new risk. When our man has halved his risk by giving up smoking, it is this new, lower risk that is halved again by his exercise programme.

When it comes to *increasing* your risks, mind you, by changing your lifestyle for the worse, you might end up with a coronary risk six times the one you started with! It's quite simple to *add* more than 100% to your risk; you might add 500%.

When you follow the advice in this book and reduce your risk, your new risk may be a small fraction of the risk you started with, but it will never get down to zero. No matter how radically you change your lifestyle, there will always be some risk attached to being alive.

◆ Simple risk scores are based on the top risk factors – cholesterol, blood pressure and smoking

◆ A big reduction in risk may mean a big change in lifestyle but, once you've adapted, your new lifestyle can be more satisfying

◆ You can reduce your risk dramatically, but not down to zero

---

Chapter 26

If you already have heart disease

'Youth is a period of missed opportunities.'

CYRIL CONNOLLY, *Journal 1928–1937,*
ed. D Pryce-Jones, 1983

◆ If you have heart disease already, you have even more to gain by reducing your risk of a future heart attack

◆ Every part of this book will help you to reduce that risk

◆ There is now evidence that, if the right changes are made, narrowed arteries can get wider again; heart disease can be reversed!

It's too late now, isn't it?

If you have already had a heart attack, or suffer from angina, what has a book on *preventing* heart disease got to offer you? Isn't it like offering a breastplate to a man who's been stabbed through the heart?

The truth is that every part of this book – from the bits on chipping away at your relative risk to the chapters on cutting it down dramatically – every part, is vital for you if you have heart disease already.

When disease in the coronary arteries has already made itself known, by a previous heart attack or the onset of angina, the chances of a future heart attack are greatly increased. Because the absolute risk of a heart attack or coronary death is so high, cutting it down by, say, 30% is *even more worthwhile* than it is for someone without heart disease!

You are no longer dealing with the risk that you might one day get heart disease – but, then again, you might not; you are dealing with the certainty that you have heart disease and there is something you can do to halt its progress – or even send it into reverse.

The cynic may think that I'm offering a ray of hope to the desperate (like William Spooner's cousin who thought that a ray of hope was a rope of hay and that he'd just be clutching at straws). No, the information in this book could be your lifeline; it's up to you whether you grasp it or not.

Doctors once thought that the best you could hope for was to slow down the growth of fatty plaques that clog up arteries. We now have good evidence that atheroma can be reversed and arteries can get wider again – especially when the blood cholesterol level is brought down really low. For many people with established heart disease, drug treatment is needed as well as lifestyle changes and I shall deal with that in this chapter.

◆ Drugs can often control the symptoms of angina

◆ In some cases angioplasty is needed to widen a narrowed coronary artery with a balloon

◆ Sometimes a bypass operation is required to get round the blocked sections of the coronary arteries

◆ After angioplasty or surgery, cholesterol should ideally be kept below 4 mmol/l (LDL-cholesterol below 2 mmol/l)

Dealing with angina

You may remember from Chapter 2 how angina occurs when the heart's oxygen supply is limited by narrowed coronary arteries. Drug treatment is used to reduce the workload of the heart while relaxing the coronary arteries, if possible, to improve the balance between work and blood supply. The aim is to control the symptoms as well as possible even if a combination of drugs is needed to achieve this.

Sometimes angina is not controlled adequately by drugs and on occasions the blockage in a coronary artery is life-threatening. This calls for a change in the plumbing.

Angioplasty involves passing a special catheter (tube) into the coronary artery and inflating a balloon at the narrow point to widen it. Usually a stent, which is a short tube made of stainless steel mesh, is inserted to keep the artery open.

A major advance has been the development of 'drug-eluting stents'; these stents are coated with a drug that reduces inflammation and damps down the healing process. With the older stents, excessive healing and formation of scar tissue led to restenosis (recurrence of the blockage) in about 10% of cases – and this used to happen within a year of stent insertion.

Angioplasty with insertion of a stent is now so successful that it is the usual way to deal with blocked coronary arteries. But surgery is still needed in some cases. A coronary artery bypass graft gives the blood another route. A length of vein from the leg or an artery inside the chest wall is used to bypass the blockage in the coronary artery. Often several blockages have to be bypassed. Whenever possible, an artery from the chest wall (the internal mammary artery) is used because it is much less likely to block up than a vein graft.

You can see why angioplasty is so popular. After stent insertion, you can usually go home the next day. Traditional bypass surgery, on the other hand, involves cutting through the breastbone to open the chest wall, and using a heart-lung machine so the heart can be stopped; it's followed by a spell in the intensive care unit and several weeks of convalescence.

But less drastic surgery is now possible. Internal mammary artery grafting can be carried out through a small incision in the chest wall while the heart is still beating! A comparison of this technique with stent insertion (to tackle a single blockage in the left anterior descending artery) was published in the *British Medical Journal* in 2007. Surgery came out very well: angina was more than twice as likely to recur after stenting. (Mind you, the studies analysed were generally using bare-metal rather than drug-eluting stents.)

If you are seriously disabled by angina, having balloon angioplasty or a bypass operation can make a huge difference and you don't want the problem to come back. So it is vital to protect the plumbing with drugs as well as diet and lifestyle, and to get the cholesterol level right down – ideally below 4 mmol/l (LDL-cholesterol below 2 mmol/l). And, of course, this will reduce your chances of having a heart attack too.

- ◆ After a heart attack, gentle walking is usually increased gradually during the first week

- ◆ It is essential to stop smoking and adopt a healthy lifestyle

- ◆ Many people make a full recovery from a heart attack

- ◆ Sometimes drugs are needed to control angina or heart failure; they should always be used to reduce the risk of a further heart attack

Heart attack!

Whenever a heart attack is suspected, perhaps because of central chest pain (see page 16), it is very important to ring for an emergency ambulance straight away. Don't waste time by phoning your doctor, or anyone else, for advice. The patient should chew an aspirin while waiting for the ambulance. Chest pain can be caused by many things including indigestion, pneumonia and muscle strain, but if a heart attack is confirmed, emergency treatment can make all the difference.

When I qualified, and we're only going back to the last century, treatment for a heart attack was largely a case of relieving pain with morphine and hoping for the best. Things are different now. We still relieve pain; in fact the ambulance crew can do that, as well as administering oxygen and taking an ECG. In many cases, damage to the heart muscle can be limited by injection of a drug to disperse the blood clot (thrombolysis). But increasingly, heart-attack victims are taken straight to specialised units where emergency angioplasty and stenting are carried out.

After a heart attack

Long gone are the days when doctors put people on bed rest for several weeks after a heart attack! We now understand how important it is to get moving again. You would normally be sitting out of bed on the second or third day after admission with a heart attack. Gentle walking is gradually increased and, before the first week is up, you may be climbing a few stairs. Of course, some heart attacks are bigger than others and some people must take it more slowly than others.

Over the next few weeks, your exercise should be stepped up gradually and a continuing exercise routine, pitched at the right level, is very important. Don't rush it. Ease up if there are any symptoms such as chest pain or nausea.

Join a rehabilitation programme if you possibly can. A well run programme is invaluable, not just for supervising your exercise plan, but also for education and confidence-building, which are so important for getting back to normal.

Here are a few tips.

- **Smoking**
  If you were a smoker before your heart attack, you must stop now. Those who continue to smoke are much more likely to have another heart attack (and that may well be the last). Don't imagine that it will take years to reap the risk reduction after giving up: some of the risk is cut very quickly because smokers are more likely to have a thrombosis.

- **Weight control**
  Losing flab reduces the strain on your heart and lowers your blood pressure. The weight control plan in this book will improve your cholesterol too.

- **Why me?**
  If you are a slim non-smoker, you are probably asking why you had a heart attack. Your doctor will be checking your lipid levels, blood pressure and other risk factors. Often the problem is that several marginal risk factors, unimpressive by themselves, are interacting with each other. Do you have the metabolic syndrome (Table 24)? You are clearly at increased risk, but the diet and lifestyle plan in this book will reduce that risk.

- **Feelings**
  You don't laugh off a heart attack. You're bound to take it to heart and it will shake your confidence. It's hardly surprising that anxiety is a normal response and it can give way to depression. The support of those close to you is so important but it's often hard for families to understand the emotional chaos that follows a heart attack. Some people wear their heart on their sleeve while others bottle it up. Sharing emotions and using relaxation techniques will help (see Chapter 23).

- **Sex**
  As emotional turmoil settles and life becomes a little more
  normal, victims of a heart attack and their partners often worry
  about the safety of becoming sexually active again. One night
  stands and secret liaisons are a serious coronary hazard. But, if
  climbing two flights of stairs is no problem, or you can walk 300
  yards briskly on level ground without discomfort, there's no
  reason why you shouldn't enjoy making love to your partner.
  Let your meal go down for a couple of hours first, avoid diving
  into cold sheets, and don't be too adventurous to start with.

- **Driving**
  Don't drive for one month after a heart attack. If you have made
  a good recovery and you feel ready to drive at that stage, you
  may do so and you need not inform the DVLA at Swansea. You
  should check that your insurance policy doesn't impose any
  restrictions after a heart attack. On the other hand, if you have
  angina at rest or at the wheel, you should see your doctor,
  inform the DVLA, and avoid driving until it's sorted out.
  However fit and confident you feel, start with short, local
  journeys and take a passenger. Professional drivers holding
  LGV and PCV licences (which have replaced HGV and PSV
  licences) should inform the DVLA and follow their instructions.

- **Flying**
  Flying (in an aeroplane) will not be a problem for most survivors
  of a heart attack – following a recovery period of at least two or
  three weeks (although the airline may allow it as early as ten
  days after an uncomplicated heart attack). A pressurised cabin is
  equivalent to an altitude of about 6000 feet (1830 m) and those
  who are not fully recovered could become breathless. If you can
  walk 100 yards briskly on the flat without any symptoms, it
  should be safe to fly (as a passenger, not a pilot). Of course,
  stresses at the airport are often more significant than those in
  the air and many can be avoided by good planning: leave plenty
  of time, use a porter for heavy baggage, and don't smuggle.

- **Work**
  Don't rush back to work before you feel ready. This may be as soon
  as six weeks after a heart attack but you may need some months
  to build up your stamina first. Some jobs are flexible enough to

allow a gradual return, while others demand 'all or nothing'. If your job is not physically taxing, you are likely to be able to go back sooner than someone returning to heavy manual work.

- **Successful recovery – or failure?**
  Many people who survive a heart attack go on to make a full recovery and the small scar in the heart muscle causes no trouble at all. Some others suffer from persistent breathlessness that cannot be improved by fitness training. This is because more extensive damage to the heart muscle has reduced its pumping power and this 'heart failure' can be improved with drugs.

What drugs are used for coronary heart disease?

Not so long ago, if you had a heart attack, your doctor couldn't do very much – except wait for you to have another one. How things have changed! Now, your doctor might prescribe anything from three to six drugs to improve your quality of life and reduce your risks.

Drugs are used to treat heart failure, to control angina and to prevent future heart attacks. Most of the drugs were described in the chapter on blood pressure, so I won't go into detail about them here.

Treating heart failure

When your heart fails to pump at the proper pace, your legs and lungs can become waterlogged and diuretics relieve this.

Research has shown that using ACE inhibitors in heart failure makes you live longer. In the light of this, the argument for using diuretics alone for heart failure no longer holds water. In fact, when a heart attack upsets the heart's main pumping chamber (the left ventricle) – even mildly and temporarily – your prognosis is improved by using an ACE inhibitor. In 2007, NICE recommended that all patients should be offered an ACE inhibitor after a heart attack. Angiotensin receptor blockers provide a useful alternative when an ACE inhibitor causes side effects.

Controlling angina

The beta-blockers and calcium channel blockers that are so often used to reduce high blood pressure are also effective against angina.

In addition, nitrate drugs bring relief to many angina sufferers. Glyceryl trinitrate (GTN) is a quick-acting drug that is absorbed from a tablet or spray under the tongue; it can be used to relieve an attack once it's started, or to prevent an attack (e.g. before climbing a hill or seeing your bank manager). Nitrates can cause headaches in some people, but frequent use may solve the problem; some sufferers find that a GTN tablet under the tongue relieves their angina so quickly that they can spit it out before a headache starts. Nitrates can also be used – in skin patches or tablets – as long-acting angina preventers.

Nicorandil is a potassium channel activator. Like nitrates, it widens arteries and veins; unlike nitrates, it doesn't seem to become less effective with continuous use.

Sometimes it is necessary to use a combination of four drugs to bring angina under control.

ACTION POINT

◆ If you have had a heart attack or suffer from angina, you should take a low dose of aspirin unless there is a good reason not to (such as aspirin allergy)

Preventing future heart attacks

Drug treatment can be used to 'prevent' future heart attacks in those who have already had a heart attack or those who are known to be at increased risk because of coronary artery disease. Please don't misunderstand me here. It is accurate, though misleading, to say that certain drugs can prevent heart attacks: they prevent some heart attacks but not others. Taking such a drug can reduce your risk of having a heart attack but it can never guarantee that you won't have one.

Aspirin is top of the list. If you have had a heart attack or suffer from angina, you should be taking a low dose of aspirin (such as 75 mg daily) unless there is a good reason not to. Good reasons would include having a stomach ulcer, haemophilia or genuine aspirin allergy. Discuss it with your doctor if you're uncertain. A drug called clopidogrel is a suitable alternative in some cases (but it, too, can irritate the stomach). After insertion of a drug-eluting stent, it's very important to take clopidogrel in addition to aspirin for a full year. You remember that these clever stents inhibit the growth of scar tissue to prevent the artery from blocking up again. As the stent doesn't get covered in tissue so quickly, there's an increased risk of clot formation on the exposed stent during the first twelve months. The combination of aspirin and clopidogrel reduces that risk. After a year, clopidogrel can be stopped, but aspirin must be continued for life (or until we come up with something better).

All doctors have patients whom they would like to put on aspirin, in view of current evidence for its benefit, but who have 'slipped through the net'.

Talking of fishing nets, you probably remember that aspirin helps to prevent clots in the circulation in a similar way to fish oil – by making platelets less ready to stick together. While we would strongly recommend consumption of oily fish (e.g. two meals a week) both to those with heart disease and those without, we cannot recommend aspirin as a preventive measure for the healthy population at large. The small risk of serious bleeding from the stomach is overshadowed by the coronary protection for those with heart disease – but not necessarily for those at low coronary risk.

The doses of aspirin used to make platelets less 'sticky' are much lower than the 300–900 mg used to treat pain. These low doses are less likely to upset the stomach. Preventive aspirin is normally taken as a dispersible tablet in water, with or straight after food. Some people get on better with 'enteric-coated' tablets, which are sealed in a coating to protect the stomach.

Beta-blockers are used to reduce the risk of a further heart attack (unless there's a good reason to avoid this group of drugs, such as a history of asthma).

In 2007, NICE supported prescription of a fish oil supplement for people who had suffered a heart attack within the last three months and were not managing to eat enough oily fish (see page 97).

It has become clear that one of the most effective ways to cut down heart attacks among those with coronary heart disease is to tackle cholesterol, and it's now routine to do that with drugs.

Drug treatment of raised cholesterol

The Lifestyle Heart Trial published in *The Lancet* in 1990 showed that with far-reaching lifestyle changes (very low-fat vegetarian diet, stopping smoking, stress management training, and moderate exercise) it was possible to improve coronary atherosclerosis – even in severe cases – within one year, without the use of cholesterol-lowering drugs.

Sceptics please note: this was a properly controlled trial in which the control group received conventional advice and made moderate lifestyle changes; their atherosclerosis got worse within the year! Although no cholesterol-lowering drugs were used, the cholesterol reductions in the experimental group were better than those often seen after drugs have been prescribed. Do you want figures? OK: in the experimental group, total cholesterol fell by 24.3% and LDL-cholesterol by 37.4%. The reductions were achieved even though these people had already reduced their fat intake to 31.5% of calories and their cholesterol consumption to 213 mg/day (on average) *before baseline testing.*

Sadly, the common experience of doctors is that most people with heart disease fail to make such radical lifestyle changes as the experimental group made in this study. I am convinced that many of them fail because they are not given the necessary information or incentive, and I hope this book will play some part in putting that right.

Trials and triumphs

Several major trials using the powerful 'statin' drugs (HMG Co-A reductase inhibitors) have now been published. They must be powerful because they have transformed the thinking of the medical profession. Even doctors who were sceptical about the value of lowering cholesterol levels accept that these drugs have a vital role in the prevention of coronary deaths among those with established heart disease – so-called 'secondary prevention'.

The Scandinavian Simvastatin Survival Study (4S), published in *The Lancet* in 1994, studied 4444 people with coronary heart disease (stable angina or previous heart attack). These were men and women with total cholesterol levels ranging from 5.5 mmol/l to 8.0 mmol/l. They were divided (at random) into a treatment group who were given simvastatin tablets and a control group who were given placebo (inactive) tablets. After 5.4 years' follow-up, the main findings were that treatment with simvastatin had:

- Reduced the death rate (all causes) by 30%;

- Reduced the coronary death rate by 42%.

Like the WOSCOPS study mentioned in Chapter 4, this trial helped to reassure doctors that lowering cholesterol levels could reduce the total death rate and not just deaths from heart disease; there had previously been fears that an increase in deaths from other causes might cancel out the benefit.

It was very helpful that this trial included women as well as men, and this is now the trend. So many earlier studies on heart disease had been restricted to men.

I am now going to explain something that might seem a little technical at first but has important implications for millions of people. The starting dose of simvastatin in the 4S study was 20 mg and this was adjusted to keep the cholesterol level between 3.0 and 5.2 mmol/l. Virtually all the people ended up on 20 or 40 mg; only two were on 10 mg! This is often not appreciated by those quoting this study. Countless people in the real world are taking just 10 mg of simvastatin daily although it has not reduced their cholesterol levels into the target range for the 4S trial. It would be quite unreasonable to expect the same relative risk reduction among these people as was achieved with 20–40 mg in the 4S study. There is a good argument for raising their doses.

So, how much were cholesterol levels lowered by these higher doses in the 4S study? Simvastatin reduced the average total cholesterol by 25% and the LDL-cholesterol by 35% – remarkably similar numbers to those in the Lifestyle Heart Trial that used no lipid-lowering drugs at all. I must point out that there is no comparison between the *numbers of people* in the Lifestyle Heart Trial (48) and the 4S study (over 4000). If you have undergone coronary angiography yourself, you will understand why a trial involving repeated angiography could hardly recruit thousands of subjects. The experimental group in the Lifestyle Heart Trial was clearly a small, highly motivated group whereas the 4S study was more representative of the general population. If they were really put in the picture, many more people could be motivated and successful.

Some years after publication of the original 4S study, follow-up indicates that the participants continuing to take simvastatin are still deriving benefit from it.

The lowest of the low

Another landmark trial was the Cholesterol and Recurrent Events (CARE) study published in the *New England Journal of Medicine* in 1996. This involved 4159 men and women who had suffered a heart attack in the previous 20 months. The age range was 21–75 but all the women were past the menopause. The novel thing about this trial was that the people had 'normal' cholesterol levels – the average being 5.4 mmol/l (well below our population average). You might pause to take that in: they had cholesterol levels that our population regards as normal; they had all had a heart attack; apparently, men in their 20s were included!

The CARE study randomly divided the people into two groups: the treatment group received 40 mg of pravastatin daily and the control group took placebo tablets. (A cholesterol-lowering resin called cholestyramine was added to pravastatin or placebo if the LDL-cholesterol level remained above 4.5 mmol/l.)

The central finding was similar to that in the 4S study: there was a 24% reduction in heart attacks (fatal and non-fatal) in the pravastatin group.

It seems that if you get heart disease despite having an average cholesterol level, you benefit from reducing the level below average. Perhaps it is somewhere near the truth to say: if you get heart disease, whatever your blood cholesterol concentration is, it's too high for you.

The CARE study raised the possibility that there may be a limit to this. Unlike the 4S study, the higher the LDL-cholesterol level at the start of the trial, the bigger the relative risk reduction produced by treatment. In fact, treatment did not seem to be of any benefit at all when the LDL-cholesterol was below 3.2 mmol/l to begin with. (Some of those who have heart attacks despite low levels of LDL-cholesterol may be at risk because of low HDL-cholesterol and high triglycerides.)

More light was thrown on this by a colossal study published in *The Lancet* in 2002. The Heart Protection Study included 20 536 men and women aged between 40 and 80 (who already had heart disease or other arterial disease or diabetes) with a **total** cholesterol level of at least 3.5 mmol/l. Taking simvastatin (40 mg) produced the expected 25% reduction in heart attacks and strokes; the same benefit was seen even in those who started off with the lowest cholesterol levels. So, if you have diseased arteries or diabetes, perhaps you will benefit from taking a statin no matter how low your cholesterol is. Other studies suggest that too.

The LIPID trial (Long-term Intervention with Pravastatin in Ischaemic Disease) recruited 9014 men and women with heart disease – many of them with 'normal' cholesterol levels. Cholesterol levels ranged from just 4 mmol/l to 7 mmol/l and these people had either had a heart attack or were admitted to hospital with unstable angina. Pravastatin treatment reduced the total death rate by 23% and deaths due to heart attack by 29%. There was also a 20% reduction in strokes.

Again, the benefit seemed to be just as big in those with the lowest cholesterol levels.

Other drugs

Statins are not the only lipid-lowering drugs available, as you can see from Table 27.

Table 27 Lipid-lowering drugs

Class	Main actions
Statins (HMG CoA reductase inhibitors) Atorvastatin Fluvastatin Pravastatin Rosuvastatin Simvastatin	Reduce cholesterol production in liver Lower LDL-cholesterol levels (May lower triglycerides and raise HDL-cholesterol)
Fibrates Bezafibrate Ciprofibrate Clofibrate Fenofibrate Gemfibrozil	Lower triglycerides Lower LDL-cholesterol Raise HDL-cholesterol
Anion-exchange resins Cholestyramine Colestipol	Bind bile acids in gut Lower LDL-cholesterol (can *raise* triglycerides)
Nicotinic acid group Acipimox Nicotinic acid	Lower LDL-cholesterol Lower triglycerides Raise HDL-cholesterol
Fish oils	Lower triglycerides (reduce platelet 'stickiness')
Soluble fibre Ispaghula husk	Increases excretion of bile acids Lowers LDL-cholesterol
Selective cholesterol absorption inhibitors Ezetimibe	Block cholesterol uptake from gut Lower LDL-cholesterol

After statins, the fibrates are the most widely prescribed. They are particularly useful for people who have very raised triglycerides. If necessary, a fibrate can be used in combination with a statin, but this increases the risk of side effects and requires careful monitoring.

Anion-exchange resins can be used with statins in people who have severely raised cholesterol levels (such as those with familial hypercholesterolaemia). Taken as a drink, they are not very palatable and are used less often now that more effective and better-tolerated agents are available.

A novel class of drugs, selective cholesterol absorption inhibitors, was launched in 2003 with the introduction of ezetimibe (Ezetrol®). Blocking the absorption of cholesterol from the intestine gets rid of some of the cholesterol made in the liver as well as cholesterol from food (see page 55). Ezetimibe blocks cholesterol absorption without interfering with the uptake of fatty acids or vitamins. It is proving extremely useful. In difficult cases, the cholesterol reduction achieved by a statin may be inadequate; addition of ezetimibe can make all the difference.

Nicotinic acid is interesting because it was promoted as an over-the-counter DIY cholesterol remedy some years ago – partly on the basis that it's 'just a vitamin'. The doses used to lower cholesterol are vastly greater than the quantities obtained from food; side effects are common and medical supervision is essential. In the past, self-medication, particularly with older slow-release preparations, led to liver damage in some cases. A superior slow-release version (Niaspan®) is now available on prescription. Its main use is to boost flagging HDL levels where other measures have failed.

The stars

The statins have stolen the show. Massive trials using simvastatin and pravastatin convinced doctors that these drugs should be prescribed routinely for people with heart disease and for those at very high risk of arterial disease (such as people with diabetes). Since those early studies, evidence for the beneficial effects of atorvastatin and rosuvastatin has accumulated.

Impressive cholesterol reductions can usually be achieved with atorvastatin and now there is good evidence from trials that it, too, saves lives. In the GREACE study (GREek Atorvastatin Coronary-heart-disease Evaluation), LDL-cholesterol was reduced to below 2.6 mmol/l with atorvastatin (usually 20 mg), producing a massive 47%

reduction in deaths from heart disease; the atorvastatin group also had 47% fewer strokes and enjoyed a drop of 43% in total mortality.

What would happen if you gave atorvastatin to people with high blood pressure, in addition to the drugs to lower their blood pressure? That was one of the questions asked by the Anglo-Scandinavian Cardiac Outcomes Trial (ASCOT). Some people received atorvastatin 10 mg daily while others were given placebo (dummy) tablets to take with their treatment for blood pressure. This part of the trial was stopped early when it became clear that atorvastatin was saving lives by preventing strokes and heart attacks.

Rosuvastatin, the youngest of the family, is the most powerful statin yet – in the sense that a 10 mg dose will produce a bigger cholesterol reduction, on average, than the same dose of any other statin. Although it is likely that rosuvastatin also has the power to prevent heart attacks and strokes (and reduce the death rate), there is no sub-stitute for direct evidence of this.

Things look promising. The ASTEROID study was an uncontrolled trial on 507 patients published in the *Journal of the American Medical Association* – and rather sensationally reported by the media – in 2006. The patients underwent angiography for suspected coronary artery disease and were given rosuvastatin 40 mg daily for the next two years when angiography was repeated. Unfortunately, only 349 of them had results suitable for analysis. To be fair, the results were quite exciting: the majority of them had a significant reduction in the volume of atheroma blocking their arteries.

Although 40 mg is a standard dose of simvastatin, it is a high dose of rosuvastatin and 49 patients dropped out of the trial because of unwanted effects.

All drugs can produce side effects in some people; side effects can be trivial or catastrophic. Theoretically, the statins could cause liver or muscle problems. The small risk of a serious reaction in the muscles increases when statins are taken at top doses or combined with fibrates; one statin (cerivastatin) was withdrawn when it became apparent that combining it with gemfibrozil was particularly haz-ardous. If you are taking a statin and have unexplained muscle pains or weakness, your doctor can arrange a simple blood test (creatine kinase) to make sure that there is no significant inflammation in your muscles.

Big studies such as the Heart Protection Study, together with the widespread use of statins in recent years, have provided considerable reassurance that these drugs are generally well tolerated and safe. Even so, remember that we are talking about lifetime treatment; so far, those treated in the large clinical trials have been followed up for some years, but not for several decades.

REVERSING HEART DISEASE

There is strong evidence for the benefit of statin drugs in people who have heart disease even when the cholesterol level is not raised.

If you've had a heart attack or suffer from angina, the narrowing of your coronary arteries has made itself known. Fatty deposits gradually build up in our arteries for many years before we find out there's a problem. Unfortunately, we can't just have a quick look in our arteries to see how they're getting on. (Perhaps it would be too frightening if we could.) Wouldn't it be good if you could have a 'decoke'?

The Lifestyle Heart Trial published in *The Lancet* in 1990 showed that a big enough change in lifestyle could actually reverse heart disease without drugs. Those who were given routine advice made moderate lifestyle changes and their coronary arteries continued to get narrower. But a programme that involved a big change in diet, stopping smoking, managing stress and taking exercise resulted in some widening of the coronary arteries after just one year. Think how much more might be achieved in ten years!

The programme in this book is carefully balanced. It isn't a gimmick; it brings together all the ways of protecting your arteries that are firmly backed up by scientific research. Focusing your efforts on one 'cure' (whether it's fish oil or exercise) while ignoring everything else, isn't likely to be very effective. So use the Action Plan to put the whole programme into effect and start unblocking those arteries right now!

What are we aiming for?

In the light of all this evidence from the big statin trials, current guidelines recommend that if you have cardiovascular disease or diabetes, you should reduce your total cholesterol level below

5 mmol/l (LDL-cholesterol below 3 mmol/l) – or achieve a 25% reduction in total cholesterol (30% reduction in LDL), whichever results in lower levels. In other words, if you have a heart attack with a total cholesterol of 4.9 mmol/l, you shouldn't congratulate yourself that your cholesterol's on target, but reduce it by at least 25% (to less than 3.7 mmol/l). And if your total cholesterol was 5.1 mmol/l when heart disease struck, you shouldn't just get it down to 4.9 mmol/l; slash it by at least 25% to 3.8 mmol/l or lower.

But it's a moving target. In 2005, the Joint British Societies issued guidelines (known as JBS 2) recommending reduction of total cholesterol to less than 4 mmol/l (or by 25%) and reduction of LDL-cholesterol to less than 2 mmol/l (or by 30%). There is no doubt that the heart-attack risk will be further reduced by getting cholesterol that low. So a lot of experts think we should work to this target.

Even so, the lower cholesterol target has not been adopted nationally as yet. The Department of Health cannot currently face the huge additional cost of pushing statin doses up enough to hit the lower target.

**'We have saved five pence.
(Pause) But at what cost?'**

———————

SAMUEL BECKETT (1906–89),
All That Fall, 1957

After all, although people with established vascular disease and those with diabetes take priority, the plan would be to offer aggressive drug therapy to lower cholesterol (and blood pressure) to everyone with a CVD risk of 20% in ten years (page 309). It would be quite possible to bring the health service to its knees by prescribing statins for everyone who might benefit – especially if you adjust therapy to meet the proposed lower target.

Not only that, but always aiming for the lower target will mean more frequently using top doses of statins and combinations of drugs; inevitably, more people will suffer from side effects. Even now, a lot of people waste the statins they are prescribed by not taking them. If the rate of side effects increases, even more patients will abandon the prescribed treatment. As more people give up on their treatment, our efforts to reach cholesterol targets become less effective. So always aiming for the lower target could prove self-defeating.

I recommend that you take all the treatment you are prescribed, but discuss any suspected side effects with your doctor. Usually, if a drug has unwanted effects, the problem can be solved by adjusting or changing the treatment. And remember, the more you achieve with diet and lifestyle, the less intensive your drug therapy will need to be.

◆ Statin drugs can reduce the risk of having a heart attack by about 30% and the overall death rate by over 20%

◆ Statins are recommended for people with cardiovascular disease or diabetes, and people with a CVD risk of 20% in 10 years

◆ The current target is to reduce total cholesterol below 5 mmol/l (LDL below 3 mmol/l) OR reduce total cholesterol by 25% (LDL by 30%) – whichever results in lower levels

◆ Risk will be reduced further by achieving the JBS 2 target: total cholesterol below 4 mmol/l (or 25% reduction); LDL below 2 mmol/l (or 30% reduction)

◆ Lifestyle changes can bring remarkable benefits, but marginal adjustments yield marginal results

Chapter 27

Looking forward

'When people are free to do as they please,
they usually imitate each other.'

ERIC HOFFER,
The Passionate State of Mind, 1955

You are free – free to choose the way you eat and the way you live. Oh, I know that some are more limited than others by lack of money or by circumstance. But there's only one person who can decide whether you smoke, or take exercise, or control your weight. There is a vast range of foods available, and there are many different ways to cook. You can choose. You are free to follow fashion – to imitate those afflicted by a lethal epidemic.

You are free – free to get fit and to flourish on a first-class diet. You can be liberated and live, or you can be a lemming.

In the last chapter, we saw how dramatically statin drugs can reduce the risk of future heart attacks in people who already have heart disease (secondary prevention). If you don't have heart disease – and, of course, you're reading this book because you want to keep it that way – you may be saying: 'What about me?'

Perhaps you're thinking: 'A good diet and healthy lifestyle are all very well but, if this statin stuff is so good, why should I wait to have a heart attack before taking it? How about a bit of primary prevention? In any case, my first heart attack might kill me!'

Do you remember the WOSCOPS study? This showed that by giving the drug pravastatin to middle-aged men who had *not* had a heart attack (but who had an average cholesterol level of 7mmol/l) you could reduce their risk of coronary death significantly. In fact, the *relative* risk went down as much as it does when you give a statin drug to people who already have heart disease.

Remember, though, that the *absolute* risk is much lower in those without heart disease, so you have to treat many more people, and spend much more money, before you save one life.

The Polypill – poppycock or panacea?

You know that joke? The one where I say, 'Why aren't there any aspirin in the jungle?' And just as you're remembering that aspirin, or acetylsalicylic acid, is derived from the willow tree (genus *Salix*), and wondering whether willows grow in the jungle, I say, 'Because the parrots-eat-'em-all.' (It's the way I tell them.) Well, if you do know the joke, you might naturally assume the Polypill is simply paracetamol (or aspirin) for parrots.

But no. It's not even a pill for people who feel sick as a parrot. It's a pill to stop people getting sick in the first place. OK, it can't quite prevent all diseases yet – just the ones that kill most of us: cardiovascular diseases. To be fair, the designers of the Polypill don't actually claim their pill would completely eradicate diseases of the heart and circulation. They reckon it would prevent 88% of heart attacks and 80% of strokes. Not bad, eh?

I suppose science fiction writers have come up with even more fantastic ideas than this in the past. But these claims were made in the *British Medical Journal*. The creators of this magic pill are not fiction writers but eminent medical scientists.

They propose that their Polypill should be given to everyone from the age of 55, as well as anyone who already has cardiovascular disease. This strategy, they claim, 'would have a greater impact on the prevention of disease in the Western world than any other single intervention'. Quite a claim.

There must be something in it

You couldn't claim results like these from dispensing pellets of Polyfilla. The Polypill must have some serious stuff in it. So what are the magic ingredients that give this pill such powers of prevention? There are six.

First, a statin is included to lower cholesterol. Then there are three different drugs used to lower blood pressure but at half their normal doses. Add a generous helping of folic acid (0.8 mg) to lower homo-cysteine, then a dash of aspirin (75 mg) to reduce the risk of blood clots, and the recipe is complete.

If you already have heart disease, you might well be taking six drugs anyway and you would probably jump at the chance of having them all in one pill. The main drawback would be the fixed doses: you could no longer adjust the doses of individual drugs to fine tune your blood pressure and cholesterol level.

Giving six drugs to people with heart disease is one thing; giving them to people at high risk of developing cardiovascular disease is a logical next step; but dishing them out to the general population is another thing altogether.

Why stop here?

I can see an expanding role for the Polypill. Perhaps it would be wise to add a drug that counteracts insulin resistance to delay the onset of diabetes. Oh, and surely we should include an appetite suppressant to stem the tide of obesity. Maybe a bit of nicotine would make it easier for smokers to quit. And why not add a stimulant to make a sedentary population more active?

If it turns out that too many people are forgetting to take their Polypill, an anticholinesterase agent (the type of drug used to treat dementia) could be included to enhance defective memories. Should this strategy fail, we can think of other ways of delivering the drugs to the population – such as putting them in the water supply. Another advantage of this approach is that prevention would begin in child-hood instead of starting at 55. Yes, it would be very expensive and some would die of side effects but, given the scale of our Western epi-demics, what else can we do?

There is, of course, another way. In the Lyon Diet Heart Study, risk was reduced by a massive 70% – simply by changing to a delicious Mediterranean diet. Just think what could be achieved with a Polypoint Lifestyle Plan.

Making it happen

If we are to spend more and more millions on statins and other drugs in the hope of preventing people from developing heart disease, should we not put some serious resources into helping them change the way they eat and live? Do we really want to put drugs in the water supply to fight a plague produced by faulty lifestyles?

As a reader of this book, you have a detailed guide telling you which changes are worthwhile and how to make them. But being told in a consultation to improve your diet (perhaps with a few supplementary instructions such as 'reduce saturates' and 'increase polyunsaturates') is a bit like being told to go and fly an aeroplane – and being left to work out the practical details for yourself. I'm not blaming doctors; they don't have enough time to practise medicine, let alone give flying lessons.

Because dietary advice makes little difference, some health professionals have been duped: they think that *diet* makes little difference. We have seen the evidence that when people make the right changes, the impact is dramatic.

Whether you take a statin or not, whether you have a 'normal' cholesterol or not, don't forget that the impact of a good diet and lifestyle goes far beyond cholesterol. Don't forget the reduced risk of cancer, the anti-ageing effects, the protection against oxidation of LDL, the reduced risk of thrombosis, the control of blood pressure and, incidentally, the sense of wellbeing.

◆ You are free to reduce your risk, or to follow harmful customs

◆ Statin drugs have less to offer those at low risk, and really long-term safety has not yet been established

◆ Drugging the whole population is a poor way to tackle epidemics resulting from faulty lifestyles

◆ Your lifestyle remains crucial, whether you take a drug to lower cholesterol or not

◆ There is only one person who can change your lifestyle

I have a deep concern. I see our nation gripped by an epidemic – a scourge that strikes at its very heart. Yet some populations, with their simple, natural ways of life, whatever else they lack, they lack the heartache of this scourge.

I am concerned that we doctors (who have little time to dwell upon our own nutrition, let alone on yours), in our eagerness to treat this epidemic with potent drugs, may overlook a simple truth: you have the power to change; you can improve the way you eat and live – and, yes, enjoy life all the more.

It's your life. It's up to you.

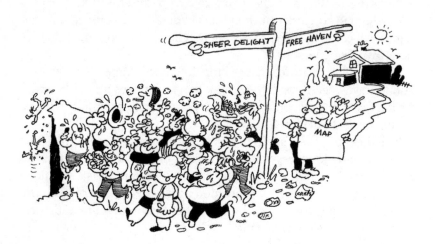

Chapter 28

The 28-day plan

TOP TIPS

◆ If you are in a small family, each eating a slice of bread a day, the bread can go stale waiting for you to eat it. Keep out what you'll eat in a couple of days and freeze the rest. If it comes to it, you can always toast frozen bread

◆ When grilling chicken for your evening meal, cook extra if you need it for a lunchtime sandwich the next day

---

Now you're ready to put it all into practice and see the results. This chapter tells you exactly how to do that.

The 28-day menu plan is supported by recipes in Chapter 29. So it's all worked out for you. But I'm now going to show you a simple, unique and completely revolutionary way to plan your daily menus that ensures you achieve the very best balance of nutrients to dump your toxic waist.

The MUNCH method

Like the pot plant in Figure 20, your diet needs to be firmly rooted in vegetables and fruit or it will be top-heavy and unbalanced. Try to have five different vegetables and three different fruits each day – and legumes (beans or lentils) most days.

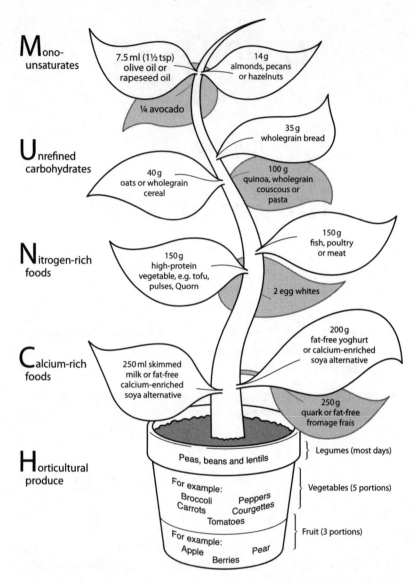

Mono-unsaturates

7.5 ml (1½ tsp) olive oil or rapeseed oil

14 g almonds, pecans or hazelnuts

¼ avocado

Unrefined carbohydrates

35 g wholegrain bread

40 g oats or wholegrain cereal

100 g quinoa, wholegrain couscous or pasta

Nitrogen-rich foods

150 g fish, poultry or meat

150 g high-protein vegetable, e.g. tofu, pulses, Quorn

2 egg whites

Calcium-rich foods

200 g fat-free yoghurt or calcium-enriched soya alternative

250 ml skimmed milk or fat-free calcium-enriched soya alternative

250 g quark or fat-free fromage frais

Horticultural produce

Peas, beans and lentils — Legumes (most days)

For example: Broccoli, Carrots, Peppers, Courgettes, Tomatoes — Vegetables (5 portions)

For example: Apple, Pear, Berries — Fruit (3 portions)

Figure 20 When planning your daily menu, use this pot plant to avoid a pot belly. Your diet should be firmly rooted in fruit and vegetables. Try to have three different fruits and five different vegetables (from Table 29) every day; pulses most days. Have two (or three) leaves from each level of the plant.

The leaves represent specified portions of vital foods. By having two leaves (up to three) from each level, you will be achieving a perfect balance. As explained in Chapter 18, this is the balance to go for if you have struggled unsuccessfully to shift abdominal fat and reverse the metabolic syndrome on a conventional low-fat, high-carbohydrate diet.

The MUNCH method **leaves** you satisfied and slim. Let's take a closer look at those leaves.

MONO-UNSATURATES (foods rich in mono-unsaturates, low in saturates)

1 7.5 ml (1½ tsp) olive oil or rapeseed oil
2 14 g almonds or hazelnuts (roughly 14 nuts), or pecans (8 or 9 halves)
3 ¼ avocado
4 10 ml (2 tsp) 59% fat olive spread
5 20 olives (but 20 olives in brine come with over 3 g salt!)

UNREFINED CARBOHYDRATE (low-GL wholegrain foods)

1 40 g porridge oats or wholegrain cereal
2 35 g slice wholegrain bread
3 100 g quinoa, wholegrain couscous, or wholegrain pasta
4 60 g brown basmati rice
5 2 wholegrain rye crispbreads (e.g. Ryvita)

NITROGEN-RICH FOODS (lean, high-protein foods)

1 150 g (100–200 g) fish, poultry or meat
2 150 g (100–200 g) tofu, soya mince/chunks (TVP), Quorn, beans or lentils
3 2 egg whites (you can have up to 1 whole egg a day, but 2 yolks a day will give you an unhelpful dose of cholesterol and fat)

CALCIUM-RICH FOODS (low-fat dairy foods and soya alternatives)

1 250 ml skimmed milk or fat-free, calcium-enriched soya alternative to milk
2 200 g fat-free yoghurt or calcium-enriched soya alternative
3 250 g quark or virtually fat-free fromage frais

HORTICULTURAL PRODUCE (vegetables and fruit)

1 5 (80-g) portions of vegetables (either including or additional to pulses)
2 3 (80-g) portions of fruit (including berries most days)

Normally, each day, have 1 and 2 from each group, i.e. the front two leaves of the plant. You can have up to three leaves from each level. Indeed, if you are a post-menopausal woman, try to have three from the calcium-rich group. It doesn't matter if you have your two or three portions of calcium-rich food in the form of skimmed milk (or fat-free soya milk fortified with calcium), i.e. 500–750 ml a day.

And if you are losing too much weight on the MUNCH plan, make a point of having three rather than two leaves from each level. Of course, by the end of the day, the poor plant will be stripped bare and uprooted, but don't worry about that: there'll be another one tomorrow.

Balance your fats

Note that almonds, hazelnuts and pecan nuts contain a high proportion of mono-unsaturates. Other nuts (e.g. walnuts) and seeds (e.g. pumpkin and sunflower seeds) are also very nutritious but they contain a high concentration of polyunsaturates. If you regularly eat large quantities of such foods, you'll find it impossible to achieve the MUNCH balance and slim your waist. Similarly, you are better off sticking with olive oil and rapeseed oil than introducing other oils like sunflower or corn oil.

On the 28-day plan, you can be confident that you are getting the right balance of the essential omega-6 and omega-3 fatty acids.

Please don't imagine for one minute that you should have your daily 7.5 ml (1½ tsp) of olive oil or rapeseed oil by pouring it onto a spoon and drinking it! Following the 28-day plan will give you the right balance: 13% of your energy intake will be coming from mono-unsaturates; less than 5% from saturates. Here's an example of how oil is consumed during the day.

		Oil intake
Lunch	15 ml (1 tbsp) salad dressing, 25% olive oil (or 7.5 ml (1½ tsp) salad dressing, 50% olive oil)	3.75 ml
Dinner	1 portion of recipe for 4 using 15 ml (1 tbsp) rapeseed oil	3.75 ml
Total		7.5 ml

Table 28 Portion sizes delivering a GL up to 10

Food	Portion size (g)	Food	Portion size (g)
BREAKFAST CEREALS		**PASTA**	
Porridge oats	40	Protein-enriched spaghetti	150
All-Bran	40	Wholewheat spaghetti	100
Muesli	35	White spaghetti	90
Shredded Wheat	20	**ROOT VEGETABLES**	
Weetabix	20	Carrots	150
BREAD		Swede (rutabaga)	150
Mixed-grain	55	Beetroot	150
Pumpernickel	50	New potatoes	135
Sourdough	45	Sweet potato	125
Wholemeal pitta	38	Yam	100
Wholemeal	35	Parsnips	100
White	30	Potatoes, general	80
White pitta	28	Cassava	70
Baguette	20	**DRIED FRUIT**	
GRAINS		Prunes	100
Couscous	150	Apricots	80
Cracked wheat (bulgar)	120	Figs	30
Quinoa	110	Dates	30
Buckwheat	100	Raisins	20
Millet	60		
Rice	60		

Table 29 Extremely low-GL vegetables

Alfalfa sprouts, raw	Cauliflower	Lettuce	Soya beans
Artichoke, globe	Celery	Mangetout	Spinach
Asparagus	Chives	Mushrooms	Spring onions
Aubergine	Courgettes	Okra	Squash, yellow
Bean sprouts	Endive	Onions	Tomatoes
Bok choy	Fennel	Peppers	Turnip
Broccoli	Green beans	Radishes	Watercress
Brussels sprouts	Kale	Rocket	
Cabbage	Kohlrabi, raw	Runner beans	
Carrots, raw	Leeks	Shallots	

The GL of many of these vegetables is negligible – too low to measure – because they contain so little digestible carbohydrate. There's no need to limit the portion size. Choose three or four vegetables from this list, ideally of three different colours, to cover half your plate. Avoid overcooking: not only does this spoil taste, texture and nutritional quality, it can also raise the GL.

Vary your vegetables

Try to get into the habit of choosing four vegetables – including three different colours wherever possible – to cover half your plate. You'll find a wide range of very low-GL vegetables in Table 29 that you can eat freely without limiting portion size. Be adventurous and try different varieties.

Did you hear about the lady who ventured to the greengrocer's to buy some vegetables? When the greengrocer came to serve her, she pointed and said, 'Man, get out'. The greengrocer looked puzzled until he realised she was pointing at the sign saying 'mangetout'. Good for her: she was presumably trying something unfamiliar.

Cooking vegetables

Most vegetables can be eaten raw, but often you'll want to cook them. You won't always have time to prepare vegetables or the inclination to use four pots to cook four different types. Don't worry. Keep bags of frozen vegetables such as soya beans, baby carrots, peas, peppers, green beans and broccoli in the freezer. You can simply bung four different vegetables together in one large microwave dish and they'll be ready in minutes.

When you have more time, steaming is an easy way to get the best out of any fresh vegetables in Table 29 that you want to cook.

It's better to keep cooking time short and enjoy raw vegetables (such as carrots, celery, broccoli and cauliflower) when you can. (All generalisations are false – including this one.) Pulses are different.

Dried beans should be soaked, rinsed and thoroughly cooked (but lentils don't have to be soaked). Tinned legumes are convenient. Go for those canned in plain water, without added salt or sugar.

Using GL as a portion guide

With high-carbohydrate foods, GL provides a useful guide to portion size. Keeping the GL of a serving down to 10 or less will help you to stay in control of your blood sugar levels. Table 28 shows the portions of common high-carbohydrate foods that will give you a GL up to 10.

Pulses
Try to include peas, beans or lentils in your menu every day. The GL of soya beans is so low that they appear in Table 29. But you can eat up to 150 g (or half a can) of any legume without worrying about GL.

Fruit
Eat plenty of berries (e.g. blackberries, raspberries, blueberries, strawberries). Raw, whole berries contain very little digestible carbohydrate so you don't need to bother about the GL; they are a useful source of fibre and are packed with antioxidants, vitamins and minerals.

You will see from Table 10 on page 71 that the GL of a portion of any other type of fresh fruit is generally no problem, but you need to limit your intake of ripe banana (a large banana weighs over 120 g).

Dried fruit is a different matter. Use Table 28 as a guide to maximum portion size.

Pasta
Despite its low GI, pasta delivers a significant GL because it is densely packed with digestible carbohydrate. It's helpful to choose a whole-grain variety, cook it *al dente* and keep portions down to 100 g cooked weight (see Table 31).

◆ The MUNCH method is a simple, unique and revolutionary way to plan your daily menu

◆ The 28-day plan precisely balances your fatty acid intake

◆ You can eat very low-GL vegetables freely: have 5 portions a day

◆ Have 3 different portions of fruit every day – berries most days

◆ Don't overcook vegetables; enjoy raw vegetables often

◆ Use GL as a guide to portion size of high-carbohydrate foods

Table 30 Useful items to keep in stock

Tinned:	Passata
Pulses, e.g. chickpeas, lentils, mixed beans (in water)	Tomato puree
Baked beans (reduced sugar and salt)	Oil – olive oil, garlic-infused olive oil, rapeseed oil
Bean sprouts (in water)	Vinegar, e.g. balsamic vinegar, wine vinegar, cider vinegar, rice vinegar
Bamboo shoots (in water)	
Tomatoes – plum and chopped	
Red peppers	Reduced-salt soy sauce
Fish, e.g. tuna (in water), salmon	Teriyaki sauce
	Mustard, e.g. Dijon
Dried beans and lentils	Crunchy peanut butter (low sugar, salt and palm oil)
Gram flour	
Arrowroot	Almond butter (100% almonds)
Wholegrain couscous	Clear honey
Quinoa	Low-salt stock cubes
Brown basmati rice	Solo or LoSalt
Wholewheat pasta	Black peppercorns
Traditional rolled oats (not instant) – for porridge and muesli	Spices, e.g. cardamom, cayenne pepper, chilli powder, coriander, cumin, curry powder, nutmeg, paprika, turmeric
All-Bran	
Nuts, e.g. almonds, hazelnuts, pecans (unsalted)	Dried herbs, e.g. basil, bay leaves, bouquet garni, dill, mixed herbs, oregano, rosemary, thyme
Ground and flaked almonds	
Dried fruit, e.g. raisins, apricots	Xylitol

Thick and fast

Using a lot of wheat flour or cornflour to thicken sauces can increase the GL of a meal significantly. This may lead to a rapid rise in blood glucose, especially when the thickener is one of a number of high-GL foods consumed together or in close succession.

GL can be reduced by using gram flour, soya flour, ground almonds or ground hazelnuts. You could even use ground groundnuts, but that's too difficult to say – and everyone thinks you have a stammer. In any case, the level of mono-unsaturates in almonds and hazelnuts is higher.

Other low-GL thickeners include vegetable purée (useful in soups), silken tofu, quark and xanthan gum.

A lot of the recipes in Chapter 29 use gram flour which is made from chickpeas. Also known as 'besan flour' and 'garbanzo flour', it provides a quick, easy, low-GL way of thickening sauces.

Xanthan gum is an alternative when you want a low-GL thickener, e.g. for sweet and sour sauce, that doesn't add the cream colour of gram flour. It's a vegetable gum (soluble fibre, in effect) purchased as a dry powder that mixes with water. You only need a pinch to thicken a sauce, so 100 g will go a long way. Add too much and you'll get sweet and sour slime.

Arrowroot is much easier to use – an excellent option when you want a completely clear sauce. Unlike cornflour, it's not upset by acidic sauces such as sweet and sour.

Sweet nothings

Artificial sweeteners, intended to add sweetness but nothing in the way of calories, have been around a long time. Products such as aspartame and sucralose can be useful.

Another option is to use a little fructose – simple fruit sugar. Fructose is sweeter than sucrose (table sugar) and imposes a lower GL. It's best used in very small quantities. For one thing, because fructose is sweeter than sucrose, you can get away with little more than half the quantity. And eating large amounts of fructose could have adverse metabolic effects which would be self-defeating. Mind you, some rumours and reports about the unwanted effects of fructose have arisen from confusing it with high-fructose corn syrup – a completely different product.

A few recipes in Chapter 29 are enhanced by **small** amounts of clear honey which contains fructose (but also other sugars).

Xylitol, a natural sugar alcohol, is a particularly useful sweetener. It tastes similar to sucrose but has a lower GI and calorie content. Unlike sugar, it doesn't attack teeth; in fact, it seems to be positively good for them! It's available from supermarkets and health food shops (Perfect Sweet™).

Bitter regret

Many of the recipes include garlic. Use as much as your social life, or your partner, can stand. Not only is it good for you (see Chapter 10), it also adds a wonderful flavour – unless you overcook it and produce a nasty bitter taste. Similarly, spices can be exquisite, but if you burn them, you will regret it.

Sauces made with tomatoes are sometimes a little sharp. You'll find grated carrot in a lot of the recipes; apart from adding useful nutrients such as vitamin A, it also balances any bitterness from the tomatoes.

A salt course for beginners

If you are used to traditional food, with loads of fat and salt, you should have no difficulty switching to low-fat cuisine. Very low-fat dishes are not necessarily any less delicious than high-fat ones and they can even be served to the uninitiated at dinner parties.

However, I don't recommend taking a sudden leap to very low-salt cooking at the same time. If you suddenly present your family with a low-sodium meal, they may well demand the saltcellar and this could create an obstacle to further progress. It is better to reduce the salt content of your food gradually, allowing the palate a period of time for adjustment. During this time, increase your skill in the use of herbs, spices and other flavourings. Use a little Solo or LoSalt where necessary.

Remember, though, that when using ingredients such as soy sauce, stock cubes and passata, you are adding salt and this should be quite enough to satisfy the average palate.

Spice power

The power of herbs, spices and similar ingredients to complement the flavour of your dishes cannot be overstated – especially when the salt content is reduced.

Use fresh herbs when you can, and in some cases, perhaps treble the quantity you would use of dried herbs. Of course, you'll always need dried herbs to fall back on; store them in tightly sealed containers or jars in a cool place out of the light.

Spices are aromatic or pungent parts of a plant – often seeds, roots or bark – used to flavour food. Store them carefully as for dried herbs. Buy both dried herbs and spices in modest quantities that you will use up over a few months as they lose their flavour when stored for years.

Peppercorns freshly ground from a peppermill give a better flavour than bought ready-ground pepper. Mixed whole peppercorns (green, black, white and pink) are an agreeable alternative to black pepper.

Game for a laugh

Frisky, frolicking animals that run (or hop) wild have far leaner, healthier bodies than sedentary residents of a farm. Anything from the ostrich to the kangaroo seems fair game these days and such creatures certainly provide a lower-fat meat and an entertaining change from regular fare.

Some people are more adventurous than others, so I haven't included less familiar species in the 28-day plan.

◆ Wheat flour and cornflour can increase the GL of a meal; gram flour and xanthan gum are low-GL thickeners; arrowroot is useful for clear sauces

◆ Xylitol is a low-GL natural sugar alcohol; it tastes like sugar and is good for teeth

◆ Burning garlic or spices ruins flavour

◆ Cut right down on salt, but do it gradually; use Solo or LoSalt when necessary

STOCK ANSWERS

Recipes frequently call for stock. If your answer is a stock cube, you are probably adding a lot of salt (and some fat). Low-salt stock cubes exist, but are not always easy to find. Vegetable bouillon powders, too, may have salt as the top ingredient; look out for the reduced-salt version.

The ideal solution is a home-made broth consisting of the ingredients you have in stock – vegetable scraps, chicken bones and so on. Water drained from cooked vegetables is always a good start. For chicken stock you might use meaty chicken bones, celery, onion, carrot, garlic, coriander, lemon grass and pepper. Cover with liquid, bring to the boil, skim off any scum, then simmer for a couple of hours. It's useful to make big batches of stock and keep some in the freezer.

Many supermarkets have ready-made refrigerated stocks (e.g. vegetable, chicken, fish) that are not salty and simply need to be diluted. Of course, if you're a bit short of stock, whether you make your own or buy it, you can always dilute it with wine, vermouth or sherry!

The grain, the whole grain and nothing but . . .

The truth is that consumers are often confused about which foods are made from whole grains. Couscous, for example, is an excellent, lower-GL alternative to rice. But the most widely available varieties are not made from whole grains. Your local supermarket might sell wholegrain couscous, but you may have to resort to a health food shop. If the packet doesn't clearly say 'wholegrain' (or 'wholewheat'), it won't be.

Quinoa, the seed of a species of goosefoot, is not technically a cereal grain (as the plant isn't a grass) but for practical purposes it is. It counts as a wholegrain food on this plan.

Unrefined carbohydrates play a crucial role in the MUNCH plan. Wherever possible, choose grains that have had nothing removed and nothing unhelpful added.

I recommend a mixed-grain bread that has visible grains within it (not just on the outside). A wholegrain product is made with whole grains which is good, but if those whole grains are then pulverised, although all the nutrients and fibre will still be present, the GI will have gone up. So when people equate 'wholegrain' with 'low-GI', there may be a grain of truth in it, but no more than that.

Wet or dry?

Another source of great confusion is the portion size of grain foods. When you read about eating 100 g of rice, for example, does this mean 100 g of the dry product from the packet or 100 g of cooked (wet) rice?

In the 28-day plan, the specified weight of couscous, quinoa, spaghetti or rice refers to the cooked weight. But, of course, you start with the dry stuff, so how do you know how much to cook? Use Table 31 which shows you the relationship between dry and cooked weights.

Table 31 Conversion of dry weight to cooked weight

FOOD	1 PORTION		4 PORTIONS	
	Dry weight (g)	Cooked weight (g)	Dry weight (g)	Cooked weight (g)
Wholegrain couscous	45	100	180	400
Quinoa	40	100	160	400
Wholewheat pasta	45	100	180	400
Brown basmati rice	25	60	100	240

Table 31 provides a practical guide based on typical values. The precise relationship between dry and cooked weights will depend on the product and the conditions of preparation.

To cook quinoa for four, rinse 160 g of quinoa and transfer it to a saucepan with 380 ml (twice the volume) of water or stock. Bring to the boil and simmer, partially covered, for 13 minutes, or until the water is absorbed.

To prepare four servings of couscous, put 180 g of couscous in a bowl, pour on 225 ml of boiling water (or stock), cover tightly and leave for five minutes.

Oat cuisine

Whole oats can boost your intake of soluble fibre and I recommend adopting them as one of your regular wholegrain foods. Traditional rolled oats are commonly cooked as porridge, but they are also great raw – in muesli or on cereal for example.

It's difficult to generalise about the GL of porridge because no two bowls of porridge are the same. You're better off with traditional rather than instant oats; after that, so much will depend on the cooking. Published data usually refer to the weight of cooked porridge, as opposed to the weight of oats and liquid used to make it.

You will find that in the 28-day plan, I have used 40 g of oats with 125 ml of skimmed milk; I just cook it for two minutes in the microwave and it produces a relatively dry porridge with identifiable oats – nothing like traditional porridge, really. That suits me fine. Once it's topped with something interesting like fat-free Greek yoghurt and berries, I'm happy.

To make traditional porridge, you need to use at least twice as much milk (or water) and cook for longer until the oats give up all hope of individuality for the common good.

If you want to make traditional porridge – either by making up the volume with water or by using 250 ml of skimmed milk or fat-free soya milk – please go ahead; I honestly don't want you to force down porridge you don't like. In fact, if you cook it slowly for 30 minutes in a double boiler, perhaps while you're getting dressed, it turns out wonderfully 'creamy', even if you use water and no milk. I suspect that my porridge will have a significantly lower GL than yours, but I don't have the laboratory evidence to prove it.

◆ Couscous won't be wholegrain unless the packet says so

◆ Choose mixed-grain bread containing visible grains (not just on the outside)

◆ Recommended portions of grain foods (e.g. couscous, quinoa, rice) refer to cooked weight – over twice the dry weight

◆ Overcooking pasta and other grain foods can raise GL

A practical plan

Try to follow the 28-day plan as closely as possible, at least until you really understand how to apply the MUNCH method to everyday life. The plan is designed for real life; it's something you can really do, not something that just looks pretty on paper.

Breakfasts have been kept deliberately simple, with an element of repetition. We don't want to think too hard at breakfast.

Each week has a different soup and that soup is on the lunch menu twice in the week. This is because it's convenient to make eight portions of soup at once. If you have a family of four, you don't want to be making a different soup before you've finished the first one. If you have a family of eight, I apologise; you'll just have to make more soup (but then you're probably used to cooking in a cauldron).

It only takes a couple of seconds to blend ingredients in a food processor – on television, in a studio. I'm guessing that you don't cook dinner in a studio. We never see the TV chef getting the food processor out of an awkward space in the cupboard, or washing it up afterwards. Food processors are invaluable, and I'm all for them. But where it's more convenient to mix ingredients in a bowl, or shake them in a sealed container, that's what I suggest.

Some ingredients, such as olive oil and reduced-salt soy sauce, are useful stock items and they turn up repeatedly in recipes. I have tried to avoid putting, for example, '1 tbsp apricot jam' in a recipe just for the fun of it. If you don't normally have apricot jam, you'll have to buy it specially; and if that recipe doesn't turn out to be one of your favourites, you're looking for ways to use up apricot jam – not very helpful if you're trying to lose weight. Similarly, I don't think it's helpful to specify a different variety every time a recipe calls for mustard.

On the other hand, if you use part of a bottle of passata (sieved tomatoes), the rest will be useful for soup and other recipes (but watch the salt content if you use a lot of it).

You'll find the marinades in these recipes are generally of very low volume. Some recipes seem to require total immersion in buckets of fluid. If it's convenient, effective and economical to use a small volume, closely applied in a plastic bag or sealed container, that's what I'd rather do. You probably feel the same way.

Recipes have been kept simple. Don't be put off if a list of ingredients looks lengthy: no complicated or drawn-out procedures are involved. It's usually just a case of throwing everything into one pot, or popping something in the oven or under the grill.

After all, if a plan isn't convenient, you won't stick to it and then it can't work.

MUNCH yourself slim

This plan has been carefully constructed to give you the energy balance illustrated in Figure 13, while being nutritionally complete and taking account of all available scientific evidence. It's designed to shift abdominal fat, reverse the metabolic syndrome, improve general health and boost energy levels.

That's an awful lot to keep in focus while translating scientific theory into everyday food – the 'ten balls' I referred to in the Preface. So many diet plans focus on one strategy and lose sight of something crucial. Why follow, for example, a low-GI diet plan that overlooks salt intake or the balance of fatty acids?

The good news is, I've done it. I've kept my eye on those ten balls, so you don't have to. Just follow the plan and the rest will take care of itself.

Of course, one factor that no diet plan should ever lose sight of (but many do) is the quality of the food itself. How appealing, varied and satisfying is it? Try to stick to a bland, restricted diet and you will inevitably fail. This plan is full of flavour, variety and deeply satisfying food.

Tastes vary, of course. There may be something I find exquisite that you don't like. If a particular meal doesn't appeal to you, swap it for one that does. Remember that each day is nutritionally balanced, but if you want to replace a meal with another in the same category, that's fine.

Every day of this plan includes a vegetarian meal – lunch or dinner – based on a good source of vegetable protein. Some foods such as Quorn or quinoa may be unfamiliar to you. Let me encourage you to give them a fair try. You may be pleasantly surprised, but sometimes the palate needs time to acquire a new taste. After all, if you didn't want to discover anything new, you wouldn't be reading this book (you'd be rereading *Noddy Goes to Toytown*).

This plan is about MUNCHing your way to success. As you enjoy three meals and three snacks a day, you will be controlling your blood sugar, reducing your adipokine levels, raising your adiponectin level, ditching toxic abdominal fat and recharging your battery.

And there's more good news. By following the plan, you will soon get a feel for the required balance of foods. Then, using the unique MUNCH method, you can go on ensuring that your daily menu delivers the right balance to keep your toxic bulge at bay.

Why not set up a MUNCH group? A circle of friends learning and making changes together can be a great encouragement to one another. Occasionally, you could have a MUNCH party where you share a meal (following MUNCH principles, of course) and exchange ideas and experiences.

What if I'm losing too much weight on the plan?

If you are overweight, the ideal rate of weight loss is one or two pounds a week. It doesn't matter if you lose more than this in the first week. After that a slow, steady loss, up to two pounds a week, helps to ensure that it's fat and not muscle you're getting rid of. Gradual loss of inches from your waist will confirm that your deadly visceral fat is disappearing.

So what if it's all happening too fast, or you've reached your target weight and waist size, but pounds and inches are still dropping off?

First, congratulations. You're following the plan and it's working. You can now eat more, but stick to the MUNCH proportions. Make sure you have three leaves from each level, rather than two (Figure 20).

If you are doing that already and still losing weight, increase portion size. Have 20 g of almonds or hazelnuts instead of 14 g. Introduce other nuts, like walnuts and pecans, and have up to three brazil nuts a day; add a tablespoon of pumpkin seeds or flax seeds most days. Make sure you are getting some olive oil or rapeseed oil (up to 15 ml/day). Put extra oats on your All-Bran and have a larger helping of muesli; have portions of up to 150 g of couscous, quinoa and pasta; have 200-g portions of high-protein foods such as fish, chicken, tofu and pulses; include extra fruit smoothies made with skimmed milk or fat-free soya milk; allow yourself more root vegetables, including new potatoes.

Don't resort to junk food. Eat more MUNCH food, in the right proportions. You're in control.

Of course, in the unlikely event that your weight fails to stabilise, you need to check that there is nothing wrong. Pay a visit to your doctor.

What if I'm not losing enough weight?

Remember, just one pound a week is fine. It may not seem dramatic at first, but it's a stone in three months; keep going at that rate and you'll be well on your way to losing four stone after a year. As long as you do it the right way, you can keep the weight off. What's the point of losing three stone rapidly only to put six back on?

What if you don't even seem to be losing a pound a week? Don't forget that muscle is heavier than fat. So if you're following the plan and losing fat while gaining muscle, the bathroom scales may not congratulate you – but you'll reap the benefit in due course. Mending your metabolism is the top priority. Does your waist measurement show progress?

Improving your metabolism isn't just about diet; exercise is essential too. Are you getting your basic minimum of 30 minutes' brisk walking a day? If you are, and your tape measure's stuck, find a way of increasing your exercise – perhaps to two 30-minute sessions a day. If you don't have any medical problems (such as heart disease), include some strength training to increase the bulk of your metabolically active muscle. You can begin simply by doing repeated arm movements (such as biceps curls) while holding cans of mixed pulses (with no added salt) from your store cupboard. If in doubt, check with your doctor first, and always follow the precautions described in Chapter 20.

Make sure you are measuring portions and not just guessing. Are you using a proper tablespoon (15 ml) or teaspoon (5 ml) to measure oil?

Are you cooking for one? If so, you need to scale down the recipes or freeze the excess for future meals. And, of course, if you are cooking for four, but the other three in your family are gerbils, that will be a problem too. Don't eat more than one portion.

Is alcohol your downfall? A little alcohol can be beneficial for some people, but if you're struggling to slim your waist, you could do without those 'empty calories' (7 calories/g of alcohol). There's a good case for cutting out alcohol altogether until you've reached your target, but if you don't want to do that, keep to a maximum of one unit every other day (see Chapter 11).

Perhaps you're sneaking some extra snacks into your daily menu. If it's crisps, cakes, ice-cream or biscuits, I really don't need to say more, do I?

But you may be supplementing the menu plan with 'healthy' snacks like muesli. After all, although the MUNCH plan lowers GL dramatically, it's not a very low-carbohydrate regime. Unrefined carbohydrate foods (such as oats, wholegrain couscous and quinoa) play a vital role. Even so, if you have already had two wholegrain foods that day, and then slip in an extra bowl of muesli, there's certainly no need to have a pile of couscous with your evening meal.

Once you've identified the problem, I am sure you'll soon be back on track. This is a truly effective plan, but the most powerful medicine in the world won't work if you don't take it.

If you're really following the plan, but the bulge refuses to budge, see your doctor to rule out problems such as thyroid deficiency.

Keeping hunger at bay

The MUNCH plan includes plenty of protein – from both animal and vegetable sources – and one of the main benefits of this is that it keeps you feeling satisfied for longer. Also, the steady control of blood glucose achieved on this plan keeps energy up and hunger down.

So what do you do if hunger strikes unexpectedly, when you're not due a meal or snack? Your first thought should be to have a glass of water, or a cup of tea or herbal tea. Sometimes a glass of water is all it takes and perhaps you're not drinking enough. These drinks don't appear in the menu plan because you can have them whenever you want. The occasional cup of coffee is fine too, as long as you don't add high-fat milk or cream. Don't drink unfiltered cafetière coffee regularly (Chapter 12).

Remember to allow that 20 minutes after a meal, a snack or a drink for your brain to get the message that you've had enough.

For those times when that just isn't enough, it is essential to have readily available snacks that won't undermine your MUNCH plan. Always keep prepared crudités – raw celery, broccoli, cauliflower, carrots and peppers, for example – in your fridge (and at work, if necessary).

When something more filling is needed, a bowl of low-calorie vegetable soup can save the day. 'Creamy tomato soup' (p. 410) is thick and satisfying. If you thin it a little with additional low-salt vegetable stock, you can always use it to fill a gap – any time of day or night.

Could I have a food allergy?

The word allergy is often used very loosely and some people even claim to be allergic to work. True allergy involves an unhelpful reaction of the body's immune system – usually to a foreign protein. (The protein is called 'foreign' because the immune system senses that it doesn't belong to the body; it's not that British eggs are safer than French.)

Severe food allergy (such as nut allergy) can result in a life-threatening reaction to tiny traces of the food. Many people have milder allergies producing less dramatic reactions.

'Food intolerance' is a much broader term covering adverse reactions to food that don't involve the immune system. I can certainly remember being intolerant of some school lunches (but that was in the bad old days). Indeed, food intolerance can produce a wide range of symptoms from migraine to irritable bowel syndrome and is often unrecognised.

Lactose intolerance is a particular example. This results from deficiency of the enzyme lactase which is needed to digest lactose (milk sugar). If you are lactose intolerant, you may tolerate small amounts of milk in food, but suffer from abdominal cramps, bloating and diarrhoea after drinking a glass of milk. Using soya alternatives to milk solves the problem.

When you suffer from symptoms suggestive of irritable bowel syndrome (such as variable bowel habit, cramps and bloating), it is usually difficult to link the symptoms to any specific food. It's well worth seeing your doctor: for one thing, it only takes a simple blood test to screen for coeliac disease (gluten sensitivity) which is often undiagnosed.

What if my cholesterol level isn't going down?

The 28-day plan will in most cases greatly improve blood cholesterol readings. Not only can you expect a significant reduction of total cholesterol, but reversal of the metabolic syndrome will improve the balance of lipids, raising HDL-cholesterol and reducing triglycerides. Carry on with the MUNCH method after the 28-day plan, and you will reap more benefit from these metabolic changes as time goes on.

If reduction of LDL-cholesterol is proving difficult, place more emphasis on your intake of soluble fibre, soya protein and almonds.

It's helpful to make fruit smoothies with fat-free soya milk and add psyllium husks. Use oat bran as well as lots of pulses and other vegetables (including okra and aubergine) to further boost your intake of soluble fibre. Also consider a daily supplement of plant sterols (e.g. one Flora pro.activ mini yoghurt drink) or stanol (e.g. one Benecol yoghurt drink).

Table 32 shows a menu plan designed to maximise reduction of LDL-cholesterol without compromising MUNCH principles. Eating a very low-fat, high-carbohydrate diet, or a diet very high in polyunsaturates, will drive down LDL-cholesterol; but if that's at the expense of pushing down HDL too, it's not the best way.

Table 32 Boosting reduction of cholesterol on the MUNCH plan

Breakfast	Oat bran porridge (20 g oats + 20 g oat bran with 250 ml fat-free soya milk); 1 Flora pro.activ mini yoghurt drink
Morning snack	Soya fruit smoothie (made with 250 ml fat-free soya milk and 2 tsp psyllium husks); 14 g almonds
Lunch	185-g can tuna in water, drained; Cannellini bean and coriander salad (p. 406), using cannellini beans and soya beans; 1 apple
Afternoon snack	Soya fruit smoothie (made with 250 ml fat-free soya milk and 2 tsp psyllium husks); 14 g almonds
Dinner	Tofu and vegetable curry (p. 397); 100 g quinoa; 80 g aubergine; 80 g okra
Evening snack	Soya fruit smoothie (made with 250 ml fat-free soya milk and 2 tsp psyllium husks)

The table shows the menu for one day in a MUNCH plan that achieves further reduction of LDL-cholesterol by increasing the intake of soya protein, soluble fibre and almonds, while adding a supplement of plant sterols (or stanol).

- ◆ The 28-day plan is easy to follow; ingredients and methods are simple, but food is varied and satisfying

- ◆ If you don't fancy a particular meal, replace it with another in the same category

- ◆ The MUNCH method is a way of life – easy to continue after the 28-day plan

- ◆ If you are losing too much weight on the plan, increase portions using the MUNCH method

Time to get a move on

Are you ready to get going and start losing those inches? Remember that activity is an essential part of this plan. Combine the MUNCH diet with movement and you'll mobilise your metabolism: tissues will respond better to insulin, blood glucose control will improve and that toxic bulge will begin to move.

The 28-day plan is designed to be combined with a minimum of 30 minutes' exercise a day (such as brisk walking). Better still, build an hour of physical activity into your daily routine – perhaps in two 30-minute sessions. Vigorous vacuum cleaning, energetic gardening and frequent fidgeting all help. But why not have some fun? Put on that CD or DVD of dance hits and go with it, in private if necessary – you know you want to.

- ◆ The plan enhances metabolism, increasing muscle and reducing toxic fat

- ◆ Wrong portions, junk snacks, alcohol and lack of exercise can all sabotage your progress

- ◆ Drink water before having an unscheduled snack; have MUNCH-friendly snacks available

- ◆ LDL-cholesterol reduction is enhanced by boosting intake of soluble fibre, soya protein, almonds and plant sterol (or stanol)

Have you cleared your fridge and cupboards of everything unhelpful that may undermine your progress? Are you stocked with useful
items (see Table 30)? Do you have everything you need for the first
two days of the plan? Right then.

Your new lifestyle begins here.

WEEK 1	Day 1	Day 2	Day 3
Breakfast	Porridge (40 g oats with 125 ml skimmed milk); 60 g 0% fat Greek yoghurt; 80 g berries (e.g. blueberries, blackberries, raspberries, strawberries)	30 g All-Bran with 125ml skimmed milk; 60 g 0% fat Greek yoghurt; 1 banana, sliced; 10 hazelnuts	½ grapefruit (with ½ tsp xylitol if required); 1 free-range egg (poached, boiled or scrambled); 1 slice wholegrain toast
Morning snack	14 almonds; 1 tbsp raisins	Fruit smoothie (p. 423)	14 almonds; 30 g dried apricots
Lunch	Tuna and orange salad (185-g can tuna in water, drained; sliced fresh orange; rocket, tomato, onion, cucumber); 1 tbsp lower-fat vinaigrette (p. 417); 1 apple	Creamy tomato soup (p. 410); 1 slice wholegrain bread (e.g. rye or mixed-grain); 1 nectarine	120 g quinoa tabbouleh (p. 388); 60 g virtually fat-free fromage frais; 80 g raspberries
Afternoon snack	Fruit smoothie (p. 423)	60 g quinoa tabbouleh (p. 388)	Fruit smoothie (p. 423)
Dinner	Chinese chickpeas (p. 391); Peas; 1 pear	Mustard lime chicken (p. 375) with mustard sauce (p. 415); Mixed green salad (p. 405); 60 g chickpeas; 2 plums	Haddock and prawns in white wine sauce (p. 383); Spinach, carrots and peas; 1 apple
Evening snack	1 slice mixed-grain bread with 1 tbsp almond butter	14 almonds; 1 tbsp raisins	60 g guacamole (p. 413); 1 wholegrain rye crispbread (e.g. Ryvita)

1 Skimmed milk and 0% fat Greek yoghurt are used extensively in this plan. Total® 0% (fat-free strained Greek yoghurt by Fage) is extremely useful; it has a relatively creamy flavour and withstands cooking. If you are intolerant of dairy products or prefer to avoid them, use calcium-enriched, fat-free and low-fat soya products instead.

2 This menu plan should be combined with exercise – a minimum of 30 minutes' brisk walking (or equivalent) a day.

Day 4	Day 5	Day 6	Day 7
30 g All-Bran with 125 ml skimmed milk; 60 g 0% fat Greek yoghurt; 80 g blackberries	Quinoa with apple and cinnamon (p. 420); 60 g 0% fat Greek yoghurt	50 g low-GL muesli (p. 420) with 125ml skimmed milk; 60 g 0% fat Greek yoghurt; 80 g berries	½ grapefruit (with ½ tsp xylitol if required); 1 piece French toast (p. 421); 1 large tomato, 60 g mushrooms (fried in 1tsp rapeseed oil)
60 g hummus (p. 412); 1 wholegrain rye crispbread (e.g. Ryvita)	60 g guacamole (p. 413); Crudités (raw celery, peppers, broccoli)	20 hazelnuts; 1 tbsp raisins	60 g virtually fat-free fromage frais; 80 g strawberries
130 g salmon pâté (p. 414) with lettuce and tomato in 2 slices mixed-grain bread or 1 wholemeal pitta; 120 g cherries	Creamy tomato soup (p. 410); 1 slice wholegrain bread; 1 orange	130 g cooked chicken with salsa (p. 413) and salad in 2 slices mixed-grain bread or 1 wholemeal pitta; 1 pear	Beans on toast (½ can beans – reduced sugar and salt – on 1 slice wholegrain toast); 14 almonds; 1 tbsp raisins
14 hazelnuts; 1 tbsp raisins	20 g pecans (12 halves); 20 g dried apricots	Fruit smoothie (p. 423)	Fruit smoothie (p. 423)
Soya goulash (p. 398); 100 g butter beans; Cauliflower and mangetout; 1 peach	Tandoori turkey (p. 379); Salad with mint and yoghurt dressing (p. 419); 60 g brown basmati rice; 60 g chickpeas; 60 g 0% fat Greek yoghurt	Chilli con Quorn (p. 389); 100 g quinoa; Peas; 2 apricots	Chicken in white wine with garlic and rosemary (p. 381); Asparagus and mangetout; Chocolate-dipped strawberries (p. 425)
Fruit smoothie (p. 423)	Fruit smoothie (p. 423)	Raw celery and broccoli	20 g dried apricots; 1 tbsp pumpkin seeds

3 Quantities shown for breakfast, lunch and snacks are for one person. Meal recipes in Chapter 29 yield four servings unless otherwise stated.

4 Recipes are suitable for children old enough to share in family meals. However, the quantities in the MUNCH plan – such as eight portions of fruit and vegetables a day – are not appropriate for tiny tummies!

5 1 tbsp = 1 level 15-ml measure; 1 tsp = 1 level 5-ml measure.

WEEK 2	Day 1	Day 2	Day 3
Breakfast	30 g All-Bran + 2 tbsp oats with 125 ml skimmed milk; 1 banana, sliced; 60 g virtually fat-free fromage frais	Porridge (40 g oats with 125 ml skimmed milk); 60 g virtually fat-free fromage frais; 80 g berries	50 g low-GL muesli (p. 420) with 125 ml skimmed milk; 60 g 0% fat Greek yoghurt; 10 hazelnuts; 40 g dried apricots, chopped
Morning snack	14 almonds; 1 tbsp raisins	14 hazelnuts; 1 tbsp raisins	Fruit smoothie (p. 423)
Lunch	Puy lentil and pepper salad (p. 406); 1 peach	Chicken pitta (100 g cooked chicken breast; 60 g guacamole (p. 413); lettuce and tomato; 1 wholemeal pitta); 1 apple	180 g tuna spread (p. 414) on 1 slice rye bread; 30 g cooked, peeled prawns; Mixed green salad (p. 405)
Afternoon snack	10 hazelnuts	Fruit smoothie (p. 423)	60 g virtually fat-free fromage frais; 80 g strawberries
Dinner	Lemon soy salmon (p. 382); ½ plate vegetables (Table 29); 100 g wholegrain couscous; 1 apple	Quornucopia (p. 395); Mangetout	Tofu and vegetable curry (p. 397); 100 g quinoa; 1 pear
Evening snack	Fruit smoothie (p. 423)	60 g hummus (p. 412); Crudités (raw broccoli and carrots)	14 almonds; 1 tbsp raisins

Day 4	Day 5	Day 6	Day 7
½ grapefruit (with ½ tsp xylitol if required); 1 free-range egg (poached, boiled or scrambled); 1 slice wholegrain toast	30 g All-Bran + 2 tbsp oats with 125 ml skimmed milk; 60 g 0% fat Greek yoghurt; 80 g blueberries	140 g fresh fruit salad (p. 423); 60 g virtually fat-free fromage frais; 1 slice wholegrain toast with 1 tbsp almond butter	½ grapefruit (with ½ tsp xylitol if required); Scrambled egg (1 egg and 30 ml skimmed milk per person); 1 large tomato and 60 g mushrooms fried in 1 tsp rapeseed oil; 1 slice wholegrain toast with 1 tsp reduced-fat olive spread
60 g virtually fat-free fromage frais; 1 tbsp pumpkin seeds	14 almonds	Fruit smoothie	14 hazelnuts
Watercress and butter bean soup (p. 410); 1 slice rye bread; 100 g cherries	TLT sandwich (100g cooked turkey breast; 1 tbsp mustard sauce (p. 415); lettuce and tomato; wholegrain bread or pitta); 1 orange	Watercress and butter bean soup (p. 410); 1 slice wholegrain bread; 2 plums	240 g coronation chicken – i.e. 125 g chicken (p. 380); Mixed green salad (p. 405); 1 tbsp vinaigrette (p. 417); 1 apple
20 hazelnuts; 3 brazil nuts	Fruit smoothie (p. 423)	14 almonds; 1 tbsp raisins	Fruit smoothie (p. 423)
Grilled tuna with orange (p. 386); Broccoli, carrots, peas and mushrooms; 100 g wholegrain couscous with pine nuts and pumpkin seeds (p. 392); 1 banana	Chickpea jalfrezi (p. 404); Courgettes, carrots and peas; 1 nectarine	Ginger lime chicken (p. 376); Mixed green salad (p. 405) with 1 carrot, grated and 1 tbsp pumpkin seeds; 100 g quinoa	Quorn Portuguese (p. 397); Peas, carrots and broccoli; 60 g chickpeas; 60 g wholegrain couscous; Raspberry fool (p. 426)
Fruit smoothie (p. 423)	20 g pecans (12 halves); 30 g dried apricots	60 g guacamole (p. 413); 1 wholegrain rye crispbread (e.g. Ryvita)	14 almonds; 1 tbsp raisins

WEEK 3	Day 1	Day 2	Day 3
Breakfast	50 g low-GL muesli (p. 420) with 125 ml skimmed milk; 60 g 0% fat Greek yoghurt	30 g All-Bran + 2 tbsp oats with 125 ml skimmed milk; 60 g 0% fat Greek yoghurt; 80 g strawberries	½ grapefruit (with ½ tsp xylitol if required); 1 free-range egg (poached, boiled or scrambled); 1 slice wholegrain toast
Morning snack	14 almonds; 1 tbsp raisins	Fruit smoothie (p. 423)	14 almonds; 1 tbsp raisins
Lunch	Smoked salmon salad (60 g smoked salmon; 60 g reduced-fat cottage cheese; mixed green salad (p. 405); lemon juice and 1 tsp olive oil); 1 slice wholegrain bread; 1 apple	Roasted vegetable soup (p. 411); 1 slice rye bread; 1 nectarine	Mixed bean and basil salad (p. 406); 1 orange
Afternoon snack	Fruit smoothie (p. 423)	20 hazelnuts; 30 g dried apricots	14 hazelnuts; 2 tbsp pumpkin seeds; 250 ml skimmed milk
Dinner	Lentils Italienne (p. 403); Peas; 100 g wholegrain couscous; 2 plums	Honey mustard chicken (p. 377) with mustard sauce (p. 415); 100 g quinoa; 100 g cannelini beans, spinach and courgettes	Cod in spicy tomato sauce (p. 385); 60 g 0% fat Greek yoghurt; 100 g wholegrain couscous; Peas, cauliflower and courgettes; 1 peach
Evening snack	14 hazelnuts	60 g guacamole (p. 413); Celery sticks	Fruit smoothie (p. 423)

Day 4	Day 5	Day 6	Day 7
Porridge (40 g oats with 125 ml skimmed milk); 60 g 0% fat Greek yoghurt; 80 g berries	30 g All-Bran + 2 tbsp oats with 125 ml skimmed milk; 1 banana, sliced; 60 g virtually fat-free fromage frais	Beans on toast (½ can baked beans – reduced sugar and salt – on 1 slice wholegrain toast); Fruit smoothie	½ grapefruit (with ½ tsp xylitol if required); 1 piece French toast (p. 421); 1 large tomato, 60 g mushrooms (fried in 1 tsp rapeseed oil)
30 g dried apricots, chopped; 250 ml skimmed milk	Fruit smoothie (p. 423)	20 hazelnuts	14 almonds; 250 ml skimmed milk
120 g smoked mackerel pâté (p. 415); 2 wholegrain rye crispbreads; 40 g cooked, peeled prawns; Wild rocket, tomato and lemon juice; 2 apricots	Roasted vegetable soup (p. 411); 1 slice wholegrain bread; 100 g cherries	Chicken curry pitta (130 g cooked chicken with 30 g curry sauce (p. 417); red pepper, spinach, red onion, and coriander; 1 wholemeal pitta); 100 g strawberries	Quinoa and mango salad (p. 407); 60 g virtually fat-free fromage frais
Fruit smoothie (p. 423)	1 wholegrain rye crispbread (e.g. Ryvita); 1 tbsp crunchy peanut butter	20 almonds	Crudités (raw carrot, and broccoli)
Chilli tomato quinoa pilaf (p. 388); 60 g 0% fat Greek yoghurt; 120 g chickpeas; Mangetout	140 g turkey escalopes with lemon and rosemary (p. 380); Tomato, red onion and basil salad; Steamed asparagus and mangetout	Sweet and sour Quorn (p. 393); 100 g wholegrain couscous; Peas, mushrooms and broccoli	Chicken tikka masala (p. 378); 60 g brown basmati rice; ½ plate salad; Baked apple with custard (p. 424)
60 g guacamole (p. 413); Crudités (raw broccoli, carrot and celery)	30 g dried apricots 20 hazelnuts	Raw carrot sticks	Fruit smoothie (p. 423)

WEEK 4	Day 1	Day 2	Day 3
Breakfast	Porridge (40 g oats with 125 ml skimmed milk); 60 g 0% fat Greek yoghurt; 80 g berries	30 g All-Bran with 125 ml skimmed milk; 60 g 0% fat Greek yoghurt; 80 g raspberries	50 g low-GL muesli (p. 420) with 125 ml skimmed milk or fat-free soya milk; 1 banana, sliced; 60 g virtually fat-free fromage frais
Morning snack	14 hazelnuts 1 tbsp raisins	Fruit smoothie (p. 423)	14 almonds
Lunch	100 g hummus (p. 412); Mixed green salad (p. 405) with romaine lettuce and fresh coriander with 1 tbsp lemon and garlic dressing (p. 418); 1 slice mixed-grain bread; 1 apple	Tuna pitta (100 g tinned tuna with red onion, lettuce and tomato; 1 tsp olive oil and lemon juice; 1 wholemeal pitta); 1 peach	Chinese chicken soup (p. 409); 1 slice wholegrain bread; 80 g grapes
Afternoon snack	Fruit smoothie (p. 423)	14 almonds; 60 g virtually fat-free fromage frais	60 g guacamole (p. 413); Raw celery sticks
Dinner	Grilled salmon (p. 384); Mangetout, carrots, peas and sweetcorn; 1 pear	Mediterranean bean-stuffed peppers (p. 402); 60 g wholegrain couscous; ½ plate salad, 1 tbsp lower-fat vinaigrette (p. 417); 2 apricots	Jollof quinoa (p. 401); Peas and spinach; 1 nectarine
Evening snack	60 g virtually fat-free fromage frais; 30 g dried apricots	20 hazelnuts	Fruit smoothie (p. 423)

Day 4	Day 5	Day 6	Day 7
½ grapefruit (with ½ tsp xylitol if required); Cheese and onion omelette (1 egg, chopped onion and 10 g grated Parmesan); 1 slice wholegrain toast	30 g All-Bran with 125 ml skimmed milk; 60 g 0% fat Greek yoghurt; 40 g dried apricots	Fruit smoothie (p. 423); 1 slice wholegrain toast with 1 tbsp crunchy peanut butter	½ grapefruit (with ½ tsp xylitol if required); 1 kipper, grilled; 1 slice wholegrain bread
14 hazelnuts; 30 g dried apricots	Fruit smoothie (p. 423)	100 g raw sugar snap peas	Carrot sticks
Spicy-chickpea salad (p. 399); 60 g 0% fat Greek yoghurt; 80 g raspberries	Chinese chicken soup (p. 409); 1 slice rye bread; 120 g cherries	Cannellini bean and coriander salad (p. 406); 1 apple	Turkey and avocado sandwich (100 g cooked turkey breast; 40 g avocado; lettuce, onion, tomato; 2 slices wholegrain bread or 1 wholemeal pitta); 1 pear
Fruit smoothie (p. 423)	10 almonds; 10 hazelnuts; 3 brazil nuts	60 g virtually fat-free fromage frais; 100 g strawberries	Fruit smoothie (p. 423)
Baked haddock on baby leaf spinach (p. 386); Parsley sauce (p. 415); Courgettes, leeks and peas; 1 orange	Quorn bolognese (p. 392); 100 g wholewheat spaghetti; Mixed green salad (p. 405) with 1 tbsp lower-fat vinaigrette (p. 417); 2 plums	Chilli lime chicken (p. 376); 60 g guacamole (p. 413); 100 g quinoa; Asparagus, broccoli and carrots; 1 nectarine	Green lentil curry (p. 400); 60 g brown basmati rice; 60 g 0% fat Greek yoghurt; Tomato, cucumber and mint salad; Grilled pineapple with honey and cinnamon (p. 426)
2 wholegrain rye crispbreads (e.g. Ryvita); 60 g reduced-fat cottage cheese	60 g tarka dhal (p. 390); Crudités (raw broccoli, carrot and celery)	14 almonds; 1 tbsp raisins	Crudités (raw broccoli, yellow pepper, sugar snap peas)

Chapter 29

Recipes

**'The discovery of a new dish
does more for the happiness of mankind
than the discovery of a new star.'**

ANTHELME BRILLAT-SAVARIN (1755–1826)
Physiologie du Goût, 1826

Ten top tips for following the recipes

1   Meal recipes yield four servings, unless otherwise stated. If there are only two in your family, scale down the quantities or freeze half for another day.

2   Ingredients are listed 'in order of appearance' – the order they crop up in the instructions. Do all the preparation (washing, peeling, deseeding, chopping) before you start cooking, otherwise you'll burn the garlic while chopping tomatoes, and cooking will be stressful instead of relaxing and therapeutic.

3   Don't overheat olive oil (it shouldn't be smoking) and don't burn garlic or spices; it ruins the flavour.

4   Chop onion quickly and put it in a covered pot, or there'll be tears.

5   Unless your hands are fireproof, I recommend gloves for chopping chillies. Even if it doesn't seem to affect you while chopping, the afterburn can be quite irritating. At the very least, wash your hands immediately after touching raw chopped chilli.

6   Some of the recipes suggest making three or four slashes in chicken breasts to enhance penetration of a marinade. This is

conveniently done with a pair of scissors; your hands don't have to touch the meat.

7 If you use tongs to transfer raw poultry to the grill, you must assume that the tongs have been coated with salmonella in the process. Having eradicated live salmonella by cooking, you don't want to put some back when you serve with those tongs. If you wash the tongs, they will become contaminated again when you turn the meat over. The best plan is to make sure that the grill thoroughly heats the tongs (the blades, not the handle) while the meat is cooking.

8 If the recipe calls for gram flour 'blended with water', gradually stir a little water into the specified quantity of flour until you have a lump-free 'slurry' that can be poured into the sauce. Use arrowroot in the same way when you want a clear sauce; two teaspoons of arrowroot will do the job of one tablespoon of cornflour or two tablespoons of wheat flour. Once a sauce has been thickened by arrowroot, stop cooking or it may start to thin again.

9 Many of the recipes use onion; it's full of flavour and flavonoids. If you can't tolerate onion, substitute a vegetable from Table 29 that you can eat (e.g. red pepper). It won't be the same – it won't taste of onion for a start – but it will still be good.

10 Good presentation makes food more appetising. A plate of brown curry will be cheered up by bright green vegetables or salad. It's hard to beat white china plates (and they don't all have to be circular).

- ◆ Meal recipes (as opposed to recipes for dressings, dips and side dishes) yield 4 servings, unless otherwise stated

- ◆ All spoon measures are level;
  tsp = teaspoon (5 ml); tbsp = tablespoon (15 ml)

- ◆ All oven cooking times are for a preheated oven

POULTRY

Quick chicken and tomato casserole

This casserole can be cooked on the hob in a large heavy-based pan (e.g. 4 litre capacity). The finely grated carrot is important to balance any bitterness from the tomatoes. My family are particularly fond of organic button mushrooms.

15 ml (1 tbsp) olive oil
4 skinless chicken breasts, cut into chunks
1 onion, finely chopped
1 garlic clove, crushed
2×400-g (14-oz) cans peeled plum tomatoes in tomato juice
200 g (7 oz) button mushrooms
1 red pepper, chopped
1 yellow pepper, chopped
1 large carrot, finely grated
1 celery stick, chopped
5 ml (1 tsp) dried oregano
2.5 ml (½ tsp) dried basil
freshly-ground black pepper
30 g (1 oz) gram flour, blended with water
150 ml (¼ pint) low-salt chicken or vegetable stock

Heat the oil in the pan and cook the chicken on medium heat until all sides are lightly browned. Add the onion and garlic and cook for about 2 minutes, stirring, before adding the tomatoes and remaining vegetables. Season with the herbs and black pepper. Bring to the boil and simmer gently, stirring and breaking down the tomatoes.

Stir in the blended gram flour. Simmer gently for 15 minutes, stirring occasionally. Serve with mangetout and baby corn.

Chicken kebabs satay-style

Malaysian or Indonesian satay usually consists of meat barbecued on skewers and served with a spicy peanut sauce. This adaptation uses a marinade to impart a spicy peanut flavour to simple chicken kebabs.

For the marinade:
45 ml (3 tbsp) crunchy peanut butter
30 ml (2 tbsp) clear honey
juice 1 lemon
15 ml (1 tbsp) reduced-salt soy sauce
15 ml (1 tbsp) rapeseed oil
30 ml (2 tbsp) 0% fat Greek yoghurt
small bunch fresh coriander, chopped
2.5 ml (½ tsp) chilli powder
freshly-ground black pepper

500 g (1 lb 2 oz) skinless chicken breast,
cut into chunks

Mix all the ingredients for the marinade in a sealable container, add the chicken, ensuring all pieces are well coated, and refrigerate for 2–48 hours.

Thread the marinated chicken pieces onto kebab skewers (over a tray to catch the drips). Cook under a moderately hot grill (over silver foil) for about 18 minutes, turning, until the chicken is cooked through. Serve with salad.

Mustard lime chicken

Even if you haven't planned ahead, you can transform meat, fish and poultry by using a rub or by marinating for just a few minutes with a winning combination of ingredients. If you can leave the marinade to work its magic for a few hours, so much the better.

4 skinless chicken breasts

For the marinade:
30 ml (2 tbsp) Dijon mustard
juice and zest 1 lime
30 ml (2 tbsp) clear honey
10 ml (2 tsp) mixed herbs
freshly-ground black pepper

Make 3 or 4 slashes in each chicken breast. Mix all the marinade ingredients. Add the chicken, making sure all surfaces – including the slashes – are well coated. Refrigerate in a sealed container or plastic bag for 2 hours or overnight.

Cook under a moderately hot grill for 8–10 minutes each side, checking that the chicken has cooked through to the centre at the thickest point.

Serve with mustard sauce (p. 415) and salad or half a plate of vegetables.

Variations

Lemon herb chicken
4 skinless chicken breasts

For the marinade:
juice 1 lemon
15 ml (1 tbsp) garlic-infused olive oil
5 ml (1 tsp) mixed herbs
freshly-ground black pepper

Chilli lime chicken
4 skinless chicken breasts

For the marinade:
juice and zest 1 lime
2.5 ml (½ tsp) chilli powder or crushed chillies
15 ml (1 tbsp) reduced-salt soy sauce
15 ml (1 tbsp) clear honey
15 ml (1 tbsp) olive oil
1 garlic clove, crushed
1 shallot or small onion, finely chopped
freshly-ground black pepper

Ginger lime chicken
4 skinless chicken breasts

For the marinade:
5 cm (2 inches) ginger root, peeled and grated
juice and zest 1 lime
30 ml (2 tbsp) rapeseed oil
1 garlic clove, grated
15 ml (1 tbsp) reduced-salt soy sauce
freshly-ground black pepper

Honey mustard chicken
4 skinless chicken breasts

For the marinade:
30 ml (2 tbsp) clear honey
30 ml (2 tbsp) Dijon mustard
15 ml (1 tbsp) garlic-infused olive oil
juice ½ lemon
2.5 ml (½ tsp) cayenne pepper
5 ml (1 tsp) oregano

Quick chicken korma

Korma is a mild, creamy curry which is sometimes flavoured with coconut. This healthy version is quick and easy. A simple way to give it a coconut flavour is to use coconut essence, but that can be hard to find and you may need to search the internet. An alternative is to replace the stock with reduced-fat coconut milk (but even the lower-fat form adds saturated fat). With or without coconut, this is a very pleasing mild curry.

15 ml (1 tbsp) rapeseed oil
1 onion, finely chopped
2 garlic cloves, crushed
2.5 cm (1 inch) ginger root, peeled and grated
5 ml (1 tsp) garam masala
5 ml (1 tsp) turmeric
2.5 ml (½ tsp) mild chilli powder
500 g (1 lb 2 oz) skinless chicken breast,
cut into bite-sized chunks
200 ml (7 fl oz) low-salt chicken or vegetable stock
15 ml (1 tbsp) sweet mango chutney
small bunch fresh coriander, chopped
45 ml (3 tbsp) ground almonds
150 g (5½ oz) 0% fat Greek yoghurt
30 ml (2 tbsp) flaked almonds, toasted
coriander leaves to garnish

Heat the oil in a pan and cook the onion until it's soft. Add the garlic, ginger and spices and cook for 1 minute, stirring, before adding the chicken and stir-frying for about 3 minutes.

Pour on the stock, stir in the mango chutney and coriander, bring to the boil and simmer for 10 minutes.

Take the pan off the heat. Mix the ground almonds and yoghurt together and stir the mixture into the pan. Return the pan to the hob and heat gently for 2 minutes, stirring. Garnish with toasted flaked almonds and fresh coriander leaves. Serve with salad and brown basmati rice, quinoa or couscous.

Chicken tikka masala

Here's an adaptation of Britain's favourite dish that you can enjoy without inducing guilt or premature death.

For the marinade:
2.5 cm (1 inch) ginger root,
peeled and grated
2 garlic cloves, peeled and grated
30 ml (2 tbsp) chopped fresh coriander
5 ml (1 tsp) chilli powder
5 ml (1 tsp) garam masala
5 ml (1 tsp) ground paprika
15 ml (1 tbsp) tomato purée
juice 1 lime
15 ml (1 tbsp) rapeseed oil
freshly-ground black pepper
pinch Solo or LoSalt

4 skinless chicken breasts, cut into chunks

For the sauce:
15 ml (1 tbsp) rapeseed oil
1 large onion, finely chopped
1 red chilli, deseeded and finely chopped
5 ml (1 tsp) turmeric
10 ml (2 tsp) ground paprika
150 ml (¼ pint) passata
15 ml (1 tbsp) clear honey
200 g (7 oz) 0% fat Greek yoghurt
30 ml (2 tbsp) chopped fresh coriander

Mix together the ingredients of the marinade, add the chicken (ensuring that all surfaces are well coated) and refrigerate in a sealed container or plastic bag for at least an hour.

Heat the oil in a pan and cook the onion and chilli for about 5 minutes until the onion is golden brown. Add the turmeric and paprika and cook for 1 minute, stirring, before adding the passata and honey. Bring to a simmer, remove from the heat and stir in the yoghurt.

Preheat the grill. Thread the chicken pieces onto kebab skewers and cook under a hot grill (over foil) for 15 minutes, turning, until the chicken is cooked through.

Slide the chicken pieces off the skewers into the sauce. Simmer for 5 minutes, stirring frequently. Serve with quinoa tabbouleh, green salad and fat-free yoghurt or raita.

Tandoori turkey

This is a very low-fat version of the popular Indian dish and works equally well with lean turkey or chicken breast. By making your own marinade instead of using a ready-made paste, you can avoid a lot of unnecessary salt as well as colouring agents.

3 garlic cloves, crushed
2.5 cm (1 inch) ginger root,
peeled and finely grated
juice ½ lemon
5 ml (1 tsp) ground cumin
5 ml (1 tsp) garam masala
2.5 ml (½ tsp) ground coriander
2.5 ml (½ tsp) turmeric
1.25 ml (¼ tsp) chilli powder
1.25 ml (¼ tsp) cayenne pepper
freshly-ground black pepper
60 ml (4 tbsp) 0% fat Greek yoghurt
600 g (1 lb 5 oz) skinless turkey breast pieces
(or 4 chicken breasts, halved)

Place the garlic, ginger, lemon juice, spices and pepper in a plastic bowl with a sealable lid and mix them thoroughly. Stir in the yoghurt to make an evenly coloured paste. Make two or three slashes in each piece of turkey breast; one by one, add each piece to the marinade paste, massaging the paste into all surfaces and the slashes. Fit the lid and marinate in the fridge for 2–24 hours.

Preheat the oven to 230°C (450°F, Gas 8). Arrange the turkey pieces on a wire rack (brushed with rapeseed oil) over a baking tray lined with foil (which saves washing up). Bake for 20–25 minutes or until the turkey is cooked through to the centre.

Serve with lemon wedges, raita and salad.

Quick coronation chicken

Authentic coronation chicken requires a good deal of preparation and contains a lot of saturated fat. This version is much better for you and makes a quick lunch if you have leftover cooked chicken.

500 g (1 lb 2 oz) cooked skinless chicken breast
300 g (10½ oz) 0% fat Greek yoghurt
10 ml (2 tsp) mild curry powder
15 ml (1 tbsp) sweet mango chutney
50 g (2 oz) sultanas
100 g (4 oz) dried apricots, finely chopped

Dice the cooked chicken. Put the Greek yoghurt in a bowl and stir in the curry powder until the colour is uniform. Mix in the mango chutney, sultanas and apricots, chopping up any large pieces of mango with scissors. Add the chicken to the coronation sauce and serve with salad, either on a plate or in a wholemeal pitta. If the sauce becomes too thick (especially after refrigeration), simply stir in a dash of skimmed milk.

Turkey escalopes with lemon and rosemary

Delicious and succulent, these escalopes take only a couple of minutes to cook. That's what I call fast food. Of course, the turkey breasts can be marinated while you're cooking vegetables or preparing a salad, but it's best not to cook them until you're almost ready to eat.

You could allow 1½ or 2 steaks per person if they weigh less than 100 g.

4 thin turkey breast steaks
juice 1 lemon
30 ml (2 tbsp) garlic-infused olive oil
15 ml (1 tbsp) dried rosemary
freshly-ground black pepper

If the turkey breast steaks are more than about 0.7 cm (¼ inch) thick , place them between two sheets of greaseproof paper and gently beat them with a rolling pin.

Mix the lemon juice, 15 ml (1 tbsp) of the olive oil and the rosemary in a bowl with a sealable lid and add the turkey steaks. Fit the lid and rotate repeatedly to make sure all surfaces of the steaks are evenly coated with the mixture. Leave to marinate for 15–30 minutes.

Heat 15 ml (1 tbsp) of olive oil in a frying pan. Cook the steaks, two or three at a time, over high heat for about 1 minute on each side.

Chicken in white wine with garlic and rosemary

What could be easier than putting all the ingredients in a casserole and leaving the oven to do the rest? There's no need to marinate before cooking; the meat will be tender and full of flavour. If it's more convenient, you can prepare the dish in advance, and keep it in the fridge until you want to cook it, as long as you use cold stock.

If you have fresh rosemary, use 45 ml (3 tbsp) of leaves in place of the dried herb.

600 g (1 lb 5 oz) skinless chicken breast,
cut into chunks
6 garlic cloves, crushed
1 small onion, finely chopped
15 ml (1 tbsp) dried rosemary
2 bay leaves
15 ml (1 tbsp) olive oil
15 ml (1 tbsp) clear honey
10 ml (2 tsp) Dijon mustard
300 ml (½ pint) white wine
300 ml (½ pint) low-salt chicken or vegetable stock
30 g (1 oz) gram flour, blended with water
freshly-ground black pepper

Mix all the ingredients together in a casserole. Fit the lid and cook in the oven at 170°C (325°F, Gas 3) for 1½ hours. Serve with vegetables of your choice from Table 29.

FISH

Cajun tuna

This recipe uses a rub to spice up the fish just before cooking. If you have more time, you could marinate the fish in oil and lemon juice before rolling it in the dry rub.

For the rub:
15 ml (1 tbsp) ground paprika
5 ml (1 tsp) cayenne pepper
5 ml (1 tsp) dried oregano
5 ml (1 tsp) dried thyme
1 garlic clove, crushed
1 small onion, finely chopped
10 ml (2 tsp) rapeseed oil
freshly-ground black pepper

4 tuna steaks

Mix all the ingredients of the rub together and work them gently into all surfaces of the tuna steaks. Cook under a moderately hot grill for 5–6 minutes each side. Serve with vegetables of your choice.

Lemon soy salmon

This recipe makes the salmon much less 'fishy' and can even convert family members who say they don't like fish.

For the marinade:
juice 1 lemon
15 ml (1 tbsp) reduced-salt soy sauce
15 ml (1 tbsp) olive oil
15 ml (1 tbsp) clear honey
1 garlic clove, crushed
freshly-ground black pepper

4 skinless, boneless salmon fillets

Mix all the ingredients of the marinade, add the salmon, ensuring all sides are well coated, and refrigerate in a sealed container or plastic bag for an hour.

Cook the fillets under a moderately hot grill for 6 minutes each side, or until they flake easily. Serve with lemon wedges and salad or a selection of vegetables.

Haddock and prawns in white wine sauce

The health benefits of eating fish are often lost because the fish is drowning in a sauce full of saturated fat and salt. Not here.

> *400 g (14 oz) skinless haddock fillets,*
> *cut into chunks*
> *15 ml (1 tbsp) rapeseed oil*
> *1 onion, finely chopped*
> *1 garlic clove, crushed*
> *1 celery stick, finely chopped*
> *100 g (4 oz) mushrooms, sliced*
> *200 ml (7 fl oz) white wine*
> *150 g (5½ oz) cooked, peeled prawns*
> *5 ml (1 tsp) mixed herbs*
> *freshly-ground black pepper*
> *30 g (1 oz) gram flour, blended with water*
> *300 g (10½ oz) 0% fat Greek yoghurt*
> *50 g (2 oz) wholemeal breadcrumbs*
> *50 g (2 oz) miniCol cheese, grated*

Arrange the fish in an ovenproof dish.

Heat the oil in a pan and cook the onions, garlic, celery and mushrooms over a moderate heat for about 4 minutes, until the vegetables are softened. Add the wine, prawns, herbs and pepper and bring to a simmer. Stir in the blended gram flour and simmer gently, stirring, until the sauce has thickened.

Remove the pan from the heat and stir in the yoghurt. Return the pan to the heat, stirring, to bring the sauce back to simmering temperature. Pour the sauce over the fish. Top with a mixture of the breadcrumbs and cheese. Bake in the oven at 220°C (425°F, Gas 7) for 25 minutes.

Serve with your choice of vegetables or mixed salad.

Grilled salmon

A fresh salmon steak or fillet is real convenience food. Only a few moments of preparation are needed to yield perfect results, but make sure you don't overcook it.

4 salmon steaks
15 ml (1 tbsp) garlic-infused olive oil
2.5 ml (½ tsp) garlic pepper
2.5 ml (½ tsp) dried dill

Brush the salmon steaks with oil and sprinkle with garlic pepper and dill. Cook under a moderately hot grill for about 7 minutes a side, or until the fish flakes easily with a fork. Remove the skin if you prefer. Serve with a selection of vegetables or salad.

Monkfish with tomato and caper sauce

Monkfish, or anglerfish, are remarkably ugly, but their tails provide excellent firm meat which has sometimes been used as a substitute for scampi.

500 g (1 lb 2 oz) monkfish fillets

For the marinade:
juice 1 lemon
15 ml (1 tbsp) olive oil
1 garlic clove, crushed
freshly-ground black pepper

For cooking the fish:
30 ml (2 tbsp) gram flour
30 ml (2 tbsp) stoneground oatmeal
15 ml (1 tbsp) olive oil

For the sauce:
5 ml (1 tsp) olive oil
½ onion, finely chopped
1 garlic clove, crushed
300 ml (½ pint) low-salt vegetable stock
400-g (14-oz) can peeled plum tomatoes in tomato juice
15 ml (1 tbsp) tomato purée
1 medium to large carrot, finely grated
1 sweet red pepper (tinned), cut into strips

30 ml (2 tbsp) capers
30 g (1 oz) gram flour, blended with water
15 ml (1 tbsp) mixed herbs
freshly-ground black pepper

Cut the fish into chunks of about 5 cm (2 inches). Mix the ingredients of the marinade and marinate the fish for 30 minutes in a sealed plastic bag.

Mix the gram flour and oatmeal in a shallow dish and completely coat the fish pieces in the mixture. Heat 15 ml (1 tbsp) of olive oil in a frying pan and cook the fish for 8–10 minutes, turning, until all sides are browned. Set the fish aside on a warm plate.

Heat 5 ml (1 tsp) of olive oil in the pan and cook the onion and garlic until soft. Add the stock, tomatoes, tomato purée, carrot, red pepper and capers; bring to a simmer and stir in the blended gram flour. Add the herbs and pepper. Simmer, stirring, for 10 minutes.

Arrange the monkfish on serving plates and pour on the sauce. Serve with vegetables of your choice.

Cod in spicy tomato sauce

The spicy tomato sauce gives this dish a subtle kick. For a really hot sauce, add more chilli powder. You could use other white fish (such as pollock, haddock or ling) or oily fish (such as mackerel or herring).

4 skinless cod fillets
juice 1 lime
freshly-ground black pepper
15 ml (1 tbsp) rapeseed oil
1 onion, finely chopped
1 garlic clove, crushed
2.5 cm (1 inch) ginger root, peeled and grated
5 ml (1 tsp) ground coriander
5 ml (1 tsp) ground cumin
5 ml (1 tsp) turmeric
2.5 ml (½ tsp) chilli powder
200 ml (7 fl oz) passata
15 ml (1 tbsp) sweet mango chutney
150 g (5½ oz) 0% fat Greek yoghurt

Arrange the fish in an ovenproof dish and sprinkle with lime juice and black pepper.

Heat the oil in a pan. Fry the onion, garlic and ginger for about 2 minutes until the onion is softening. Add the spices and cook, stirring, for 1 minute. Stir in the passata and bring to a simmer. Remove the pan from the heat; stir in the yoghurt; return to a low heat until simmering again.

Pour the sauce over the fish, cover with foil and cook in the oven at 220°C (425°F, Gas 7) for 25 minutes. Serve with yoghurt and salad or vegetables.

Grilled tuna with orange

Unlike tinned tuna, fresh tuna is rich in omega-3 fatty acids. It only takes a few minutes to cook under the grill or in a pan.

For the marinade:
30 ml (2 tbsp) pure orange juice
(no added sugar)
juice ½ lemon
15 ml (1 tbsp) reduced-salt soy sauce
15 ml (1 tbsp) olive oil
1 garlic clove, crushed
5 ml (1 tsp) dried dill
2.5 ml (½ tsp) dried oregano
freshly-ground black pepper

4 fresh tuna steaks
1 orange, cut into wedges, to serve

Mix all the ingredients of the marinade, add the tuna steaks and leave in a sealed container or plastic bag for 30 minutes – or transfer to the fridge and marinate for longer.

Cook the tuna under a moderately hot grill for 5–8 minutes each side, depending on the thickness of the steaks and how well done you want them; traditionally, tuna steak is served pink in the centre.

Serve with orange wedges and mixed salad or vegetables of your choice.

Baked haddock on baby leaf spinach

Baking fish in foil packets is quick and easy; the house doesn't smell of fish and you save on washing up. It's also a lovely way to ensure the fish is moist and infused with flavour. Instead of chopping fresh herbs, it's convenient to throw a bunch of herbs into the parcel and remove it before serving.

Haddock is suggested here, but you could use any white fish.

4 skinless, boneless haddock steaks
180 g (6½ oz) baby leaf spinach
4 spring onions, chopped
15 ml (1 tbsp) olive oil
45 ml (3 tbsp) white wine
3 garlic cloves, crushed
freshly-ground black pepper
25 g (1 oz) fresh thyme

Wash and dry the haddock. Prepare four sheets of kitchen foil approximately 37 cm (14½ inches) wide by 40 cm (16 inches) long. Place a haddock steak on a bed of spinach in the middle of each sheet and top this with a portion of chopped spring onion.

In a bowl, mix together the olive oil, white wine, garlic and black pepper. Pour an equal quantity of the dressing onto each piece of haddock, and crown with some sprigs of fresh thyme.

Turn each foil sheet into a sealed packet by folding the edges together tightly, leaving plenty of air space above the contents. Place the parcels side by side on a baking tray and cook in the oven at 200°C (400°F, Gas 6) for 25 minutes.

Serve with parsley sauce (p. 415) and peas.

VEGETARIAN

Quinoa tabbouleh

Tabbouleh is a Lebanese dish, traditionally made with bulgar (cracked wheat). Many variations on the authentic dish are possible and quinoa – a good source of quality protein – works very well. Why not make larger quantities and keep some in the fridge for lunch?

160 g (5½ oz) quinoa
380 ml (13 fl oz) low-salt vegetable stock
10 cherry tomatoes, finely chopped
¼ cucumber, finely chopped
1 carrot, grated
6 spring onions, finely chopped
bunch flat-leaf parsley, chopped
bunch fresh mint, chopped
15 ml (1 tbsp) olive oil
juice 1 lemon
freshly-ground black pepper
pinch Solo or LoSalt

Rinse the quinoa thoroughly in a sieve and drain well. Transfer it to a saucepan with the stock, bring to the boil and simmer, partially covered, for about 13 minutes – until all the liquid is absorbed. Allow the quinoa to cool. Empty it into a large bowl and mix with all the other ingredients. Ideally, leave in the fridge for several hours, allowing flavours to blend. Bring to room temperature before serving.

Chilli tomato quinoa pilaf

This is a colourful way to enjoy quinoa with a kick, either for lunch or as an accompaniment to a main meal.

15 ml (1 tbsp) olive oil
½ onion, finely chopped
1 red chilli, finely chopped

1 red pepper, diced
1 celery stick, diced
2 carrots, diced
160 g (5½ oz) quinoa, rinsed and drained
200 ml (7 fl oz) passata
200 ml (7 fl oz) low-salt vegetable stock
100 g (4 oz) frozen peas
freshly-ground black pepper

Heat the olive oil in a saucepan; add the onion, chilli, pepper, celery and carrot; cook for 5 minutes, stirring frequently. Add the quinoa to the vegetables; cook for about 2 minutes while stirring. Pour in the passata and stock. Stir well, cover and simmer on a low heat for 15 minutes, or until the liquid is absorbed. Stir in the peas and season with black pepper. Cover and simmer for 1 minute. Serve with 0% fat Greek yoghurt and salad.

Chilli con Quorn (6 servings)

This is a robust vegetarian version of the meaty Mexican (or American) classic. Don't mention the Quorn and committed carnivores won't bat an eyelid.

15 ml (1 tbsp) olive oil
1 large onion, finely chopped
6 garlic cloves, crushed
350 g (12 oz) Quorn mince
15 ml (1 tbsp) chilli powder
5 ml (1 tsp) ground cumin
5 ml (1 tsp) ground coriander
150 ml (¼ pint) low-salt vegetable stock
2×400-g (14-oz) cans chopped tomatoes in tomato juice
15 ml (1 tbsp) tomato purée
15 ml (1 tbsp) reduced-salt soy sauce
5 ml (1 tsp) oregano
1 carrot, finely grated
1 green pepper, finely diced
1 red pepper, diced
1 can red kidney beans in water, drained
1 can soya beans in water, drained
230 g (8 oz) mushrooms, sliced

30 g (1 oz) gram flour, blended with water
freshly-ground black pepper

Heat the oil in a heavy-based pan (4 litre capacity). Gently fry the onions and garlic until just softened.

Add the Quorn and spices and cook for 2 minutes before stirring in the stock, tomatoes, tomato purée, soy sauce, oregano, carrot, peppers, beans and mushrooms.

Bring back to simmering temperature. Stir in the blended gram flour, season with black pepper and simmer gently for 30 minutes.

Serve with couscous and 0% fat Greek yoghurt.

Tarka dhal

If you've had tarka dhal in an Indian restaurant, it was probably swamped with ghee. Here's a delicious dhal that will do you nothing but good. It also makes a tasty spread or dip, for example with pitta bread, when cold.

225 g (8 oz) split red lentils
2.5 ml (½ tsp) turmeric
seeds 2 green cardamom pods, crushed
2.5 cm (1 inch) ginger root, peeled and grated
900 ml (1½ pints) low-salt vegetable stock
30 ml (2 tbsp) rapeseed oil
1 small onion, finely chopped
2 garlic cloves, crushed
15 ml (1 tbsp) ground cumin
15 ml (1 tbsp) ground coriander

Rinse the lentils in a fine sieve under cold, running water. Transfer the washed lentils to a saucepan and add the turmeric, cardamom, ginger and stock. Bring to the boil and simmer gently uncovered for about 20 minutes until the lentils are soft. Add more boiling water from a kettle if necessary to prevent the lentils from drying out and sticking to the bottom of the saucepan before cooking is complete.

Heat the oil in a separate pan. Cook the onion and garlic for about 2 minutes until the onion is softening. Add the cumin and coriander and cook for a further 2 minutes, taking care not to burn the spices. Stir this hot spiced oil (tarka) into the cooked lentils and cover until serving.

Chinese chickpeas

Although the list of ingredients is lengthy, this is a really simple dish with a short cooking time on the hob. When preparing, it's convenient to put all the liquid ingredients (not the cooking oil!) in one bowl so they can be poured into the pan together; make sure you don't discard the pineapple juice. If you don't have arrowroot, you can use 15 g (½ oz) of gram flour, blended with water, but it will give the sauce a more opaque, cream colour.

15 ml (1 tbsp) rapeseed oil
1 large onion, finely chopped
3 garlic cloves, crushed
5 cm (2 inches) ginger root, peeled and grated
1 red pepper, deseeded and sliced
1 yellow pepper, deseeded and sliced
2 medium carrots, finely sliced
2×400-g (14-oz) cans chickpeas in water, drained
220-g (8-oz) can water chestnuts, drained and sliced
220-g (8-oz) can pineapple chunks in own juice
juice ½ lemon
30 ml (2 tbsp) sherry
30 ml (2 tbsp) rice vinegar
30 ml (2 tbsp) tomato purée
30 ml (2 tbsp) xylitol (or clear honey)
15 ml (1 tbsp) reduced-salt soy sauce
150 ml (¼ pint) low-salt vegetable stock
freshly-ground black pepper
10 ml (2 tsp) arrowroot, blended with water

Heat the oil in a large (e.g. 4-litre) heavy-based pan and cook the onion on medium heat for about 4 minutes until soft.

Add the garlic, ginger, peppers and carrots and stir-fry for about 3 minutes.

Add all the remaining ingredients, except the blended arrowroot. Bring to the boil and simmer for 15 minutes. Stir in the blended arrowroot and cook until the sauce has thickened. Serve with mangetout or peas.

Quorn Bolognese

Named after Bologna in Italy, Bolognese sauce is traditionally made with beef. Quorn mince is an excellent vegetarian alternative. For a meaty low-fat sauce, use lean turkey mince.

15 ml (1 tbsp) olive oil
1 large onion, finely chopped
2 garlic cloves, crushed
350 g (12 oz) Quorn mince
10 ml (2 tsp) mixed herbs
1 large carrot, finely grated
1 celery stick, finely chopped
400-g (14-oz) can chopped tomatoes in tomato juice
15 ml (1 tbsp) tomato purée
1 can sweet red peppers, drained and diced
150 ml (¼ pint) red wine
150 ml (¼ pint) low-salt vegetable stock
15 ml (1 tbsp) fresh thyme leaves
1 bay leaf
3 drops Tabasco
freshly-ground black pepper
30 g (1 oz) gram flour, blended with water

Heat the oil in a large heavy-based pan and fry the onion and garlic until softened. Add the Quorn, herbs, carrot and celery and cook for about 2 minutes, stirring, before adding all the remaining ingredients. Stir well, cover and simmer gently for 30 minutes, stirring occasionally. Serve with wholewheat spaghetti (up to 100 g cooked weight per person) or couscous.

Couscous with toasted pine nuts and pumpkin seeds

Couscous couldn't be easier to 'cook'; you just need to pour on the right volume of boiling water. I always use stock for extra flavour. It's a lovely low-GL alternative to rice or pasta.

180 g (6½ oz) wholegrain couscous
225 ml (8 fl oz) boiling, low-salt vegetable stock
30 ml (2 tbsp) fresh mint, chopped
25 g (1 oz) pine nuts
25 g (1 oz) pumpkin seeds

Put the couscous in a large bowl and pour on the stock. Stir in the fresh mint. Cover with a lid or plate and leave to stand for 5 minutes. In the meantime, put the pine nuts and pumpkin seeds in a dry saucepan and heat on the hob, tossing frequently, until they just start browning. Remove the saucepan from the heat. Once the couscous is ready, add the pine nuts and pumpkin seeds and stir before serving.

Sweet and sour Quorn

You can enjoy this satisfying Chinese dish without worrying about an overdose of sodium or fat. Quorn chicken-style pieces provide an excellent vegetarian option. Extend the cooking time if you use real chicken.

If you don't have arrowroot, use 15 g (½ oz) of gram flour, blended with water; the sauce will take on a cream colour, but will taste just as good.

For the marinade/sauce:
juice from 220-g (8-oz) can pineapple chunks
15 ml (1 tbsp) reduced-salt soy sauce
60 ml (4 tbsp) sherry
30 ml (2 tbsp) rice vinegar
30 ml (2 tbsp) clear honey
juice ½ lime
15 ml (1 tbsp) tomato purée
freshly-ground black pepper

Other ingredients:
350 g (12 oz) Quorn chicken-style pieces
15 ml (1 tbsp) rapeseed oil
2 shallots or 1 small onion, finely chopped
2 garlic cloves, grated
5 cm (2 inches) ginger root, peeled and grated
1 yellow pepper, deseeded and diced
220-g (8-oz) can pineapple chunks in own juice,
drained (using juice for marinade)
220-g (8-oz) can water chestnuts, sliced
220-g (8-oz) can bamboo shoots (not bean sprouts)
10 ml (2 tsp) arrowroot, blended with water

Put all the ingredients of the marinade in a plastic bowl with a sealable lid and mix thoroughly with a fork or whisk. Add the Quorn pieces, fit the lid tightly and turn the bowl upside down repeatedly to ensure all Quorn pieces are thoroughly coated. Allow to stand for about 30 minutes, turning occasionally.

Heat the oil in a large pan (e.g. 4 litre capacity) and cook the shallots, garlic and ginger for about 2 minutes, stirring, before adding the Quorn and any marinade left in the bowl. Stir and cook for another 2 minutes, then add all the remaining ingredients, except the blended arrowroot.

Stir thoroughly, cover and simmer gently on a very low heat for 10 minutes, making sure the sauce doesn't stick on the bottom of the pan. Add the blended arrowroot and stir until the sauce has thickened.

Serve with peas and couscous, quinoa or brown basmati rice.

Fried teriyaki tofu

If you've had a bad experience of tofu, fried marinated tofu could change your view.

> *500 g (1 lb 2 oz) firm tofu (not silken)*
> *60 ml (4 tbsp) teriyaki marinade*
> *1 free-range egg (e.g. Columbus)*
> *15 ml (1 tbsp) skimmed milk*
> *60 ml (4 tbsp) stoneground oatmeal*
> *60 ml (4 tbsp) gram flour*
> *15 ml (1 tbsp) curry powder*
> *15 ml (1 tbsp) cayenne pepper*
> *freshly-ground black pepper*
> *30 ml (2 tbsp) rapeseed oil*

Cut the tofu into slices, roughly ½ inch (1.3 cm) thick; lay these flat on absorbent kitchen towel; cover with at least five layers of kitchen towel and compress this sandwich gently under a chopping board to squeeze out excess moisture. Repeat the process with dry kitchen towel. It is often convenient to leave the tofu compressed by a weight on the chopping board. Cut the tofu slices in half to produce bite-sized pieces.

Lay the tofu pieces side by side in a plastic bag, add the teriyaki marinade and seal the bag, excluding as much air as possible to keep the marinade in close contact with the tofu. Rotate the bag to ensure all the tofu is covered in marinade. Marinate for 15–30 minutes, or for longer in the fridge.

Beat the egg and skimmed milk together in a bowl. Mix the oatmeal, gram flour, curry powder, cayenne and black pepper in a shallow dish, ensuring the curry powder is evenly distributed.

Dip each tofu piece in the egg and milk before rolling it in the oatmeal mixture.

Heat the oil in a frying pan over medium heat. Fry the tofu pieces, turning with tongs every 10–15 seconds until all sides are golden brown. Allow to drain on kitchen towel. Serve with lemon wedges, curry sauce (p. 417), fresh coriander and salad.

Quornucopia (6 servings)

The title of this recipe may be a bit Quorny, but it truly is a horn of plenty: with an abundance of vegetables and pulses, and a choice vegetarian alternative to chicken, it's a complete meal in one pot. As the legend of the cornucopia emerged from Greek mythology, it's appropriate that this dish is enhanced with oregano which means 'joy of the mountains' in Greek, and thyme, a symbol of courage in ancient Greece.

15 ml (1 tbsp) olive oil
1 large onion, finely chopped
3 garlic cloves, crushed
350 g (12 oz) Quorn chicken-style pieces
5 ml (1 tsp) oregano
2.5 ml (½ tsp) thyme
1 celery stick, finely chopped
2 medium courgettes, sliced
3 peppers (1 red, 1 yellow, 1 orange), thinly sliced
300 ml (½ pint) white wine
300 ml (½ pint) low-salt vegetable stock
400-g (14-oz) can chickpeas in water, drained
400-g (14-oz) can cannellini beans in water, drained
50 g (2 oz) gram flour, blended with water (p. 373)
80 g (3 oz) frozen peas
80 g (3 oz) frozen sweetcorn kernels
freshly-ground black pepper
pinch Solo or LoSalt to taste

Heat the oil in a large heavy-based pan (e.g. 4 litre capacity) and cook the onion until soft. Add the garlic, Quorn and herbs and cook for about 2 minutes, stirring, before adding the other ingredients up to and including the gram flour. Stir well and simmer gently on a very low heat, covered, for 15 minutes. Stir in the peas, sweetcorn and black pepper (and Solo or LoSalt if required). Simmer for a further 5 minutes.

Tofu and vegetable stir-fry

A stir-fry can be a great way of enjoying a variety of fresh vegetables with a good source of protein such as tofu. Recipes often include vast quantities of salt (from soy sauce) and fat (oil). You don't need much fat to cook the vegetables: they should be steamed rather than deep-fried. Buying bags of prepared vegetables saves time. There are lots of ways that you can vary this recipe. You may prefer to marinate the tofu and fry it separately (p. 394). Why not try a sweet and sour sauce, as in the Quorn recipe on p. 393, or use Five Spice powder (p. 419)?

30 ml (2 tbsp) rapeseed oil
500 g (1 lb 2 oz) firm tofu, cut and dried (p. 394)

Sauce:
15 ml (1 tbsp) reduced-salt soy sauce
15 ml (1 tbsp) rice vinegar
15 ml (1 tbsp) clear honey
30 ml (2 tbsp) sherry
8 drops Tabasco
150 ml (¼ pint) low-salt vegetable stock
15 ml (1 tbsp) gram flour, mixed with water (p. 373)

1 onion, finely chopped
2 garlic cloves, grated
5 cm (2 inches) ginger root, peeled and grated
500 g (1 lb 2 oz) mixed vegetables (e.g. peppers, bok choy, broccoli,
mushrooms, carrots), cut into small pieces
100 g (4 oz) bean sprouts
220-g (8-oz) can water chestnuts, sliced
freshly-ground black pepper

Heat the oil in the wok and fry the tofu (in batches) until golden; transfer the tofu to a warm plate. Mix the sauce ingredients in a saucepan and bring to a simmer, stirring, until the sauce thickens. Remove from the heat. Put the onion, garlic and ginger in the wok and stir-fry for about 2 minutes until the onion starts to soften. Add the remaining vegetables and stir-fry for 4 minutes or until the vegetables just begin to wilt.

Serve the tofu on a bed of stir-fried vegetables and pour on the sauce.

Quorn Portuguese

If you use fresh chillies for this recipe, even mild ones, don't forget to use gloves to chop them. You can always turn up the heat with chilli powder or crushed chillies.

15 ml (1 tbsp) olive oil
1 onion, finely chopped
350 g (12 oz) Quorn chicken-style pieces
3 garlic cloves, crushed
2 moderately hot chillies, deseeded and finely chopped
5 ml (1 tsp) dried oregano
5 ml (1 tsp) ground paprika
juice and zest 1 lime
200 ml (7 fl oz) red wine
200 ml (7 fl oz) low-salt vegetable stock
15 ml (1 tbsp) tomato purée
1 medium to large courgette, sliced
30 g (1 oz) gram flour, blended with water
freshly-ground black pepper
pinch Solo or LoSalt to taste

Heat the oil in a large, heavy-based pan (e.g. 4 litres), add the onion and cook until it starts to soften. Add the Quorn, garlic, chilli, oregano and paprika; cook, stirring, for about 3 minutes.

Add all the remaining ingredients and bring to the boil. Stir well and simmer gently, covered, for 10 minutes. Serve with your choice of vegetables and couscous or quinoa.

Tofu and vegetable curry

Tofu haters won't notice the small pieces of tofu that silently pack some quality protein into this delicious but mild vegetarian curry.

15 ml (1 tbsp) rapeseed oil
1 large onion, finely chopped
2.5 cm (1 inch) ginger root, peeled and grated
6 green cardamom pods, lightly crushed

3 garlic cloves, crushed
5 ml (1 tsp) ground cumin
5 ml (1 tsp) ground coriander
5 ml (1 tsp) turmeric
5 ml (1 tsp) chilli powder
500 g (1 lb 2 oz) firm tofu, dried (p. 394
and cut into cubes, about 1 cm (½ inch)
300 ml (½ pint) low-salt vegetable stock
300 ml (½ pint) passata
1 cauliflower, cut into florets
2 celery sticks, finely chopped
2 carrots, grated
170 g (6 oz) green beans, sliced
30 g (1 oz) gram flour, blended with water
100 g (4 oz) frozen peas
5 ml (1 tsp) garam masala
freshly-ground black pepper
pinch Solo or LoSalt to taste

Heat the oil in a large, heavy-based pan (e.g. 4 litre capacity). Fry the onion until soft. Add the ginger, cardamom, garlic and spices and cook for 1–3 minutes over low heat, stirring; make sure you don't burn the garlic or spices.

Now add the tofu and stir for about 30 seconds before adding the stock, passata and vegetables. Bring to a simmer and stir in the blended gram flour. Simmer gently for 30 minutes, covered.

Add the frozen peas and stir in the garam masala. Simmer for a further 5 minutes and season with black pepper. Serve with couscous, quinoa or brown basmati rice (60 g cooked weight per person).

Soya goulash (6 servings)

Traditionally, Hungarian goulash is made with beef, red peppers and lots of paprika. Other meats such as veal or lamb are also used and seasonal vegetables added. This version uses soya mince. I find that large soya chunks are less popular than mince as they have a tougher texture. You could equally well use Quorn or extra-lean turkey mince.

The manufacturer's instructions typically recommend soaking soya mince in hot water for five minutes; using stock (or reduced-salt vegetable bouillon) increases the depth of flavour.

15 ml (1 tbsp) olive oil
2 large onions, finely chopped
3 garlic cloves, crushed
100 g (4 oz) soya mince (dry weight),
soaked in stock and drained
30 ml (2 tbsp) ground paprika
10 ml (2 tsp) mixed herbs
2.5 ml (½ tsp) freshly-ground black pepper
2 bay leaves
1 medium carrot, sliced
2 peppers (1 red, 1 green), diced
100 g (4 oz) mushrooms, sliced
400-g (14-oz) can chopped tomatoes in tomato juice
15 ml (1 tbsp) tomato purée
150 ml (¼ pint) red wine
150 ml (¼ pint) low-salt vegetable stock
30 g (1 oz) fresh parsley, finely chopped
30 g (1 oz) gram flour (or soya flour), blended with water
pinch Solo or LoSalt to taste

Heat the oil in a large heavy-based pan (e.g. 4 litre capacity). Fry the onions over high heat, stirring, for about 2 minutes until softening. Add the garlic, soya mince, paprika, herbs, black pepper, bay leaves, carrot, peppers and mushrooms and stir well over medium heat for about 2 minutes, making sure that nothing burns or sticks to the bottom of the pan.

Add the tomatoes, tomato purée, wine, stock and most of the parsley, keeping some parsley back as a garnish. Bring to the boil, stirring, and simmer gently over low heat for 15 minutes. Stir in the blended flour and simmer for another 2 minutes. Serve with 0% fat Greek yoghurt and garnish with chopped parsley.

Spicy-chickpea salad

Here's a quick way to spice up some tinned chickpeas for a lunchtime salad.

2×400-g (14-oz) cans chickpeas, drained
300-g (10½-oz) bag mixed salad leaves
12 cherry tomatoes, sliced
1 carrot, grated

1 green pepper, deseeded and diced
60 ml (4 tbsp) vinaigrette dressing (p. 417)
15 ml (1 tbsp) garlic-infused olive oil
1 small red onion, finely chopped
15 ml (1 tbsp) medium curry powder
10 ml (2 tsp) crushed chillies
10 ml (2 tsp) ground paprika

Rinse the chickpeas in a sieve, allow them to drain and pour them into a bowl lined with kitchen towel to dry.

Put the salad leaves, tomatoes, carrot and green pepper in a bowl and toss them in the vinaigrette.

Heat the oil in a frying pan and cook the onion until it starts to soften. Stir in the curry powder, chilli and paprika and cook for 30 seconds before adding the chickpeas. Cook for 4 minutes. Add the chickpeas to the salad, toss and serve.

Green lentil curry

This nutritious vegetarian curry is quick and easy to make. Green lentils keep their shape much better than red lentils; they have a lovely flavour, perfectly complemented by the curry spices.

250 g (9 oz) green lentils
600 ml (1 pint) low-salt vegetable stock
30 ml (2 tbsp) rapeseed oil
1 large onion, finely chopped
2.5 cm (1 inch) ginger, peeled and grated
3 garlic cloves, crushed
45 ml (3 tbsp) medium curry powder
5 ml (1 tsp) chilli powder
400-g (14-oz) can chopped tomatoes in tomato juice
15 ml (1 tbsp) tomato purée
2 medium carrots, finely grated
1 red pepper, deseeded and diced
freshly-ground black pepper

Wash the lentils in a sieve under cold running water, transfer them to a large saucepan with the stock and bring to the boil. Cover and simmer on a low heat for 20 minutes, adding a little boiling water if necessary, until the lentils are soft (but not mushy).

In the meantime, heat the oil in a separate pan and cook the onion over high heat, stirring, until golden brown. Add the ginger and garlic and cook for 2 minutes. Add the curry and chilli powders and stir for 30 seconds before adding the remaining ingredients. Simmer over low heat until the lentils are ready.

Mix the lentils and curry sauce together (in whichever pan is larger) and simmer for 5 minutes.

Serve with couscous and peas.

Jollof quinoa

Jollof rice is a popular West African dish. It takes many different forms, but its other name 'benachin' means 'one pot' and a characteristic feature of the dish is that the tomatoes colour the rice. In this vegetarian version, the glycaemic load is reduced by using quinoa, and the protein content is boosted with soya.

The vegetables make a significant contribution to the liquid taken up by the quinoa; if you use different vegetables, you may need to adjust the quantity of stock.

> 100 g (4 oz) dry soya mince
> 600 ml (1 pint) low-salt vegetable stock, hot
> 15 ml (1 tbsp) rapeseed oil
> 2 red onions, finely chopped
> 1 red pepper, diced
> 1 aubergine, diced
> 2 medium courgettes, sliced
> 100 g (4 oz) mushrooms, sliced
> 1 large carrot, finely grated
> 2 bay leaves
> 15 ml (1 tbsp) dried thyme
> 2.5 ml (½ tsp) cayenne pepper
> 2.5 ml (½ tsp) ground nutmeg
> 3 garlic cloves, crushed
> 400-g (14-oz) can chopped tomatoes in tomato juice
> 15 ml (1 tbsp) tomato purée
> 200 g (7 oz) quinoa, rinsed
> freshly-ground black pepper
> pinch Solo or LoSalt to taste

Soak the soya mince in the hot vegetable stock for at least 5 minutes.

Heat the oil in a large (e.g. 4-litre), heavy-based pan and cook the onion on high heat until softening. Add the red pepper, aubergine, courgettes and mushrooms and cook for 5 minutes, stirring.

Add the soya mince, grated carrot, bay leaves, thyme, cayenne pepper, nutmeg and garlic. Cook for 5 minutes, stirring.

Stir in the chopped tomatoes, tomato purée and quinoa. Cover and simmer for 15 minutes. If there is still any free liquid, cook for a little longer, uncovered, until all the sauce is taken up. Season with black pepper and a little Solo or LoSalt to taste. Remove the bay leaves.

Serve with mangetout, green beans or peas.

Mediterranean bean-stuffed peppers

Peppers are stuffed with all kinds of things, but in this wholesome vegetarian dish, pulses are used to pack them with protein. And with tomatoes, olive oil and oregano, they're packed with flavour too.

> *4 peppers (e.g. 2 red, 2 yellow), washed and dried*
> *15 ml (1 tbsp) olive oil*
> *1 onion, finely chopped*
> *2 garlic cloves, crushed*
> *400-g (14-oz) can chickpeas, drained and rinsed*
> *400-g (14-oz) can red kidney beans, drained and rinsed*
> *400-g (14-oz) can chopped tomatoes in tomato juice*
> *15 ml (1 tbsp) tomato purée*
> *1 medium carrot, finely grated*
> *60 g (2 oz) mushrooms, finely sliced*
> *15 ml (1 tbsp) balsamic vinegar*
> *10 ml (2 tsp) dried oregano*
> *2.5 ml (½ tsp) dried basil*
> *freshly-ground black pepper*
> *pinch Solo or LoSalt to taste*
> *40 g (1½ oz) Parmesan (or miniCol) cheese, grated*

Cut each pepper in half lengthways, bisecting the stalk and leaving it attached (although it won't be eaten). Remove the seeds. Lightly wipe the outer surface of each pepper half with olive oil and place, cut surface uppermost, on a baking tray lined with kitchen foil.

Heat the oil in a pan and fry the onion and garlic until the onion is softening. Add all the remaining ingredients except the cheese. Bring to the boil, stir, and simmer for 10 minutes.

Remove the pan from the heat, allow it to cool a little, and carefully spoon the filling into each pepper half; unless you have extra small or large peppers, there should be just enough for a heaped filling in each half. Top this with the grated cheese.

Bake in the oven at 200°C (400°F, Gas 6) for 20 minutes. Serve two pepper halves to each person (e.g. 1 red, 1 yellow) with wholegrain couscous and salad or vegetables of your choosing.

Lentils Italienne

Lentils provide protein, iron, zinc, B vitamins and fibre. Unlike dried beans, they don't have to be soaked before cooking. Here's an easy way to enjoy the satisfying flavour of green lentils. It's convenient to cook the lentils (for just 15 minutes) while preparing the other ingredients.

250 g (9 oz) green lentils
600 ml (1 pint) low-salt vegetable stock
15 ml (1 tbsp) olive oil
1 large onion, finely chopped
3 garlic cloves, crushed
2 peppers (1 red, 1 yellow), deseeded and diced
15 ml (1 tbsp) dried oregano
400-g (14-oz) can chopped tomatoes in tomato juice
30 ml (2 tbsp) tomato purée
1 large carrot, finely grated
1 medium courgette, sliced
100 g (4 oz) mushrooms, sliced
freshly-ground black pepper

Wash the lentils thoroughly in a fine sieve under cold running water. Transfer them to a saucepan with the stock, bring to the boil and simmer for 15 minutes, adding a little boiling water if they become too dry.

Heat the olive oil in a large, heavy-based pan. Add the onion, garlic, peppers and oregano and stir-fry until the onion is soft.

Add all the remaining ingredients and the lentils, stir thoroughly, bring to the boil and simmer for 20 minutes.

Serve with peas and wholegrain couscous or quinoa.

Chickpea jalfrezi

Jalfrezi dishes are stir-fried in very little sauce. Chicken jalfrezi is usually cooked with onion, tomatoes, green peppers and green chillies – a fresh, hot dish with a small amount of thick sauce clinging to the meat and vegetables. In this vegetarian jalfrezi, the green pepper is added towards the end of cooking to retain its fresh colour and texture.

Don't forget to wear gloves to chop the chilli (or at least, wash your hands immediately afterwards). You can always add more chillies, if you're a fire-eater, but remember that one chilli goes a long way in a small volume of sauce.

15 ml (1 tbsp) rapeseed oil
1 onion, finely chopped
2 garlic cloves, peeled and finely chopped
1 green chilli, deseeded and finely chopped
15 ml (1 tbsp) medium curry powder
2.5 ml (½ tsp) cayenne pepper
15 ml (1 tbsp) tomato purée
2×400-g (14-oz) cans chickpeas, drained
2 plum tomatoes, chopped
150 ml (¼ pint) low-salt vegetable stock
1 green pepper, deseeded and sliced
5 cm (2 inches) ginger root, peeled and grated
45 ml (3 tbsp) fresh coriander leaves, chopped
5 ml (1 tsp) garam masala

Heat the oil in a large frying pan and cook the onion, garlic and chilli for about 3 minutes, to soften the onion without burning the garlic.

Add the curry powder, cayenne pepper and tomato purée and stir-fry for about 30 seconds. Take care not to burn the spices.

Stir in the chickpeas, chopped tomatoes and stock. Bring to the boil and simmer for 6 minutes to reduce the sauce, stirring frequently.

Add the green pepper, ginger, coriander and garam masala. Stir and simmer for 2 minutes. Serve with salad or vegetables and fat-free yoghurt or raita.

SALADS

Mixed green salad

Making a mixed salad gives you the opportunity to blend a wonderful variety of tastes and textures in every mouthful. What a contrast to the isolated lettuce leaf and naked tomato that puts so many children off salad for life!

Here is a simple recipe using common salad vegetables. The variations are endless. For a start, we have a marvellous choice of leaves such as baby spinach, cos, iceberg, lamb's lettuce, little gem, mizuna, radicchio, rocket and watercress. Then there are herbs like basil, mint and parsley. Sometimes you will want to add beetroot, broccoli, carrots, or celeriac, chicory, mushrooms, radishes or peas. Why not throw in a few chives or capers or sprinkle your salad with toasted pine nuts or pumpkin seeds?

Generally, all salad vegetables should be carefully washed in clean, cold water and dried in a salad spinner or tea towel (as water doesn't make a very interesting dressing). Bags of prepared salad leaves are a great convenience.

A good dressing can transform an interesting collection of vegetables into a sensational salad. If you like your salad well dressed, avoid traditional vinaigrette (typically two-thirds oil) and use a lower-fat version (p. 417).

200 g (7 oz) mixed salad leaves, torn where necessary
3 plum tomatoes, sliced
1 green pepper, deseeded and cut into strips
1 yellow pepper, deseeded and cut into strips
1 celery stick, finely chopped
¼ cucumber, diced
6 spring onions, chopped
60 ml (4 tbsp) salad dressing (p. 417)

Toss all the ingredients together in a bowl and serve. If preparing the salad in advance, add the dressing just before serving; leaves start to wilt once the dressing is applied.

Puy lentil and pepper salad

Traditionally grown in the volcanic soils of le Puy in France, Puy (pronounced 'pwee') lentils are considered topnotch. They retain their shape and have a distinctive peppery taste. Dried Puy or green lentils don't have to be soaked, and cook in 20 minutes. Even so, the canned products are extremely convenient when you want to make a quick salad.

2×400-g (14-oz) cans Puy lentils, drained and rinsed
1 green pepper, deseeded and diced
1 yellow pepper, deseeded and diced
¼ cucumber, diced
1 carrot, coarsely grated
1 small red onion, finely chopped
25 g (1 oz) fresh mint, chopped
60 ml (4 tbsp) lower-fat vinaigrette dressing (p. 417)

Toss all the ingredients together in a bowl.

Cannellini bean and coriander salad

In this vegetarian salad, protein-packed cannellini beans are perfectly complemented by coriander and capers. One portion (a quarter) of this salad is a good lunch by itself. It also goes well with tinned tuna and makes a fine accompaniment for a hot dinner.

2×400-g (14-oz) cans cannellini beans,
drained and rinsed
1 small red onion, finely chopped
60 g (2 oz) mixed salad leaves, washed and torn
60 g (2 oz) fresh coriander leaves, washed and chopped
1 celery stick, chopped
16 cherry tomatoes, halved
30 ml (2 tbsp) capers, drained
60 ml (4 tbsp) lower-fat vinaigrette (p. 417)

Toss the ingredients together and serve.

Mixed bean and basil salad

A can of mixed beans in water (with no added sugar or salt), containing perhaps nine different varieties of beans, is a really excellent product – just the thing when you want to knock up a quick, high-protein vegetarian salad.

There's nothing like the smell of fresh basil. Simply tear the basil if you want a leafier salad; chopping it finely distributes it more evenly.

2×400-g (14-oz) cans mixed beans, drained and rinsed
25 g (1 oz) fresh basil leaves, finely chopped
1 green pepper, deseeded and diced
1 medium carrot, coarsely grated
1 celery stick, finely chopped
12 cherry tomatoes, halved
6 spring onions, chopped
60 ml (4 tbsp) vinaigrette
or lemon and garlic dressing (p. 418)

Gently mix all the ingredients without breaking up any beans. A convenient way to do this is to put all the vegetables and dressing in a large bowl with a sealable lid. Make sure the lid is fitted securely and rotate the bowl repeatedly like a concrete mixer.

Quinoa and mango salad

You may not have thought of putting mango in a salad. I find most people are pleasantly surprised by this combination. If your mango is juicy, some liquid may collect after the salad has been resting in the fridge. This simply adds to the dressing and doesn't make it any less delicious.

160 g (5½ oz) quinoa
380 ml (13 fl oz) low-salt vegetable stock
1-cm (½-inch) slice ginger root
seeds 4 green cardamom pods,
ground in a pestle and mortar
1 mango, peeled and chopped
8 cherry tomatoes, finely chopped
1 celery stick, finely chopped
1 yellow pepper, deseeded and diced
¼ cucumber, diced
juice 1 lemon
15 ml (1 tbsp) olive oil
freshly-ground black pepper

Rinse the quinoa in a sieve under cold, running water. Put it in a saucepan with the stock, ginger and ground cardamom seeds. Bring to the boil and simmer, partially covered, for 13 minutes – uncovering if necessary for the last couple of minutes to ensure there is no excess liquid at the end of the cooking time. Remove the ginger and allow the quinoa to cool.

Transfer the quinoa to a bowl and mix it with all the remaining ingredients. Ideally, cover and refrigerate for an hour or more to allow all the flavours to blend.

SOUPS

Chinese chicken soup (8 servings)

This soup takes very little time to prepare and only about 15 minutes to cook. It makes a lovely oriental lunch. If you don't need 8 servings straightaway, refrigerate the remainder and use it within two days, making sure you reheat it thoroughly.

> *800 g (1¾ lb) skinless chicken breast*
> *15 ml (1 tbsp) reduced-salt soy sauce*
> *15 ml (1 tbsp) rice vinegar*
> *15 ml (1 tbsp) clear honey*
> *2.5 ml (½ tsp) crushed chillies*
> *freshly-ground black pepper*
> *15 ml (1 tbsp) rapeseed oil*
> *6 spring onions, chopped*
> *2 lemongrass stalks*
> *1 garlic clove, crushed*
> *5 cm (2 inches) ginger root, peeled and grated*
> *2 litres (4¼ pints) low-salt vegetable or chicken stock*
> *50 g (2 oz) mushrooms, finely sliced*
> *400-g (14-oz) can bean sprouts, drained*
> *225-g (8-oz) can bamboo shoots, drained*

Cut the chicken into thin strips about 0.5 cm (¼ inch) thick and no more than 5 cm (2 inches) long and place in a plastic bowl with a sealable lid. Add the soy sauce, vinegar, honey, crushed chillies and black pepper; fit the lid and shake, making sure the chicken pieces are thoroughly mixed with the marinade; this is a low-volume marinade which will be completely taken up by the chicken.

Heat the oil in a 4-litre, heavy-based pan and fry the onions, lemongrass, garlic and ginger for about 2 minutes. Add the chicken and stir-fry for 2–3 minutes.

Pour in the stock and bring to the boil. Stir in the mushrooms, bean sprouts and bamboo shoots. Simmer gently for 10 minutes. Remove the lemongrass and serve, ensuring each bowl gets a fair share of chicken.

Watercress and butter bean soup (8 servings)

This is a really satisfying soup that only takes a few minutes to prepare and cook if you use bags of ready-washed watercress. You might like to try two bags of watercress with one of spinach, or spinach and rocket.

Using a hand blender in the saucepan is so much quicker and easier than transferring the soup to a blender.

30 ml (2 tbsp) rapeseed oil
1 large onion, finely chopped
2 litres (4¼ pints) low-salt vegetable stock
2×400-g (14-oz) cans butter beans, drained
300 g (10½ oz) watercress
350 g (12 oz) silken tofu, roughly chopped
freshly-ground black pepper

Heat the oil in a 4-litre, heavy-based pan and fry the onion for about 5 minutes until soft and lightly browned. Add the stock and butter beans and bring to the boil.

Add the watercress, tofu and black pepper. Simmer for 5 minutes. Remove the pan from the heat and use a hand blender to produce a lump-free soup.

Any excess soup can be kept in the fridge for up to 3 days.

Creamy tomato soup (8 servings)

Here's a healthy tomato soup, made 'creamy' with silken tofu. Smoothly satisfying to grown-ups, it's also loved by children who would normally run away from vegetables or anything with lumps in it.

A soup like this – consisting mainly of low-carbohydrate vegetables and water – makes a good lunch but also a great gap-filler at any time of day. Always having it available can keep you going and keep you on track.

You could further reduce the salt content by replacing the passata with four 400-g (14-oz) cans of plum tomatoes in tomato juice (perhaps adding a little basil), but I prefer it with passata.

30 ml (2 tbsp) rapeseed oil
1 large onion, roughly chopped
4 large carrots, peeled and chopped
3 celery sticks, chopped

2 red peppers, deseeded and chopped
4 garlic cloves, crushed
2×700-g (25-oz) jars passata
600 ml (1 pint) low-salt vegetable stock
350 g (12 oz) silken tofu, roughly chopped
freshly-ground black pepper

Heat the oil in the pan and cook the onion, carrots, celery and red peppers over medium heat for 5 minutes, stirring frequently. Add the garlic and cook for another 3 minutes until all the vegetables have softened.

Pour in the tomatoes and stock, bring to the boil and simmer, covered, for 20 minutes. Add the tofu and simmer for 5 minutes. Turn off the heat and use a hand blender to liquidise all the lumps. Season and serve.

Roasted vegetable soup (8 servings)

The oven does most of the work in this recipe, roasting extra flavour into the vegetables, and there's very little for you to do. Using one bulb of fennel adds a subtle aniseed-like flavour; if that's not to your liking, leave it out – it's scrumptious either way.

1 butternut squash, peeled and deseeded
1 fennel bulb, trimmed
2 peppers (e.g. 1 red, 1 orange), stalks and seeds removed
2 red onions, quartered
6 garlic cloves, whole
2 large carrots, peeled
15 ml (1 tbsp) olive oil
freshly-ground black pepper
2 litres (4¼ pints) low-salt vegetable stock
350 g (12 oz) silken tofu, roughly chopped
pinch Solo or LoSalt to taste

Cut all the vegetables into chunks no bigger than 5 cm (2 inches) and arrange them in a baking tray wiped with oil. Drizzle olive oil over the vegetables, season with black pepper and roast in the oven at 200°C (400°F, Gas 6) for 30 minutes.

Transfer the vegetables to a 4-litre, heavy-based pan. Add the stock and tofu, bring to the boil and simmer for 10 minutes. Remove the pan from the heat and use a hand blender to break down all the lumps until the soup is completely smooth.

DIPS and DOLLOPS

Dips, Sauces, Spreads and Dressings

Hummus

Popular as a dip in the Middle East, hummus makes a tasty high-protein snack and versatile spread. It's often spoilt by excessive levels of salt or oil.

400-g (14-oz) can chickpeas,
drained and rinsed
45 ml (3 tbsp) tahini (sesame-seed paste)
juice 2 lemons
2 garlic cloves, crushed
15 ml (1 tbsp) olive oil
pinch Solo or LoSalt to taste
1.25 ml (¼ tsp) ground paprika

Put all the ingredients except the paprika in a food processor and blend until smooth. Transfer to a serving bowl and sprinkle with the paprika. Serve with crudités (e.g. raw carrot, celery, pepper or broccoli) or pitta bread. You can keep it in the fridge for up to 3 days or freeze it for up to 3 months.

Tzatziki

This classic Greek dip is normally made with full-fat yoghurt, drained overnight in muslin. Here's a quick low-fat version. Use dill rather than mint if you are making a sauce to accompany fish.

200 g (7 oz) 0% fat Greek yoghurt
½ cucumber, peeled
15 ml (1 tbsp) lemon juice
10 ml (2 tsp) olive oil
15 ml (1 tbsp) finely chopped mint or dill

Drain any excess fluid from the yoghurt. Cut the cucumber in half lengthwise and scrape out the seeds with a teaspoon. Coarsely grate the cucumber into a fine sieve, allow liquid to drain for a few minutes and squeeze with kitchen towel. Mix all the ingredients in a bowl. Cover and refrigerate for 30 minutes before serving. To make a tzatziki sauce rather than a dip, you could add extra lemon juice. You can always add a little xylitol if you prefer it sweeter.

Guacamole

Many variations of this Mexican dish are possible. I like to give it a mild kick, without overwhelming the buttery subtlety of the avocado. You can use it as a dip, but also as a spread or sauce.

Unusually for a fruit, the avocado contains a lot of fat – but it's mainly mono-unsaturated fat and a lot of useful nutrients come with it. And if you use avocado in place of mayonnaise, you'll be halving the fat and calories.

You need ripe avocados for guacamole. If they feel too firm, leave them in a paper bag to ripen for two or three days.

2 ripe avocados
juice 1 lime
1 shallot, finely chopped
1 garlic clove, crushed
1 mild red chilli, deseeded and chopped
80 g (3 oz) tomatoes, chopped
2.5 ml (½ tsp) cayenne pepper
freshly-ground black pepper
pinch Solo or LoSalt to taste

Cut the avocados in half, remove the stones, scoop the flesh into a bowl and discard the skin. (If you have children, they may like to try growing avocado plants from the stones.) Add the lime juice, mash the avocado with a fork and mix in the other ingredients. You can always use a food processor if you want a smoothly blended sauce. Unless you are using it straight away, refrigerate in a sealed container. The lime (or lemon) juice helps to stop it discolouring.

Quick salsa

Throw the ingredients of this salsa together, let them mingle in the fridge, and you can add instant zing to any meal, snack or sandwich.

> *400-g (14-oz) can chopped tomatoes in tomato juice*
> *½ can sweet red peppers, drained and chopped*
> *2 mild chillies, finely chopped*
> *1 small onion, finely chopped*
> *bunch parsley (or coriander), finely chopped*
> *juice 1 lime*
> *freshly-ground black pepper*

Drain most of the tomato juice from the can of chopped tomatoes and reserve it to add back later if it won't make the salsa too sloppy. Mix all the ingredients together, cover and refrigerate for an hour before serving.

Salmon pâté

Packed with protein, calcium and omega-3, this scrumptious pâté is so easy to make you'll wonder why you ever bought ready-made sandwich fillers. Try it with salad in wholemeal pitta, or add fat-free Greek yoghurt to use it as a dip.

> *400-g (14-oz) can salmon, drained*
> *100g (4oz) quark (virtually fat-free soft cheese)*
> *1 garlic clove, crushed*
> *juice 1 lemon*
> *30ml (2 tbsp) chopped fresh chives*
> *freshly-ground black pepper*

Mix all the ingredients in a bowl until the consistency is smooth (and the garlic is evenly distributed). Cover and chill in the fridge for at least 30 minutes before serving.

Tuna spread

Here's another chance to produce a brilliant blend of flavours in minutes without having the food processor to wash up.

> *2×185-g (6½-oz) cans tuna in water, drained*
> *15ml (1 tbsp) garlic-infused olive oil*
> *1 small red onion, finely chopped*
> *juice 1 lemon*
> *freshly-ground black pepper*

Mix the ingredients in a bowl. Either use immediately in salad or sandwiches, or cover and refrigerate before serving. You can also blend it with quark to produce a tuna pâté or with fat-free Greek yoghurt to make a dip.

Smoked mackerel pâté

Some recipes for mackerel pâté add large quantities of unnecessary saturated fat in the form of butter. You can make lovely pâté without adding fat. Mackerel, of course, is a good source of omega-3 fatty acids, but smoking's bad for fish too: a lot of salt is added in the process. So just have this occasionally, or in small quantities.

You can use quark instead of yoghurt for a stiffer pâté – or a mixture of quark and yoghurt.

225 g (8 oz) smoked mackerel fillets
225 g (8 oz) 0% fat Greek yoghurt
30 ml (2 tbsp) horseradish sauce
juice 1 lemon
freshly-ground black pepper

Skin the mackerel and use a fork to flake the fish in a large bowl, taking care to remove any bones. Add the other ingredients and mix to form a pleasantly coarse pâté. (Use a food processor if you want it really smooth.)

Serve with lemon wedges and rye crispbreads or toasted triangles of wholemeal pitta.

Mustard sauce

Why buy sauces and dips, full of unwanted ingredients, when they can be this simple to make? This is great on the plate, e.g. with mustard lime chicken (p. 375) or in a pitta or sandwich.

45 ml (3 tbsp) 0% fat Greek yoghurt
15 ml (1 tbsp) Dijon mustard

Mix the two ingredients in a bowl until the colour is even.

Parsley sauce

White sauce can be used as a basis for a wide variety of sauces, sweet and savoury, and is usually made with a roux (fat and flour paste).

Simply using a thickener, such as cornflour, with skimmed milk produces a virtually fat-free sauce.

Here, parsley is added to make a traditional accompaniment for white fish. Parsley sauce has a gentle flavour, so be careful not to overwhelm it with pepper.

20 ml (4 tsp) cornflour
300 ml (½ pint) skimmed milk
60 ml (4 tbsp) finely chopped curled-leaf parsley
LoSalt or Solo and pepper to taste

Put the cornflour in a basin and mix it with a dash of the cold milk to make a smooth paste; stir in a little more milk – just enough to produce a lump-free liquid.

Heat the remaining milk in a saucepan to near boiling point. Gradually stir this hot milk into the cornflour mixture.

Return the contents of the basin to the saucepan and gently bring to the boil, stirring continuously.

Remove from the heat, stir in the parsley and season.

Mint sauce

Mint sauce traditionally accompanies roast lamb, but there's no reason why you shouldn't enjoy it with poultry, new potatoes or vegetables. It's also a convenient starting point if you want to produce a quick mint and yoghurt dressing (p. 419). Making your own mint sauce gives you full control over the ingredients. The best way to have fresh mint available when you want it is to grow it yourself.

bunch fresh mint, say 100 g (4 oz), washed
15 ml (1 tbsp) xylitol
60 ml (4 tbsp) boiling water
60 ml (4 tbsp) white wine vinegar

Strip the leaves off the mint, place them in a bowl with the xylitol and chop finely with scissors (unless you are a champion chopper, in which case sprinkle xylitol over the leaves before chopping on a board and transferring to a bowl). Pour on the boiling water, stir and allow to cool. Stir in the vinegar. You can adjust the taste with a little more xylitol or vinegar. Store the sauce in a sealed jar in the fridge.

Curry sauce

This low-fat sauce only takes a few minutes to prepare. You can use it as a dip or as an accompaniment to meals like fried teriyaki tofu (p. 394).

300 g (10½ oz) 0% fat Greek yoghurt
15 ml (1 tbsp) medium curry powder
30 ml (2 tbsp) sweet mango chutney

Mix the ingredients in a bowl to make a smooth sauce. If there are any lumps of mango in the chutney, chop them into small pieces with scissors.

Mint raita

This very simple raita is a good accompaniment for any curry, especially a hot one. You can add more or less xylitol according to taste. If you find it too thick and prefer it to be of pouring consistency, add a dash of skimmed milk.

150 g (5½ oz) 0% fat Greek yoghurt
60 ml (4 tbsp) finely chopped fresh mint leaves
15 ml (1 tbsp) lime juice
15 ml (1 tbsp) xylitol

Mix the ingredients together.

Lower-fat vinaigrette

Vinaigrette dressing typically contains more oil than anything else so, if you're not careful, a salad can become a high-fat meal. In this tasty dressing, olive oil makes up just under a quarter of the volume; if you have 15 ml (1 tbsp) on your salad, you know you're getting less than 4 ml of olive oil. A variation is to use vegetable stock instead of fruit juice to dilute the oil.

Of course, you can make up a larger quantity, using the same proportions, and keep it in the fridge.

15 ml (1 tbsp) garlic-infused olive oil
15 ml (1 tbsp) balsamic vinegar
15 ml (1 tbsp) cider vinegar
15 ml (1 tbsp) orange juice

> *2.5 ml (½ tsp) clear honey*
> *2.5 ml (½ tsp) Dijon mustard*
> *freshly-ground black pepper*

Put all the ingredients in a jar or plastic container, fit the lid tightly and shake vigorously. Store any excess dressing in the fridge.

Lemon and garlic dressing

Lemons vary in size and juiciness, but you can often get more than 60 ml of juice from one large lemon. The xylitol is optional but you may well find it too sharp without sweetening.

This recipe provides 8 servings of 15 ml (1 tbsp); each serving gives you 7.5 ml (1½ tsp) of oil.

> *60 ml (4 tbsp) lemon juice*
> *60 ml (4 tbsp) olive oil*
> *2 garlic cloves, crushed*
> *2.5 ml (½ tsp) Dijon mustard*
> *5 ml (1 tsp) xylitol*
> *freshly-ground black pepper*

Shake all the ingredients together in a sealed container.

Mustard and honey dressing

This is the ideal dressing to bring out the flavour of lamb's lettuce, but if you like mustard, you'll enjoy it on any salad. And 15 ml (1 tbsp) of this dressing gives you just 5 ml (1 tsp) of olive oil – half the quantity in traditional vinaigrette. Remember your daily limit is 3 teaspoons of oil from all salad dressings and recipes.

> *15 ml (1 tbsp) Dijon mustard*
> *15 ml (1 tbsp) clear honey*
> *30 ml (2 tbsp) cider vinegar*
> *30 ml (2 tbsp) olive oil*
> *1 garlic clove, crushed*
> *freshly-ground black pepper*

Shake all the ingredients together in a sealed jar.

Mint and yoghurt dressing

This tasty low-fat dressing takes moments to prepare if you already have the mint sauce (p. 415). If you use bought mint sauce, it will be sweetened with lots of sugar so you may not need to add xylitol to the dressing. This is the ideal dressing for a salad accompanying tandoori turkey or chicken tikka.

100 g (4 oz) 0% fat Greek yoghurt
30 ml (2 tbsp) mint sauce
juice ½ lemon
15 ml (1 tbsp) garlic-infused olive oil
15 ml (1 tbsp) xylitol
freshly-ground black pepper

Put all the ingredients in a bottle, jar or other suitable container, seal on the lid and shake. Use immediately or store in the fridge for up to a week.

Five-spice powder

Five-spice powder is a convenient way of adding a little Chinese charm to marinades and stir-fries. The trouble with ready-made versions on sale is that they are normally laden with salt. Here is a simple recipe to make your own; you can always add some Solo or LoSalt if you want.

The proportions can be varied according to taste: if you like a dominant aniseed flavour, add more star anise. Once you're happy with the balance, you can mix up a larger quantity and keep it in an air-tight jar. Either buy ground spices or grind them yourself in a spice grinder or pestle and mortar.

10 ml (2 tsp) ground cinnamon
10 ml (2 tsp) ground cloves
10 ml (2 tsp) ground fennel seeds
5 ml (1 tsp) ground star anise
5 ml (1 tsp) ground black peppercorns

Thoroughly mix the ingredients and store in a jar with a close-fitting lid. Typically, you would use 5 ml (1 tsp) in a recipe for four people.

BREAKFASTS

Quinoa with apple and cinnamon

Having this as an alternative to breakfast cereal gets your daily protein intake off to a good start. Fat-free Greek yoghurt is the ideal foil for the sweetness.

150 g (5½ oz) quinoa
300 ml (½ pint) apple juice (no added sugar)
50 g (2 oz) raisins
25 g (1 oz) walnuts, chopped
1 apple, thinly sliced
5 ml (1 tsp) ground cinnamon

Rinse the quinoa in a fine sieve and transfer to a saucepan adding the apple juice, raisins, walnuts, apple and cinnamon. Bring to the boil, stirring. Cover and simmer for 13 minutes, or until the liquid is absorbed. Serve with 0% fat Greek yoghurt.

Low-GL muesli

Muesli can be a delicious source of whole grains and some of the ready-made versions are very appealing. It's best to avoid those with added salt or sugar. Even then, your muesli might still deliver a high GL. Excessive portions of a muesli, full of apparently wholesome ingredients, could sabotage your plan to lose those pounds and inches.

Making your own muesli puts you in control. Here's a simple low-GL version. The recipe provides 12 servings.

240 g (8½ oz) rolled oats
180 g (6½ oz) oat bran
60 g (2 oz) flaked almonds
60 g (2 oz) hazelnuts
30 g (1 oz) pumpkin seeds
30 g (1 oz) dried apricots, chopped

Mix all the ingredients, serve with skimmed milk or fat-free soya alternative to milk and top with berries (e.g. strawberries, raspberries, blackberries or blueberries) and 0% fat Greek yoghurt.

French toast

Often descriptively called 'eggy bread', French toast is usually served as a savoury dish in the UK, but sweet versions (e.g. with sugar and cinnamon) are popular elsewhere.

If you want to have it for breakfast every day, you can avoid the saturated fat and cholesterol by simply using 1 egg white with 15 ml (1 tbsp) of skimmed milk per slice of bread.

3 free-range eggs (e.g. Columbus)
60 ml (4 tbsp) skimmed milk
freshly-ground black pepper
pinch Solo or LoSalt to taste
4 slices mixed-grain bread
10 ml (2 tsp) rapeseed oil

Beat the eggs, milk and seasoning together in a shallow bowl and soak each slice of bread in the mixture.

Heat 5 ml (1 tsp) of the oil in a non-stick frying pan and cook the first two slices (one at a time if necessary) over medium heat for about a minute each side, until golden brown. Heat the other 5 ml of oil in the pan and repeat for the second two slices. Serve with a dash of tomato ketchup – or with cinnamon and apple, or strawberries.

Low-fat mushroom and onion omelette

This omelette is made with two egg whites and no yolk; it's packed with good quality protein, but has none of the saturated fat and cholesterol that come in the yolk. The 28-day plan includes the occasional whole egg. If you use two egg whites instead of a whole egg, there is absolutely no reason why you shouldn't have egg every day.

Because this omelette is full of juicy flavour, you won't miss the yolk.

10 ml (2 tbsp) rapeseed oil
2 egg whites
15 ml (1 tbsp) skimmed milk
30 g (1 oz) mushrooms, finely sliced

¼ red onion, finely chopped
5 ml (1 tsp) grated Parmesan cheese
freshly-ground black pepper
pinch Solo or LoSalt to taste

Heat the oil in a non-stick frying pan. Whisk all the other ingredients together in a bowl with a fork and pour into the hot pan, tilting the pan as necessary to take the mixture evenly to the edges. Cook briefly on a high heat, freeing the edges with a slice, until the omelette can be turned over without disintegrating. Cook the second side for about 30 seconds and then start rolling the omelette up, ensuring it is adequately cooked as you go, and serve.

DESSERTS

Fruit salad

Fruit salads are often dressed in syrup made with a large quantity of sugar. Using xylitol and some fruit juice (in this case from the tinned pineapple) reduces the GL.

You can use any fruits that take your fancy. Always wash fresh fruit (in cold water) no matter how clean it looks. It's convenient to make a large quantity of fruit salad (not just four servings) and keep the excess in the fridge. You can have a ladle of fruit salad in place of a piece of fresh fruit after a meal.

> *2 apples, cored and chopped*
> *3 nectarines, pitted and chopped*
> *400 g (14 oz) strawberries, halved*
> *400 g (14 oz) blueberries*
> *425-g (15-oz) can pineapple chunks in own juice*
> *juice 1 lime*
> *30 ml (2 tbsp) brandy*
> *60 ml (4 tbsp) xylitol*
> *5 ml (1 tsp) ground ginger or cinnamon (optional)*

Put the fruit in a large serving bowl, but tip the juice from the pineapple chunks into a small bowl and mix it with the lime juice, brandy, xylitol and ginger (or cinnamon); make sure the xylitol has dissolved. Pour this dressing into the serving bowl and toss the fruit gently. Ideally, leave the flavours to blend for a couple of hours before serving.

Fruit smoothie

This is a good way to knock up a refreshing and nutritious snack, packed with protein, calcium and antioxidants. On a cholesterol-lowering plan, smoothies can be used to boost your intake of soya protein and provide a vehicle for psyllium husks. You can even bump up the content of soya protein with soft tofu (or dairy protein with quark). Experiment and find a blend that suits you. Adding a little cranberry juice makes the smoothie less thick and modifies the flavour.

It's convenient to use a small blender that's always on hand and easy to wash up, rather than a big food processor – especially if you want to make smoothies often.

If you use large fruits like bananas and nectarines, it's best to cut them into chunks before freezing.

150 g (5½ oz) frozen berries (e.g. blueberries,
blackberries, raspberries, strawberries)
or
1 banana, peach or nectarine, cut into chunks and frozen
250 ml (½ pint) skimmed milk or fat-free soya milk

Place the ingredients in a blender and process until smooth.

Baked apples with custard

Traditionally, Bramley cooking apples are used for baking, but sweeter eating apples such as Golden Delicious bake beautifully too.

There's no reason why you shouldn't have small amounts of custard (especially when it's made with skimmed milk and xylitol). Here I have suggested just ½ pint for four people – enough to dress the apple, but not enough for apple bobbing. If you want to double the quantity, that's fine (but you will, of course, get double the quantity of cornflour from the custard powder).

4 eating apples, washed and dried
40 g (1½ oz) sultanas
25 g (1 oz) pecan nuts, chopped
5 ml (1 tsp) ground allspice (or cinnamon)
10 ml (2 tsp) clear honey
30 ml (2 tbsp) water

For the custard:
18 g (2 level tbsp) custard powder
7.5 ml (1½ tsp) xylitol
300 ml (½ pint) skimmed milk

Remove the apple cores with a corer; if necessary, extend the hole a little to cut out any remaining hard bits or pips. Using a knife point, score a horizontal line through the apple skin at the 'equator'. (The apple will expand when cooking and a neat separation of the skin in the middle is more attractive than uncontrolled volcanic eruptions.)

Mix together the sultanas, chopped pecan nuts and allspice and stuff the mixture into the apples. Push the stuffing down firmly to leave a small well at the top and pour 2.5 ml (½ tsp) of clear honey into this well on each apple.

Stand the apples in an ovenproof dish and pour in the 30 ml (2 tbsp) of water. Bake in the oven at 190°C (375°F, Gas 5) for 25 minutes.

Follow the manufacturer's instructions to make the custard, using the xylitol instead of sugar and skimmed milk instead of whole milk. Note that when manufacturers refer to '1 tablespoon', they often mean a heaped rather than a level tablespoon, and weight may be a better guide to the quantity of custard powder required.

Chocolate-dipped strawberries

The combination of succulent ripe strawberries and good quality dark chocolate is a delight to the eye and the palate.

Make sure the strawberries are absolutely dry (a drop of water can make the chocolate separate) and take care not to overheat the chocolate. If you use Lindt dark chocolate, 60 g is six 'squares'.

400 g (14 oz) fresh strawberries
60 g (2 oz) dark chocolate (85% cocoa solids)

Wash the strawberries gently under cold, running water and dry them thoroughly with paper towel. Don't remove the green caps or stalks.

Prepare a tray lined with greaseproof paper to receive the strawberries once they've been dipped.

Break the chocolate into small pieces and place it in a glass basin in a saucepan of water. Heat the water, but there's no need to bring it to the boil. Once the chocolate **starts** melting, turn off the heat. The chocolate will go on melting; stir it a few times with a spatula until there are no lumps.

One at a time, hold each strawberry by the stalk and dip it into the chocolate, leaving the upper third uncovered. Tilt the basin to increase the depth of chocolate. Place the dipped strawberries on the prepared tray. When there is very little chocolate left, use the spatula to transfer the residue to the last strawberry.

Put the tray in the fridge and leave it for up to half an hour to make sure the chocolate is set, but keep the dipped berries at room temperature before serving.

Raspberry fool

This delightfully simple adaptation of the classic dessert fits perfectly into the MUNCH plan. Enjoyment of a fruit fool is normally tempered by the knowledge that you're overdosing on saturated fat and sugar. You can round off your meal with this one, or variations using other berries, knowing that it's doing you a power of good.

300 g (10½ oz) fresh raspberries
30 ml (2 tbsp) xylitol
400 g (14 oz) 0% fat Greek yoghurt

Rinse the raspberries gently in a sieve under cold, running water and allow them to drain. Transfer the berries to a bowl, sprinkle the xylitol over them, and crush them with a fork.

Mix the crushed raspberries and yoghurt together, ideally leaving a slightly marbled effect, rather than mixing thoroughly enough to produce a uniform pink (but don't worry about it because the little bits of raspberry add visual interest anyway). Spoon the mixture into four wine glasses or small dessert dishes. Chill in the fridge before serving (and don't forget to refrigerate the dessert as well). Garnish with a whole raspberry and a sprig of fresh mint.

Grilled pineapple with honey and cinnamon

Here's a quick dessert using tinned pineapple. Always buy it in its own juice, not in syrup. Use fresh pineapple when you have time.

425-g (15-oz) can pineapple slices, drained
5 ml (1 tsp) clear honey
2.5 ml (½ tsp) ground cinnamon
240 g (8½ oz) 0% fat Greek yoghurt
20 ml (4 tsp) xylitol
20 g (2 'squares') dark chocolate (85% cocoa solids)

Brush the pineapple slices with the honey, and sprinkle with cinnamon. Cook under a moderately hot grill for 6–8 minutes until the slices are browned, but not burnt.

Stir the xylitol into the yoghurt and mix thoroughly. Divide the grilled pineapple and sweetened yoghurt between four plates. Top the yoghurt with grated dark chocolate.

Chapter 30

Action checklist

Where do you start? You want to tackle all your important risk factors. You know it's not very effective to put all your energy into one risk factor and ignore the others.

That doesn't mean it's practical to tackle everything at once. Then again, if you start with one risk factor, you have to be careful not to forget about the others and lose your motivation as time goes by.

Use the checklist (Table 33) to see what changes you need to make. Every tick in the **NO** column shows you that action is needed. Don't be overwhelmed if you've ticked every box! The 28-day plan will soon get you into a new routine.

It's a good idea to tick the boxes with a pencil – then you can rub out your tick under **NO** and place one under **YES** when you've put something right. How satisfying it will be to see the **NO** column empty and the **YES** column fill up! Not only will this signify a huge reduction in risk, but also an improvement in your health: you will look, feel and function so much better.

The beauty of this system is that you don't lose track of what you've achieved and what remains to be tackled.

It's a good idea to enter an annual review date in your calendar or diary, to make sure you haven't slipped back. You could link this to getting your blood pressure checked every year.

It's only once a week, Doc

Of course, if your **NO** column is empty because you have high-fat dairy products, eat salted snacks, and polish off a pound of chocolate almost once a week, there's a lot of room for improvement!

Perhaps your tradition of a cooked breakfast on Sunday morning is important to you. Fair enough. At least use a good pan, requiring the minimum of rapeseed oil or olive oil; have mushrooms, tomatoes, baked beans and smoked turkey rashers or lean bacon – not sausage, streaky bacon, egg and greasy fried bread.

When it comes to such things as pork crackling, full-fat cheese, cream and confectionery, it's very much easier not to spend the week looking forward to the one day when these will be allowed. Otherwise, not only do you end up with a 'moderate diet' that has disappointing results, but you also enjoy your food less – always hankering after forbidden fruits. Simply fill your menu with an appetising abundance of helpful foods; you will then feel free to enjoy those other items on rare occasions that are genuine exceptions to your routine.

Priorities, practicalities and precautions

If you are a smoker, giving up should be your top priority. There's little point in fine tuning your dairy products while smoking 30 a day. Read Chapter 21 again and work out your timetable for Ready, Steady, Stop.

If you regularly eat lunch in a staff canteen, it's worth meeting the catering staff to make sure something suitable is always available. In restaurants, too, be specific: why shouldn't you have your fish cooked in olive oil instead of butter?

Don't forget that the positive goals (such as eating more pulses and fish) are just as important as the negative ones (such as eating less processed meat). In fact, they go hand in hand: processed meat will be replaced by pulses and fish.

If your only regular exercise at the moment is lifting a knife and fork, remember to increase very gradually, starting with gentle walking before you get too frisky. Read Chapter 20 again. Build up the intensity until half an hour's brisk walking a day is routine.

Unless you live in splendid isolation, this living and eating business is a family affair. It's hard to give up smoking in a household of smokers; it's hard to eat a good diet when the cupboards are crammed with high-fat processed foods. So clear your kitchen of everything that threatens your success and stock up using Chapters 28 and 29 as a guide. Getting the right balance of nutrients is the key, and this is made easy by the 28-day plan; it will soon come naturally. Once your metabolism is on the mend, you won't want to go back to your old ways.

Table 33 Action Checklist for you to fill in.

	Action Needed (NO)	OK (YES)
Am I a non-smoker?	☐	☐
Was my last blood pressure reading:		
Within the last year?	☐	☐
Normal?	☐	☐
Have I had my urine checked (for diabetes)?	☐	☐
Have I had a cholesterol check?	☐	☐
Was my total cholesterol below 5.0 mmol/l?		
(Or LDL-cholesterol below 3.0 mmol/l)	☐	☐
Was my HDL-cholesterol at least 1.0 mmol/l		
and my triglyceride level below 1.7 mmol/l?	☐	☐
Is my waist circumference normal?		
(Below 80 cm for a woman; below 94 cm for a man)	☐	☐
Do I have 20 minutes continuous exercise a day?		
(Or 30 minutes 5 days a week)	☐	☐
Have I got stress under control?	☐	☐
Have I discussed drug therapy (e.g. aspirin, statin)		
with my doctor in the last year?	☐	☐
Do I eat two servings of wholegrain foods (e.g. porridge,		
muesli, mixed-grain bread) each day?	☐	☐
Do I watch the quality and quantity of carbohydrate foods		
to keep the GL of one portion below 11?	☐	☐

Table 33 Action Checklist (*cont'd*).

	Action Needed (NO)	OK (YES)
Do I eat at least 5 portions of fruit and vegetables a day?	☐	☐
At main meals, do I cover half my plate with vegetables of three different colours?	☐	☐
Do I avoid fatty red meat or always trim off visible fat?	☐	☐
Do I avoid fatty minced meat or always drain off the fat?	☐	☐
Do I have sausages, meat pies, pâtés or other processed meat products less than once a week?	☐	☐
Do I avoid fatty poultry (e.g. goose, duck with skin)?	☐	☐
Do I always remove skin from chicken and turkey?	☐	☐
Do I eat fish at least twice a week?	☐	☐
Do I eat oily fish once a week (or take fish oils)?	☐	☐
Do I eat at least 5 servings of pulses (peas, beans, lentils, chickpeas, etc.) a week?	☐	☐
Do I eat other good sources of vegetable protein (e.g. tofu, Quorn, quinoa) most days?	☐	☐
Do I keep to a maximum of 1 egg yolk a day?	☐	☐
Do I avoid butter, and fat spreads that are not high in mono-unsaturates or fortified with stanol/sterol?	☐	☐
Do I avoid full-fat mayonnaise, salad dressing or sauces?	☐	☐
Do I avoid cooking oils/fats high in saturates?	☐	☐

Table 33 Action Checklist (*cont'd*).

	Action Needed (NO)	OK (YES)
Do I have up to 3 teaspoons (15 ml) a day of an oil high in mono-unsaturates (olive oil, rapeseed oil) in recipes and salad dressing?	☐	☐
Do I have a few nuts (e.g. almonds) most days?	☐	☐
When baking, do I avoid butter, lard, suet or unsuitable shortening?	☐	☐
Do I eat bought cakes and biscuits less than once a week? (The alternative is home-made, not stolen)	☐	☐
Do I eat fatty/sugary sweets (fudge, toffee, milk chocolate, etc.) less than once a week?	☐	☐
Do I eat high-fat puddings/ice-cream less than once a week?	☐	☐
Do I use skimmed milk or low-fat soya milk (calcium enriched) instead of whole milk?	☐	☐
Do I have higher-fat dairy products less than once a week? (e.g. full-fat yoghurts, cream)	☐	☐
Do I have cheese (other than cottage cheese, quark, etc.) less than once a week?	☐	☐
Have I stopped adding salt in the kitchen (other than a pinch of Solo or LoSalt occasionally) and at the table?	☐	☐
Do I check the sodium content of processed foods?	☐	☐
Do I have salted snacks (nuts, crisps, etc.) less than once a week?	☐	☐
Do I use low-salt stock and limit the use of salty seasonings like soy sauce?	☐	☐
Do I have fried food less than once a week?	☐	☐

Table 33 Action Checklist (*cont'd*).

	Action Needed (NO)	OK (YES)
Do I make sauces with skimmed milk or soya products and without a roux (butter and flour)?	☐	☐
Do I drain off meat/poultry fat before making gravy?	☐	☐
Do I eat in a canteen/restaurant (without knowing about fat and salt used) less than once a week?	☐	☐
Do I eat takeaway food (other than chicken kebab) less than twice a month?	☐	☐
Do I avoid having cafetière coffee every day?	☐	☐
Do I drink 6 glasses or more of water a day? (or other low-fat, low-sugar drink)	☐	☐
Do I drink less than 3 units of alcohol a day?	☐	☐
Have I considered taking psyllium husks and/or oat bran to boost my intake of soluble fibre ?	☐	☐

Glossary

ACE inhibitors A class of drugs (which act on the renin–angiotensin system) used to treat high blood pressure and heart failure.

adipokines Protein messengers released by abdominal fat, many of which produce damaging changes in body chemistry.

adiponectin A beneficial protein messenger released by fat cells but produced in smaller quantities when there is excess abdominal fat.

aerobic exercise Repetitive movement of large muscles (e.g. running) resulting in an increased supply of oxygen to the muscles.

alpha-blockers A class of drugs that lower blood pressure by relaxing muscle in artery walls. They can be used to relieve prostate symptoms by relaxing muscle round the bladder outlet.

alpha-linolenic acid An essential polyunsaturated fatty acid in the omega-3 family that can be converted by the body to other omega-3 fatty acids (such as EPA and DHA which are found in fish). Walnuts are a rich source.

anaerobic exercise Muscles straining against resistance for short periods (e.g. tug of war), without an increased supply of oxygen.

aneurysm An abnormally wide section of an artery, resulting from a weakness in the artery wall.

angina (or angina pectoris) A 'tight' or 'heavy' pain and/or breathlessness caused by an inadequate supply of oxygen to the heart muscle – often triggered by exercise, stress or cold weather. Pain is typically felt across the chest, but may occur in the jaw, shoulder or arm. Unlike a heart attack, it doesn't damage the heart muscle and pain settles quickly.

angiogram An X-ray examination of blood vessels, after injecting a substance opaque to X-rays. Coronary angiography examines the coronary arteries supplying the heart.

angiotensin receptor blockers A class of drugs used to treat high blood pressure and heart failure, especially when ACE inhibitors are not tolerated.

antioxidant A chemical that neutralises the damaging effects of free radicals. Notable examples are vitamins C, E, and beta-carotene.

aorta The main artery that carries oxygen-rich blood from the heart to all the other arteries.

arrhythmia Any abnormal rhythm of the heartbeat.

arteriole A small artery that leads to capillary blood vessels.

artery A blood vessel that carries blood *away* from the heart.

atheroma Fatty deposits that build up on the lining of arteries.

atherosclerosis The process in which fatty and fibrous deposits cause narrowing and hardening of arteries.

atorvastatin A statin drug launched after simvastatin and pravastatin which, unlike previous statins, works just as well if taken in the morning rather than the evening.

beta-blockers A class of drugs that slow the heart and lower blood pressure.

biofeedback A technique in which a signal feeds back information to a person about some unconscious body function (such as blood pressure). With training, it is possible to exert control over the function (e.g. to lower the blood pressure).

blood pressure The pressure of the blood in the arteries expressed as the maximum (systolic) over the minimum (diastolic) pressure in millimetres of mercury (mmHg).

body mass index (BMI) Your body weight in kilograms divided by the square of your height in metres. A BMI between 20 and 25 is considered normal.

brachial artery The major artery in the arm, used for measuring blood pressure.

C-reactive protein A protein in the blood which is found in higher concentrations during inflammation. Raised levels are linked with an increased risk of coronary heart disease.

calcium channel blockers A class of drugs used to treat angina and high blood pressure. These drugs relax artery walls by blocking the passage of calcium through cell membranes.

capillaries The smallest blood vessels, which allow oxygen to pass from the blood to body cells (and waste products from cells to the blood).

cardiac arrest A complete halt in the pumping action of the heart.

cardiomyopathy A disease of the heart muscle that reduces the heart's pumping efficiency. There are various causes but often the cause is unknown.

cardiovascular disease A disease of the heart or circulation (such as coronary heart disease or stroke).

carotid arteries The major arteries in the neck.

central obesity The condition of having excess abdominal fat – a feature of the metabolic syndrome.

CHD Coronary heart disease.

cholesterol A lipid – or fatty substance – found in the blood and cells of animals but not found in plants.

cilia (pronounced 'sillier') Microscopic, hair-like structures. Movement of cilia in the lungs results in a cleansing flow of mucus that is brought to a standstill by smoking.

claudication Pain in the leg(s) on walking as a result of inadequate blood flow to the exercising muscles; it is relieved by rest.

climacteric The 'change of life', also known as the perimenopause; the time around the menopause during which a woman has symptoms due to falling oestrogen levels.

clinical trial A scientific experiment to test the value of a medical treatment. The best clinical trials are controlled, randomised, and double-blind. For example, if an active drug is being compared with a placebo (control), whether a patient receives the drug or the placebo is decided at random (like tossing a coin) and both patient and doctor are 'blind' to the truth until the end of the trial. In a single-blind trial, the doctor knows which patients are having active treatment; results may be affected by bias.

coronary arteries The arteries supplying blood to the heart.

coronary heart disease Heart disease resulting from atheroma of the coronary arteries; it may cause angina, a heart attack, or sudden death.

coronary thrombosis Formation of a blood clot in a coronary artery – a heart attack.

CRP C-reactive protein.

DHA Docosahexaenoic acid.

diabetes (diabetes mellitus) The medical condition in which blood glucose levels rise as a result of inadequate production of (or response to) insulin.

diastole The period in which the heart muscle relaxes between beats.

diastolic blood pressure The pressure of blood in the arteries during diastole. It is the minimum pressure and is written underneath the systolic when blood pressure is recorded.

diuretic A drug that stimulates production of urine.

docosahexaenoic acid An omega-3 polyunsaturated fatty acid notably found in fish oil.

dyslipidaemia An unfavourable balance of blood lipids including low HDL-cholesterol and raised triglycerides.

eicosapentaenoic acid An omega-3 polyunsaturated fatty acid notably found in fish oil.

embolus (plural: emboli) An abnormal particle, usually a blood clot, that is carried along in the circulation. A fragment of blood clot may move downstream until it lodges in a narrower part of the blood vessel, causing an obstruction (embolism).

endometrium The layer of tissue lining the uterus (womb).

endothelium The thin layer of cells forming a smooth lining to arteries and all other blood vessels.

EPA Eicosapentaenoic acid.

essential hypertension High blood pressure for which no specific cause is found.

extrinsic sugar Sugar that has been extracted from the plant cells in which it occurs naturally.

ezetimibe A selective cholesterol absorption inhibitor which lowers blood cholesterol levels by blocking the uptake of cholesterol in the small intestine – most of which is cholesterol made by the liver. It is commonly combined with a statin, but is useful by itself when statins are not tolerated.

familial hypercholesterolaemia An inherited condition causing very high blood cholesterol levels; it affects about 1 in 500 people. Fatty lumps (xanthomas) may develop under the skin, especially round tendons. Drug treatment (in addition to lifestyle management) is essential to prevent early death from heart disease.

familial hyperlipidaemia Any of several inherited disorders causing high levels of blood lipids (e.g. cholesterol and/or triglycerides).

fatty acids The chemical units that make up a fat, usually in combination with glycerol to form triglycerides.

fatty streaks Fatty deposits on the lining of artery walls that can lead on to atheroma.

fibrinogen A protein (in the blood) involved in the formation of blood clots; high levels of fibrinogen increase the risk of a heart attack.

flavonoids A group of over 3000 antioxidant compounds occurring in apples, onions, coloured fruits and vegetables, red wine, and tea.

foam cell A scavenging white blood cell that has become laden with cholesterol and may contribute to the development of fatty streaks.

folic acid A B vitamin that helps to lower blood homocysteine levels.

Rich sources are: green, leafy vegetables; Brussels sprouts; blackeye beans.

free radical An unstable chemical that causes damage (e.g. to lipids, proteins, DNA) by oxidation.

fructose A simple (monosaccharide) sugar known as 'fruit sugar' which occurs naturally in fruit and is sometimes used as a low-GI alternative to sucrose (table sugar).

gamma-linolenic acid A polyunsaturated fatty acid in the omega-6 family, abundant in evening primrose oil.

GI Glycaemic Index.

GL Glycaemic Load.

glycaemic index A number indicating how fast the carbohydrate in a food is converted to blood glucose.

glycaemic load A measure of the effect on blood glucose levels of one portion of food, derived by multiplying the GI of the food by the available carbohydrate in the portion (in grams) and dividing by 100.

gram flour A flour made from ground chickpeas with a lower GI than wheat flour or cornflour.

HDL-cholesterol High-density lipoprotein cholesterol. Cholesterol in this form is being transported away from artery walls. It is often called 'the good cholesterol' because higher levels of HDL-cholesterol are linked with lower risk of heart disease.

heart attack Blockage of a coronary artery resulting in death of an area of heart muscle.

heart block A fault in the heart's natural pacemaker causing the heart to beat abnormally slowly (e.g. 30 beats per minute).

homocysteine A breakdown product of the amino acid methionine. There is a link between high blood levels of homocysteine and coronary heart disease. Homocysteine may play a part in atherosclerosis and thrombosis.

hormone replacement therapy Replacement of the female hormone oestrogen (with or without progestogen) after output from the ovaries has declined or stopped.

HRT Hormone replacement therapy.

hypercholesterolaemia High level of cholesterol in the blood.

hyperlipidaemia Raised levels of blood lipids (e.g. cholesterol, triglycerides).

IHD Ischaemic heart disease.

infarction The death of body tissue (e.g. brain, heart muscle) that occurs when the blood supply is cut off (e.g. by a clot or embolus).

insulin resistance Insensitivity of body tissues to insulin which causes the pancreas to release higher levels of insulin and may lead on to Type 2 diabetes.

intrinsic sugar Sugar that is still in the plant cell where nature put it (e.g. the sugar in an apple).

ischaemia Inadequate blood flow to an area of the body.

ischaemic heart disease Another term for coronary heart disease.

larynx The 'voice box' in the neck. You can feel the carotid pulse to one side of the larynx.

LDL-cholesterol Low-density lipoprotein cholesterol. Cholesterol in this form is sometimes called 'bad cholesterol' because it can be deposited in plaques, and higher levels are linked with higher death rates from coronary heart disease.

linoleic acid An omega-6 polyunsaturated fatty acid abundant in oils such as safflower oil, corn oil, and sunflower oil.

lipids Fatty substances such as cholesterol and triglycerides. Lipids do not dissolve in water but are soluble in organic solvents.

lipoprotein lipase An enzyme that releases triglycerides from the lipoproteins which transport them; it also raises HDL levels. The rise in HDL-cholesterol that occurs with regular exercise may be the result of increased lipoprotein lipase activity in trained muscles.

lipoproteins Lipid particles linked with protein. This is the form in which cholesterol is transported in the bloodstream.

maximum heart rate The number of heartbeats per minute given by subtracting your age in years from 220. At age 50, the maximum heart rate would be 170 beats per minute; the *target* range for exercise could be 65–75% of the maximum (110–127 at age 50).

menopause A woman's last menstrual period.

metabolic syndrome The association of excess abdominal fat with insulin resistance, raised blood pressure and dyslipidaemia which increases the risk of diabetes and heart disease.

metabolism All the complex chemical processes within the human body (or other organisms) necessary to maintain life – including the chemical reactions that convert food into energy for movement.

MI Myocardial infarction.

mmol/l A measure of concentration – the number of millimoles (mmols) of a substance in one litre (1l) of a fluid. A millimole is the molecular weight (or atomic weight) in milligrams (mg). In the

UK, cholesterol levels are expressed as millimoles of cholesterol in one litre of serum. In the USA, they measure mg/dl – milligrams per decilitre (one-tenth of a litre). To convert a cholesterol measurement in mmol/l to mg/dl you multiply by 39. A cholesterol level of 5.2 mmol/l is just over 200 mg/dl.

mono-unsaturated fatty acids (mono-unsaturates) Fatty acids in which only one area of the molecule is not saturated with hydrogen. Replacing saturates with mono-unsaturates helps to lower LDL-cholesterol without reducing HDL-cholesterol.

myocardial infarction A heart attack.

myocardium The heart muscle.

oesophagus (or gullet) The muscular tube that carries food and drink from the throat to the stomach.

oestrogen The major female hormone (or, strictly, group of hormones) produced by the ovaries before the menopause. Natural oestrogens (e.g. oestradiol) are used for HRT but synthetic versions are available (such as ethinyl oestradiol which is used in the contraceptive pill).

omega-3 fatty acids Polyunsaturated fatty acids such as EPA and DHA that are particularly abundant in fish oils.

omega-6 fatty acids Polyunsaturated fatty acids such as linoleic acid found, for example, in vegetable oils and nuts.

ORAC Oxygen radical absorbance capacity.

oxygen radical absorbance capacity A laboratory measurement of the antioxidant power of a food.

pacemaker The group of cells in the heart (or an electronic device) that starts off the electrical wave which causes a heartbeat. The heart's natural pacemaker (sinoatrial node) normally regulates the heart rate. When this system fails, an artificial, electronic pacemaker is sometimes used.

placebo A 'dummy' drug containing no active ingredients but designed to pass off as the real thing. Administering a placebo normally has some benefit. For example, giving a placebo painkiller to someone in pain usually produces some relief (the 'placebo effect'). Placebos used in clinical trials should look, smell and taste like the real drug so no one can tell who's having the active treatment until the code is broken at the end of the trial.

plaque A deposit (consisting of fatty substances such as cholesterol, hardened with fibrous matter and calcium) in an artery affected by atherosclerosis.

platelets (thrombocytes) The smallest of the blood cells. Platelets plug damaged areas in blood vessels and are a vital part of the blood-clotting system.

polyunsaturated fatty acids (polyunsaturates) Fatty acids in which more than one area of the molecule is not saturated with hydrogen. Replacing saturates with polyunsaturates lowers LDL-cholesterol, but HDL-cholesterol falls as well.

pravastatin One of the statin drugs. Pravastatin was used to lower cholesterol in the WOSCOPS and CARE studies.

primary prevention Measures taken to prevent someone developing a disease (e.g. changing your lifestyle to reduce your coronary risk, before there are any signs of heart disease).

progesterone The female hormone produced by the ovaries in the second half of the menstrual cycle (after ovulation). Synthetic versions (progestogens) are used with oestrogen when HRT is prescribed for women who still have a uterus.

radial pulse The pulse in the radial artery, which can be felt on the thumb side of the wrist.

renin An enzyme in the kidney that sets off a chain reaction to produce angiotensin II and raise blood pressure.

rosuvastatin A potent statin drug, launched in the UK in 2003.

satiety The feeling that you have eaten enough.

saturated fatty acids (saturates) Fatty acids in which the molecule has no room for any more hydrogen atoms. A diet high in saturated fatty acids raises blood cholesterol levels and increases the risk of thrombosis.

sclerosis Hardening of some part of the body (as in atherosclerosis).

secondary hypercholesterolaemia High blood cholesterol levels caused by an underlying medical condition (such as thyroid or liver disease).

secondary prevention Measures taken to limit the effects or progress of a disease once it has occurred (e.g. giving a statin drug to someone with heart disease).

serum the clear yellowish fluid that is left after extracting all the solid components (e.g. red and white cells) from blood.

simvastatin A statin drug used to lower blood cholesterol levels. Simvastatin was used in the 4S study.

sphygmomanometer An instrument used to measure blood pressure.

stanols Substances derived from sterols which, like plant sterols, can be added to fatty foods to reduce absorption of cholesterol from the intestine.

statins A class of drugs used to lower blood cholesterol levels. The formal name for statins (HMG CoA reductase inhibitors) describes the way they work, which is to block the activity of an enzyme involved in cholesterol production.

sterols A group of naturally occurring compounds which includes cholesterol – a sterol found only in animals. Plant sterols can be added to a fat spread to lower blood cholesterol by reducing cholesterol absorption in the intestine.

stroke Damage to part of the brain resulting from a breakdown in the blood supply (which can be caused by a thrombus, an embolus or a bleed). The consequences reflect the area of brain damaged and may include defects of speech, vision, sensation and movement.

systole The period in which a heart chamber is contracting. With every heartbeat, the upper chambers (atria) contract first, squeezing blood into the ventricles below them. This 'atrial systole' is followed immediately by contraction of the main pumping chambers (ventricular systole).

systolic blood pressure The maximum pressure in the arteries as blood is forced out of the heart in ventricular systole. The systolic pressure is written above the diastolic.

target range The heart-rate range (such as 65–75% of your maximum rate) that you aim to stay within during a session of aerobic exercise.

thermic effect of food The energy (calories) the body uses to process the food. Protein has a higher thermic effect – i.e., the body uses more calories to process it – than fat, which is more easily utilised and stored.

thrombosis The formation of a blood clot within the circulation. Thrombosis in an artery can result in a heart attack or stroke; deep vein thrombosis can send an embolus to the lungs (pulmonary embolism).

thrombus A blood clot that develops *within* the circulation (unlike the blood clot that develops *outside* the circulation when you graze your knee).

trans fatty acids Unsaturated fatty acids in which the molecule is 'twisted' into a different shape from the normal (cis) form. (In the cis isomer, the two hydrogen atoms on each side of the double bond are on the same side of the molecule; in the trans isomer they are on opposite sides, as shown on page 40.) Trans fatty acids have the same unwanted effects as saturated fatty acids. Hard margarines and hydrogenated vegetable oils are likely to contain high levels of trans fatty acids.

triglycerides Fats in which three fatty acids are bonded to a glycerol molecule. The fat in our food and the fat we store in our bodies is generally in this form. The blood triglyceride concentration is measured in a fasting lipid test but is less clearly linked with heart disease than cholesterol levels are. Very high blood triglyceride levels raise the risk of pancreatitis.

visceral fat Fat within abdominal organs (e.g. the liver) where it is particularly linked with the metabolic syndrome and increased risk.

xanthan gum A vegetable (polysaccharide) gum used as a thickening agent in food.

xanthelasmas (or xanthelasmata) Yellowish, fatty deposits in the eyelids that are *sometimes* linked with high levels of blood cholesterol.

xanthomas (or xanthomata) Fatty lumps under the skin, often associated with various types of hyperlipidaemia. In familial hypercholesterolaemia, xanthomas are typically on tendons (e.g. the Achilles tendon in the heel).

xylitol A natural sugar alcohol with a similar taste to sucrose; its lower GI and calorie content, and its positive effect on teeth, make it an attractive alternative to table sugar.

Appendix 1

Useful organisations

If you write for information from any of these organisations, it is helpful to enclose a large, self-addressed envelope.

Al-Anon Family Groups
61 Great Dover Street
London SE1 4YF
Tel: 020 7403 0888
Fax: 020 7378 9910
Website: www.al-anonuk.org.uk
World-wide organisation offering support to families and friends of problem drinkers; has nearly 1000 local groups. Alateen, part of Al-Anon, is dedicated to helping teenagers with an alcoholic relative.

Alcohol Concern
64 Lemon Street
London E1 8EU
Tel: 0207264 0510
Fax: 020 7488 9213
Website: www.alcoholconcern.org.uk
National charity working against alcohol misuse. Members receive regular magazine and have access to extensive information and training services.

Alcoholics Anonymous (Scotland) (AA)
Baltic Chambers
50 Wellington Street
Glasgow G2 6HJ
Helpline: 0845 769 7555
Tel: 0141 226 2214
Website: www.alcoholics-anonymous.org.uk
Northern office of worldwide charity which offers information and support, via local groups, to people with an alcohol problem who want to stop drinking.

Alcoholics Anonymous (AA)
PO Box 1
Stonebow House
Stonebow
York YO1 7NJ
Helpline: 0845 769 7555
Tel: 01904 644 026
Fax: 01904 629 091
Website: www.alcoholics-anonymous.org.uk
Headquarters of worldwide organisation which offers information and support, via local groups, to people with alcohol problems who want to stop drinking.

**ASH
(Action on Smoking and Health)**
144–5 Shoreditch High Street
London E1 6JE
Helpline: 0800 169 0169
Tel: 020 7739 5902
Fax: 020 7613 0531
Website: www.ash.org.uk
*National organisation with local
branches. Campaigns on antismoking
policies. Offers free information on
website or for sale from HQ.
Catalogue on request.*

ASH in Wales
ASH Wales Ltd
2nd Floor
8 Museum Place
Cardiff CF10 3BG
Fax: 02920 641 045
Website: www.ashwales.co.uk
*National organisation with local
branches. Campaigns for antismoking
policies. Has free leaflets plus range of
publications and videos for sale.*

ASH Northern Ireland
Ulster Cancer Foundation
40–44 Eglantine Avenue
Belfast BT9 6DX
Tel: 02890 663 281
Fax: 02890 668 715
Website: www.ulstercancer.org
*National organisation with local
groups. Campaigns for antismoking
policies. Range of publications and
videos for sale.*

ASH Scotland
8 Frederick Street
Edinburgh EH2 2HB
Helpline: 0800 169 0169
Tel: 0131 225 4725
Fax: 0131 225 4759
Website: www.ashscotland.org.uk
*National organisation with local
branches. Campaigns for antismoking
policies. Free information on website
and for sale from HQ. Catalogue on
request.*

**British Association
for Cardiac Rehabilitation (BACR)**
c/o British Cardiac Society
9 Fitzroy Square
London W1T 5HW
Tel: 020 7383 3887
Fax: 020 7383 7388
Website: www.bcs.com/bacr
*Holds national register of cardiac
rehabilitation programmes. Health
professionals and non-professionals
with bona fide interest in rehab of
cardiac patients can become members
of the BACR.*

**British Cardiac Patients Association
(BCPA)**
6 Rampton End
Willingham
Cambridge CB24 5JB
Helpline: 01223 846845
Tel: 01954 260731
Website: www.bcpa.co.uk
*Supports heart patients and their
carers. Publishes regular magazine.*

British Heart Foundation (BHF)
14 Fitzhardinge Street
London W1H 6DH
Helpline: 08450 708070
Tel: 020 7935 0185
Fax: 020 7486 5820
Website: www.bhf.org.uk
Funds research, promotes education
and raises money to buy equipment to
treat heart disease. List of
publications, posters and videos; send
stamped addressed envelope. Their
helpline, HeartstartUK, can arrange
training in emergency life-saving
techniques for lay people.

British Hypertension Society
Website: www.bhsoc.org

British Nutrition Foundation
High Holborn House
52–54 High Holborn
London WC1V 6RQ
Tel: 020 7404 6504
Fax: 020 7404 6747
Website: www.nutrition.org.uk
Professional association. Authoritative
publications and information sheets
available on request: stamped
addressed envelope requested as no
telephone advice is available.

Cardiomyopathy Association
40 The Metro Centre
Tolpits Lane
Watford
Herts WD18 9SB
Helpline: 0800 0181 024
Tel: 01923 249977
Fax: 01923 249987
Website: www.cardiomyopathy.org
Offers information for health
professionals; also support and
information for people with
cardiomyopathy and their families.

**Chest, Heart and Stroke Association
(N. Ireland)**
21a Dublin Road
Belfast BT2 7HB
Helpline: 08457 697 299
Tel: 02890 320 184
Fax: 02890 333 487
Website: www.nichsa.com
Funds research and provides
information on chest, heart and
stroke-related illnesses.

Chest, Heart and Stroke Scotland
65 North Castle Street
Edinburgh EH2 3LT
Tel: 0131 225 6963
Fax: 0131 220 6313
Website: www.chss.org.uk
Funds research and provides
information on chest, heart and
stroke-related illnesses.

Citizens Advice
(National Association – NACAB)
Myddleton House
115–123 Pentonville Road
London N1 9LZ
Tel: 020 7833 2181
Fax: 020 7833 4371
Website: www.citizensadvice.org.uk
HQ of national charity offering a
wide variety of practical, financial
and legal advice. Network of local
branches throughout the UK listed in
phone books and in Yellow Pages
under Counselling and Advice.

Consumers' Association
2 Marylebone Road
London NW1 4DF
Helpline: 0845 307 4000
Tel: 020 7770 7000
Fax: 020 7770 7600
Website: www.which.co.uk
Campaigns on behalf of consumers
and produces reports on products
including foods.

Department of Health
(DoH)
PO Box 777
London SE1 6XH
Helpline: 08701 555 455
Tel: 020 7210 4850
Fax: 01623 724 524
Textphone: 020 7210 5025
Website: www.dh.gov.uk
Produces literature about health
issues, available via helpline.
A more technical site with National
Service Frameworks available from
internet e.g. www.doh.gov.uk/nsf

Diabetes UK
10 Parkway
London NW1 7AA
Helpline: 0845 120 2960
Tel: 020 7424 1000
Fax: 020 7424 1001
Textline 020 7424 1031
Website: www.diabetes.org.uk
Provides advice and information on
diabetes; has local support groups.

Diabetes UK
Distribution Centre
PO Box 3030
Swindon SN3 4WN
Helpline: 0800 585 088
Part of Diabetes UK, separate from
London HQ for ordering publications.

Drinkline
(National Alcohol Helpline)
Essentia Group
Lower Ground
Sky Park
72 Finneston Square
Glasgow G3 8ET
Helpline: 0800 917 8282
Fax: 0141 568 4001
Funded by Department of Health,
provides educational material for
schools, health professionals and
general information on drink, sex
and drugs issues. Refers to local
agencies for support.

Emmi UK Limited
MBC
Ashfield Avenue
Mansfield
Nottinghamshire, NG18 2AE
Helpline: 01244 893155
Email: info.minicol@uk.emmi.ch
Website: www.emmi-minicol.ch
Manufacturers of miniCol cheese.

Health Development Agency
Holborn Gate
330 High Holborn
London WC1V 7BA
Helpline: 0870 121 4194
Tel: 020 7430 0850
Fax: 020 7061 3390
Website: www.hda-online.org.uk
*Formerly Health Education
Authority; now only deals with
research. Publications on health
matters can be ordered via helpline.*

Heart UK
7 North Road
Maidenhead SL6 1PE
Helpline: 0845 450 5988
Fax: 01628 628 698
Website: www.heartuk.org.uk
*Will help anyone at high risk of heart
attack, but specialises in inherited
conditions causing high cholesterol
(i.e. familial hypercholesterolaemia).
(Was Family Heart Association.)*

Irish Heart Foundation
4 Clyde Road
Ballsbridge
Dublin 4
Tel: 00353 1 668 5001
Fax: 00353 1 668 5896
Website: www.irishheart.ie
*Offers information, publications,
training and support in prevention of
heart disease. Collaborates with other
heart-related organisations and has
some local support groups.*

**MIND (National Association
for Mental Health)**
Granta House
15–19 Broadway
London E15 4BQ
Helpline: 0845 766 0163
Tel: 020 8519 2122
Fax: 020 8522 1725
Website: www.mind.org.uk
*Mental health organisation working
for a better life for everyone
experiencing mental distress.
Offers support via local branches.
Publications available on
020 8221 9666.*

NHS Direct
Helpline: 0845 4647
Tel: 020 8867 1367
Website: www.nhsdirect.nhs.uk
*NHS Direct is a 24-hour helpline
offering confidential healthcare
advice, information and referral
service 365 days of the year. A good
first port of call for any health advice.
Textphone for people with a hearing
impairment 0845 606 4647.*

Quit
211 Old Street
London EC1V 9NR
Helpline: 0800 002200
Tel: 020 7251 1551
Fax: 020 7251 1661
Website: www.quit.org.uk
*Offers advice to stop smoking in
English and Asian languages; also
to schools, and on pregnancy.
Runs training courses for health
professionals. Can put people in
touch with local support groups.*

Relate
Premier House
Carolina Court
Lakeside
Doncaster DN4 5RA
Tel: 01302 347 747
Fax: 01302 366 287
Website: www.relate.org.uk
Offers relationship counselling via local branches. Relate publications on health, sexual, self-esteem, depression, bereavement and remarriage issues available from bookshops, libraries or via website.

Sport England
3rd Floor
Victoria House
Bloomsbury Square
London WC1B 4SE
Tel: 0845 8508 508
Fax: 020 7383 5740
Website: www.sportengland.org
Government agency promoting sport in England with a wide variety of activity programmes.

Sport Scotland
Caledonia House
1 Redheughs Rigg
South Gyle
Edinburgh EH12 9DQ
Tel: 0131 317 7200
Fax: 0131 317 7202
Website: www.sportscotland.org.uk
Government agency in Scotland promoting sport with a wide range of activity programmes.

Sports Council for Northern Ireland
House of Sport
Upper Malone Road
Belfast BT9 5LA
Tel: 02890 381 222
Fax: 02890 682 757
Website: www.sportni.net
Government agency promoting sport in Northern Ireland with a wide variety of activity programmes.

Sports Council for Wales
Sophia Gardens
Cardiff CF11 9SW
Tel: 0845 045 0904
Fax: 0845 846 0014
Website: www.sports-council-wales.org.uk
Headquarters for national network of local clubs who arrange integrated projects to bring disabled and able-bodied people together. Promotes sport in Wales and distributes lottery funding. Supports Paralympic athletes.

Stroke Association
Stroke House
240 City Road
London EC1V 2PR
Helpline: 0845 303 3100
Tel: 020 7566 0300
Fax: 020 7490 2686
Website: www.stroke.org.uk
Funds research and provides information now specialising in stroke only. Publications can be ordered from 01933 400 604.

**Vegetarian Society
of the United Kingdom**
Parkdale
Dunham Road
Altrincham
Cheshire WA14 4QG
Tel: 0161 925 2000
Fax: 0161 926 9182
Website: www.vegsoc.org
*Offers information on the vegetarian
way of life, day and residential
training courses at own Centre.
Provides literature for GCSE projects,
advice to school caterers. Food
manufacturers and restaurants can
apply for vegetarian accreditation.*

Women's Health Concern (WHC)
Whitehall House
41 Whitehall
London SW1A 2BY
Tel: 020 7451 1376
Fax: 020 7925 1505
Helpline: 0845 123 2319
Website: www.womens-health-concern.org
*National charity that offers help to
women, particularly on questions
of hormone health, HRT and
gynaecology.*

Yorktest Laboratories Ltd
York Science Park
York YO10 5DQ
Tel: 0800 458 2052
Website: www.yorktest.com
*Yorktest supply testing kits, such as
the 113 food SCAN food intolerance
test, by mail order.*

Appendix 2

Useful publications

Cooking and Eating

Cooking for a Healthy Heart, by Jacqui Lynas, published by Hamlyn (2002) ISBN 0 600 60570 1

The Everyday Diabetic Cookbook, by Stella Bowling, published by Grub Street/British Diabetic Association (1995) ISBN 1 898697 25 6

The Everyday Light-Hearted Cookbook, by Anne Lindsay, published by Grub Street/British Heart Foundation (1994) ISBN 0 948817 78 X

The Light-Hearted Cookbook: Recipes for a Healthy Heart, by Anne Lindsay, published by Grub Street/British Heart Foundation (1999) ISBN 1 902304 15 2

Low Fat, Low Cholesterol: recipes for a healthy heart, by Christine France, published by Southwater (2000) ISBN 1 84215 093 6

Quick Children's Meals, by Annabel Karmel, published by Ebury Press (1997) ISBN 0 09 185189 0

Sue Kreitzman's Complete Low-Fat Cookbook, by Sue Kreitzman, published by Piatkus (1996) ISBN 0 7499 1661 3

The Ultimate Low Fat Low Cholesterol Cookbook, by Christine France, published by Lorenzo Books (1996) ISBN 1 859672 37 X

Stopping Smoking

Allen Carr's Easy Way to Stop Smoking, by Allen Carr, published by Penguin (1999) ISBN 0 14 027763 3

How to Stop Smoking and Stay Stopped for Good, by Gillian Riley, published by Vermilion (2003) ISBN 0 09 188776 3

Stop Smoking for Good, by Robert Brynin, published by Hodder & Stoughton (1995) ISBN 0 340 63240 2

General Health

Type 2 Diabetes: Answers at your fingertips by Dr Charles Fox and
Dr Anne Kilvert, published by Class Publishing (2007)
ISBN 978 1 85959 176 5

The New Glucose Revolution, by Dr Anthony Leeds, Assoc. Prof.
Jennie Brand Miller, Kaye Foster-Powell and Dr Stephen Colagiuri,
published by Avalon Publishing Group (2003) ISBN 1 56924 506 1

Heart Health – the 'at your fingertips' guide, (Third edition)
by Dr Graham Jackson, published by Class Publishing (2004)
ISBN 1 85959 097 X

High Blood Pressure – the 'at your fingertips' guide (Third edition),
by Dr Tom Fahey, Professor Deidre Murphy with Dr Julian Tudor
Hart, published by Class Publishing (2004) ISBN 1 85959 090 X

Stress

Understanding Stress, by Professor Greg Wilkinson, published by
Family Doctor Publications (2000) ISBN 1 898205 91 4.

The Family Doctor Series covers around 27 titles including
cholesterol, stress and high blood pressure. Published by FDP,
10 Butchers Row, Banbury, Oxon OX16 8JH (Tel: 01295 276627).
Many of the organisations listed in the previous section publish
advisory leaflets, which are available on application.

Index

Numbers in *italics* refer to Figures and Tables. The letter *g* after the number indicates a glossary entry.

The *Class Health* Feedback Form

We hope that you found this *Class Health* book helpful. We always appreciate readers' opinions and would be grateful if you could take a few minutes to complete this form for us.

❶ How did you acquire your copy of this book?

From my local library ☐

Read an article in a newspaper/magazine ☐

Found it by chance ☐

Recommended by a friend ☐

Recommended by a patient organisation/charity ☐

Recommended by a doctor/nurse/advisor ☐

Saw an advertisement ☐

❷ How much of the book have you read?

All of it ☐

More than half of it ☐

Less than half of it ☐

❸ Which chapters have been most helpful?

....

....

❹ Overall, how useful to you was this *Class Health* book?

Extremely useful ☐

Very useful ☐

Useful ☐

❺ What did you find most helpful?

....

....

❻ What did you find least helpful?

....

....

7 Have you read any other health books?

Yes ☐   No ☐

If yes, which subjects did they cover?

....

....

....

How did this *Class Health* book compare?

Much better   ☐

Better   ☐

About the same   ☐

Not as good   ☐

8 Would you recommend this book to a friend?

Yes ☐   No ☐

Thank you for your help. Please send your completed form to:

Class Publishing, FREEPOST, London W6 7BR

Surname _____ First name _____

Title Prof/Dr/Mr/Mrs/Ms _____

Address _____

_____

Town _____ Postcode _____ Country _____

☐ Please add my name and address to receive details of related books
[*Please note, we will not pass on your details to any other company*]

Have you found **Dump Your Toxic Waist!** useful and practical?
If so, you may be interested in other books from Class Publishing.

Heart Health:
Answers at your fingertips £17.99
Dr Graham Jackson

This practical handbook, written by a leading cardiologist, answers all your questions about heart conditions. It tells you all about you and your heart; how to keep your heart healthy, or if it has been affected by heart disease – how to make it as strong as possible.

> *'Those readers who want to know more about the various treatments for heart disease will be much enlightened.'*
> **Dr James Le Fanu**
> *The Daily Telegraph*

Type 2 Diabetes:
Answers at your fingertips £14.99
Dr Charles Fox and Dr Anne Kilvert

The latest edition of our bestselling reference guide on diabetes has now been split into two books covering the two distinct forms of the disease. These books maintain the popular question and answer format to provide practical advice for patients on every aspect of living with the condition.

> *'I have no hesitation in commending this book.'*
> **Sir Steve Redgrave**
> Vice President, Diabetes UK

Type 2 Diabetes in Adults
of All Ages £19.99
Dr Charles Fox and Dr Ragnar Hanas

This practical, easy-to-read book tells you everything you need to know to become an expert on your own diabetes. Bestselling authors Charles Fox and Ragnar Hanas have produced a comprehensive, no-nonsense manual that shows you how to regain control of your life. Whether you have been living for years with Type 2 diabetes, or have only just been diagnosed, you will find much here that is positive and helpful.

High Blood Pressure:
Answers at your fingertips £14.99
Dr Tom Fahey, Professor Deirdre Murphy with Dr Julian Tudor Hart

The authors use all their years of experience as blood pressure experts to answer your questions on high blood pressure, in order to give you the information you need to bring your blood pressure down – and keep it down.

> *'Readable and comprehensive information'*
> **Dr Sylvia McLaughlan**
> Director General, The Stroke Association

Stroke:
Answers at your fingertips £17.99
Dr Anthony Rudd, Penny Irwin and Bridget Penhale

This essential guidebook tells you all about strokes – most importantly how to recover from them.

As well as providing clear explanations of the medical processes, tests, and treatments, the book is full of practical advice, including recuperation plans. You will find it inspiring.

Beating Depression £17.99
Dr Stefan Cembrowicz and Dr Dorcas Kingham

Depression is one of most common illnesses in the world – affecting up to one in four people at some time in their lives. *Beating Depression* shows sufferers and their families that they are not alone, and offers tried and tested techniques for overcoming depression.

> *'All you need to know about depression, presented in a clear, concise and readable way.'*
> **Ann Dawson**
> World Health Organization

PRIORITY ORDER FORM

Cut out or photocopy this form and send it (post free in the UK) to:

Class Publishing   **Tel: 01256 302 699**
FREEPOST 16705   **Fax: 01256 812 558**
Macmillan Distribution
Basingstoke RG21 6ZZ

Please send me urgently   *Post included price*
(tick below)   *per copy (UK only)*

☐ **Dump Your Toxic Waist!** (ISBN 978 1 85959 191 8)   £17.99

☐ **Heart Health: Answers at your fingertips** (ISBN 978 1 85959 157 4)   £20.99

☐ **Type 2 Diabetes – Answers at your fingertips**
(ISBN 978 1 85959 176 5)   £17.99

☐ **Type 2 Diabetes in Adults of All Ages** (ISBN 978 1 85959 153 6)   £23.99

☐ **Beating Depression** (ISBN 978 1 85959 150 5)   £20.99

☐ **High Blood Pressure: Answers at your fingertips**
(ISBN 978 1 85959 090 4)   £17.99

☐ **Stroke: Answers at your fingertips** (ISBN 978 1 85959 113 0)   £20.99

TOTAL _____

Easy ways to pay

Cheque: I enclose a cheque payable to Class Publishing for £ _____

Credit card: Please debit my   ☐ Mastercard   ☐ Visa   ☐ Amex

Number _____ Expiry date _____

Name _____

My address for delivery is _____

_____

Town _____ County _____ Postcode _____

Telephone number (*in case of query*) _____

Credit card billing address if different from above _____

_____

Town _____ County _____ Postcode _____

Class Publishing's guarantee: remember that if, for any reason, you are not satisfied with these books, we will refund all your money, without any questions asked. Prices and VAT rates may be altered for reasons beyond our control.